Recent Advances in Long-Acting Drug Delivery and Formulations

Recent Advances in Long-Acting Drug Delivery and Formulations

Editors

Hamdy Abdelkader
Adel Al-Fatease

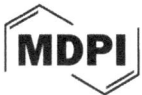

Basel • Beijing • Wuhan • Barcelona • Belgrade • Novi Sad • Cluj • Manchester

Editors
Hamdy Abdelkader
Pharmaceutics Department
King Khalid University
Abha
Saudi Arabia

Adel Al-Fatease
Pharmaceutics Department
King Khalid University
Abha
Saudi Arabia

Editorial Office
MDPI
St. Alban-Anlage 66
4052 Basel, Switzerland

This is a reprint of articles from the Special Issue published online in the open access journal *Pharmaceutics* (ISSN 1999-4923) (available at: www.mdpi.com/journal/pharmaceutics/special_issues/465G0LZD61).

For citation purposes, cite each article independently as indicated on the article page online and as indicated below:

Lastname, A.A.; Lastname, B.B. Article Title. *Journal Name* **Year**, *Volume Number*, Page Range.

ISBN 978-3-0365-9439-2 (Hbk)
ISBN 978-3-0365-9438-5 (PDF)
doi.org/10.3390/books978-3-0365-9438-5

© 2023 by the authors. Articles in this book are Open Access and distributed under the Creative Commons Attribution (CC BY) license. The book as a whole is distributed by MDPI under the terms and conditions of the Creative Commons Attribution-NonCommercial-NoDerivs (CC BY-NC-ND) license.

Contents

Adel Al Fatease and Hamdy Abdelkader
Recent Advances in Long-Acting Drug Delivery and Formulations
Reprinted from: *Pharmaceutics* **2023**, *15*, 2519, doi:10.3390/pharmaceutics15112519 1

Heba S. Abd-Ellah, Ramesh Mudududdla, Glen P. Carter and Jonathan B. Baell
Novel Perspectives on the Design and Development of a Long-Acting Subcutaneous Raltegravir Injection for Treatment of HIV—In Vitro and In Vivo Evaluation
Reprinted from: *Pharmaceutics* **2023**, *15*, 1530, doi:10.3390/pharmaceutics15051530 4

Patrick Pan, Darren Svirskis, Geoffrey I. N. Waterhouse and Zimei Wu
Hydroxypropyl Methylcellulose Bioadhesive Hydrogels for Topical Application and Sustained Drug Release: The Effect of Polyvinylpyrrolidone on the Physicomechanical Properties of Hydrogel
Reprinted from: *Pharmaceutics* **2023**, *15*, 2360, doi:10.3390/pharmaceutics15092360 27

Maria Abedin Zadeh, Raid G. Alany, Leila Satarian, Amin Shavandi, Mohamed Abdullah Almousa and Steve Brocchini et al.
Maillard Reaction Crosslinked Alginate-Albumin Scaffolds for Enhanced Fenofibrate Delivery to the Retina: A Promising Strategy to Treat RPE-Related Dysfunction
Reprinted from: *Pharmaceutics* **2023**, *15*, 1330, doi:10.3390/pharmaceutics15051330 47

Sravani Emani, Anil Vangala, Federico Buonocore, Niousha Yarandi and Gianpiero Calabrese
Chitosan Hydrogels Cross-Linked with Trimesic Acid for the Delivery of 5-Fluorouracil in Cancer Therapy
Reprinted from: *Pharmaceutics* **2023**, *15*, 1084, doi:10.3390/pharmaceutics15041084 63

Cleildo P. Santana, Brock A. Matter, Madhoosudan A. Patil, Armando Silva-Cunha and Uday B. Kompella
Corneal Permeability and Uptake of Twenty-Five Drugs: Species Comparison and Quantitative Structure–Permeability Relationships
Reprinted from: *Pharmaceutics* **2023**, *15*, 1646, doi:10.3390/pharmaceutics15061646 82

Heba A. Abou-Taleb, Mai E. Shoman, Tarek Saad Makram, Jelan A. Abdel-Aleem and Hamdy Abdelkader
Exploration of the Safety and Solubilization, Dissolution, Analgesic Effects of Common Basic Excipients on the NSAID Drug Ketoprofen
Reprinted from: *Pharmaceutics* **2023**, *15*, 713, doi:10.3390/pharmaceutics15020713 104

Karema Abu-Elfotuh, Amina M. A. Tolba, Furqan H. Hussein, Ahmed M. E. Hamdan, Mohamed A. Rabeh and Saad A. Alshahri et al.
Anti-Alzheimer Activity of Combinations of Cocoa with Vinpocetine or Other Nutraceuticals in Rat Model: Modulation of Wnt3/β-Catenin/GSK-3β/Nrf2/HO-1 and PERK/CHOP/Bcl-2 Pathways
Reprinted from: *Pharmaceutics* **2023**, *15*, 2063, doi:10.3390/pharmaceutics15082063 119

Saima Mahmood, Nauman Rahim Khan, Ghulam Razaque, Shefaat Ullah Shah, Memuna Ghafoor Shahid and Hassan A. Albarqi et al.
Microwave-Treated Physically Cross-Linked Sodium Alginate and Sodium Carboxymethyl Cellulose Blend Polymer Film for Open Incision Wound Healing in Diabetic Animals—A Novel Perspective for Skin Tissue Regeneration Application
Reprinted from: *Pharmaceutics* **2023**, *15*, 418, doi:10.3390/pharmaceutics15020418 146

Yahia Alghazwani, Krishnaraju Venkatesan, Kousalya Prabahar, Mohamed El-Sherbiny, Nehal Elsherbiny and Mona Qushawy
The Combined Anti-Tumor Efficacy of Bioactive Hydroxyapatite Nanoparticles Loaded with Altretamine
Reprinted from: *Pharmaceutics* **2023**, *15*, 302, doi:10.3390/pharmaceutics15010302 . . . . **169**

Anand Kumar, Priyanka Prajapati, Gurvinder Singh, Dinesh Kumar, Vikas Mishra and Seong-Cheol Kim et al.
Salbutamol Attenuates Diabetic Skeletal Muscle Atrophy by Reducing Oxidative Stress, Myostatin/GDF-8, and Pro-Inflammatory Cytokines in Rats
Reprinted from: *Pharmaceutics* **2023**, *15*, 2101, doi:10.3390/pharmaceutics15082101 . . . . **181**

Meghana Goravinahalli Shivananjegowda, Umme Hani, Riyaz Ali M. Osmani, Ali H. Alamri, Mohammed Ghazwani and Yahya Alhamhoom et al.
Development and Evaluation of Solid Lipid Nanoparticles for the Clearance of A in Alzheimer's Disease
Reprinted from: *Pharmaceutics* **2023**, *15*, 221, doi:10.3390/pharmaceutics15010221 . . . . **205**

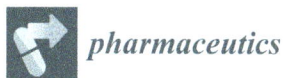

Editorial

Recent Advances in Long-Acting Drug Delivery and Formulations

Adel Al Fatease and Hamdy Abdelkader *

Pharmaceutics Department, College of Pharmacy, King Khalid University, Abha 62223, Saudi Arabia; afatease@kku.edu.sa
* Correspondence: habdelkader@kku.edu.sa

1. Introduction

Conventional immediate-release delivery systems are simple, industrially reproducible, acceptable, and easy-to-use by most patients. Nevertheless, these dosage forms have received critique for not being able to consistently provide optimum therapy for chronic disease conditions, as well as for their potential to induce adverse effects. This is primarily due to the typical rapid, pulse-release and absorption patterns of their drug cargo leading to rapidly fluctuating systemic drug concentration [1].

Long-acting drug delivery systems (LADDS) encompass a range of formulations and technologies that can be used to precisely deliver drug molecules into target tissues. These operate either through systemic circulation or via localized organs/tissues (e.g., skin, eye, and specific lesions) to treat chronic diseases like diabetes, cancer, and brain disorders, as well as for age-related eye diseases. LADDS have been shown to prolong drug release from several hours up to 3 years depending on characteristics of the drug, disease and delivery system [2,3]. LADDS include oral sustained release systems, injectable implants, in situ forming implants, inserts, wafers, transdermal patches, microspheres and nanoparticles [1,4,5]. A number of potential drug classes could be good candidates for LADDS: these include pain killers, biopharmaceuticals, anticancer drugs and centrally acting drugs [2,6].

The Special Issue, entitled "Recent Advances in Long-Acting Drug Delivery and Formulations", encompasses versatile and innovative research domains of oral, ocular, brain and topical delivery systems and chemical approaches (e.g., prodrugs), highlighting the progress made in identifying excipients (e.g., basic amino acids to ameliorate gastric side effects of non-steroidal anti-inflammatory drugs (NSAIDs)), polymers, and molecular targets to achieve a more effective sustained release systems and safer medicine. A total of 78 authors have contributed to this publication, with 11 original research articles, spanning five contents (Asia, Europe, Africa, North America and Australasia) providing important insights into the pharmaceutical sciences. I would like to encourage the readers to go through each paper and imbibe deeply the published state-of-the-art work in the field; before that, I will to summarize key research findings of interest.

2. Overview of the Published Articles

One fascinating paper in this Special Issue concerned the exploration of three basic amino acids (trometamine, lysine and arginine). These were used to form three salts with ketoprofen (one of commonly prescribed NSAIDs for chronic pain and inflammation). Analgesic activity was significantly enhanced and proceed for these acids in the following order Tris >> lysine > arginine > ketoprofen base. The least severe gastric side effects were experienced by patients treated with lysine and arginine salts.

Abd-Ellah et al. [7] investigated a novel chemical approach (aminoalkoxycarbonyloxymethyl (amino-AOCOM) ether prodrug concept) in order to design a long-acting subcutaneous raltegravir injection for the treatment of HIV.

The corneal permeability in three animal models—rabbit, pigs, and cows— was studied for 25 drugs in an attempt to relate corneal permeability to drug physicochemical properties and tissue thickness via the analysis of quantitative structure permeability relationships (QSPRs) [8]. These twenty-five drugs comprised various drug classes including NSAIDs, β-blockers and corticosteroids commonly prescribed for treating different diseases of the anterior segment of the eye.

One study tested a microwave-treated, physically cross-linked polymer blend film (sodium alginate and carboxymethyl cellulose sodium), prepared via the solvent casting method, for its potential to optimize microwave treatment time. This procedure also allowed researchers to testing for physicochemical attributes and wound healing potential in diabetic animals [9]. The study concluded that the microwave-treated polymer blend films have sufficiently enhanced physical properties, making them an effective candidate for ameliorating the diabetic wound healing process and hastening skin tissue regeneration.

Hybrid gels of hydroxyl propyl methylcellulose (HPMC) and polyvinylpyrrolidone (PVP) were studied in order to enable sustained release topical skin delivery with unique features of superior adhesiveness, spreading ability, and greater cosmetic acceptability than homopolymers alone. These binary hydrogels showed low viscosity, but high bioadhesiveness. Indeed, they still can be applied on the skin comfortably, while providing for the controlled release of the drug over extended periods of time.

Drug repurposing is useful a method for accelerating the drug development process by finding a new clinical use for a substance already on the market and registered for a different indication. On this front, two articles were published that sought to repurpose salbutamol and fenofibrate for treatment of muscle atrophy and retinal diseases, respectively [10,11].

Kumar et al. studied the repurposing potential of the bronchodilator drug salbutamol (β2-receptor agonist) for a beneficial role in diabetics with muscle atrophy. The oral administration of salbutamol increased voluntary muscle strength in diabetic rat models.

In diabetic rats, salbutamol greatly boosted lean muscle mass and grip strength. Additionally, salbutamol therapy increased antioxidant levels in muscles, decreased muscular atrophy and inflammatory markers, and restored muscle damage biomarkers, all of which suggested salbutamol's potential to lower muscle inflammation and oxidative stress.

Novel 3D polymeric scaffold implantable systems were investigated for intraocular injection in order to retinal diseases. The 3D scaffolds, comprising alginate (ALG) and bovine serum albumin (BSA) containing fenofibrate, were prepared via the freeze-drying technique.

Alzheimer's disease is a brain ailment that gradually impairs thinking and memory abilities as well as the capacity to perform even the most basic tasks. The majority of Alzheimer's patients exhibit their initial symptoms later in life. Various estimates show that more than 6 million Americans, the majority of whom are 65 or older, may be affected by Alzheimer's disease. In this Special Issue, two studies covering novel treatment strategies of Alzheimer's disease are published. Memantine HCl and Tramiprosate-loaded solid lipid nanoparticles (SLNs) were prepared and characterized for the clearance of Aβ on SHSY5Y cells in a rat hippocampus. Additionally, the neuroprotective effects of cocoa, either alone or in combination with other nutraceuticals, were discussed in the context of an animal model of aluminum-induced Alzheimer's disease.

In terms of sustained release, forming polymer chitosan has shown superior mechanical properties when cross-linked with trimesic acid. 5-fluorouracil (5-FU)-loaded hydrogels crosslinked with trimesic acid demonstrated the most sustained release profile among the formulations studied in a 3 h period, with 35 to 50% release.

3. Limitations and Future Perspectives

In conclusion, LADDS hold promise for the treatment of a variety of chronic diseases, offering safer and more efficient alternatives to the traditional (immediate-release) medication administration method. By creating APIs (small drug molecules or biologics) using long-acting drug delivery systems (LADDS), both efficacy and safety can be improved.

LADDS provide advantages that are acknowledged and supported by regulatory bodies, medical professionals, and patients. For individuals who would often need lifelong treatment for debilitating chronic ailments such eye diseases, diabetes, cancer, and brain disorders, LADDS can offer both lasting systemic and local effects.

The cost and accessibility of the biomaterials used to create LADDS, the complexity of some LADDS' complex systems, and the dependence of some LADDS' drug carriers on external stimuli (such as light, lasers, and the application of magnetism) to achieve consistent drug release are just several of the hurdles that require resolution. These problems make some LADDS ineligible for regulatory approval. The skyrocketing cost of biomaterials, inadequate scientific knowledge, and a dearth of excipients suitable for recently developing technologies like 3D printing and microneedle systems also hinder the advancement of this technology. The majority of novel long-acting anticancer drug delivery system concepts have been tested in animal models; nevertheless, regulatory organizations have voiced strong ethical and technological objections to translating such success in animal models to clinical phases.

Finally, the guest editors of this Special Issue extend their sincere appreciation for all the authors and reviewers who responded to our invitation. Your willingness to share the outcomes of your outstanding research has greatly enriched this collection, and your contributions have been invaluable in the meticulous evaluation of the manuscripts.

Conflicts of Interest: The authors declare no conflict of interest.

References

1. Abdelkader, H.; Fathalla, Z.; Seyfoddin, A.; Farahani, M.; Thrimawithana, T.; Allahham, A.; Alani, A.; Al-Kinani, A.; Alany, R. Polymeric long-acting drug delivery systems (LADDS) for treatment of chronic diseases: Inserts, patches, wafers, and implants. *Adv. Drug Deliv. Rev.* **2021**, *177*, 113957. [CrossRef] [PubMed]
2. Chappel, E. Implantable drug delivery devices. In *Drug Delivery Devices and Therapeutic Systems*; Elsevier: Amsterdam, The Netherlands, 2021; pp. 129–156.
3. Turner, J.G.; White, L.R.; Estrela, P.; Leese, H.S. Hydrogel-Forming Microneedles: Current Advancements and Future Trends. *Macromol. Biosci.* **2021**, *21*, e2000307. [CrossRef] [PubMed]
4. Wright, J.C.; Hoffman, A.S. Historical overview of long acting injections and implants. In *Long Acting Injections and Implants*; Wright, J.C., Burgess, D.J., Eds.; Springer: New York, NY, USA, 2012; pp. 11–24.
5. Wright, J.C.; Sekar, M.; Osdol, W.V.; Su, H.C.; Miksztal, A.R. In Situ Forming Systems (Depots). In *Long Acting Injections and Implants*; Wright, J.C., Burgess, D.J., Eds.; Springer: New York, NY, USA, 2012; pp. 153–166.
6. Majcher, M.J.; Babar, A.; Lofts, A.; Leung, A.; Li, X.; Abu-Hijleh, F. In situ-gelling starch nanoparticle (SNP)/O-carboxymethyl chitosan (CMCh) nanoparticle network hydrogels for the intranasal delivery of an antipsychotic peptide. *J. Control. Release* **2021**, *330*, 738–752. [CrossRef] [PubMed]
7. Abd-Ellah, H.; Mudududdla, R.; Carter, G.; Baell, J. Novel Perspectives on the Design and Development of a Long-Acting Subcutaneous Raltegravir Injection for Treatment of HIV—In Vitro and In Vivo Evaluation. *Pharmaceutics* **2023**, *15*, 1530. [CrossRef] [PubMed]
8. Santana, C.; Matter, B.; Patil, M.; Silva-Cunha, A.; Kompella, U. Corneal Permeability and Uptake of Twenty-Five Drugs: Species Comparison and Quantitative Structure–Permeability Relationships. *Pharmaceutics* **2023**, *15*, 1646. [PubMed]
9. Mahmood, S.; Mahmood, S.; Khan, N.; Razaque, G.; Shah, S.; Shahid, M.; Albarqi, H.; Alqahtani, A.; Alasiri, A.; Basit, H. Microwave-Treated Physically Cross-Linked Sodium Alginate and Sodium Carboxymethyl Cellulose Blend Polymer Film for Open Incision Wound Healing in Diabetic Animals—A Novel Perspective for Skin Tissue Regeneration Application. *Pharmaceutics* **2023**, *15*, 418. [PubMed]
10. Wright, A.D.; Dodson, P.M. Medical management of diabetic retinopathy: Fenofibrate and ACCORD Eye studies. *Eye* **2011**, *25*, 843–849. [CrossRef] [PubMed]
11. Kumar, A.; Prajapati, P.; Raj, V.; Kim, S.; Mishra, V.; Raorane, C.; Raj, R.; Kumar, D.; Kushwaha, S. Salbutamol ameliorates skeletal muscle wasting and inflammatory markers in streptozotocin (STZ)-induced diabetic rats. *Int. Immunopharmacol.* **2023**, *124*, 110883. [CrossRef] [PubMed]

Disclaimer/Publisher's Note: The statements, opinions and data contained in all publications are solely those of the individual author(s) and contributor(s) and not of MDPI and/or the editor(s). MDPI and/or the editor(s) disclaim responsibility for any injury to people or property resulting from any ideas, methods, instructions or products referred to in the content.

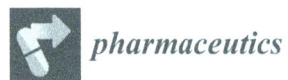

Article

Novel Perspectives on the Design and Development of a Long-Acting Subcutaneous Raltegravir Injection for Treatment of HIV—In Vitro and In Vivo Evaluation

Heba S. Abd-Ellah [1,2], Ramesh Mudududdla [1,*], Glen P. Carter [3] and Jonathan B. Baell [1,4,*]

1. Medicinal Chemistry, Monash Institute of Pharmaceutical Sciences, Parkville, VIC 3052, Australia; hebasaleh.chem@gmail.com
2. Medicinal Chemistry Department, Faculty of Pharmacy, Minia University, Minia 61519, Egypt
3. Microbiology and Immunology Department, Peter Doherty Institute for Infection and Immunity, The University of Melbourne, Parkville, VIC 3001, Australia; glen.carter@unimelb.edu.au
4. School of Pharmaceutical Sciences, Nanjing Tech University, No. 30 South Puzhu Road, Nanjing 211816, China
* Correspondence: ramesh.mudududdla@monash.edu (R.M.); jonathan.baell@njtech.edu.cn or jbaell29@gmail.com (J.B.B.); Tel.: +61470330093 (R.M.); +61402194571 (J.B.B.)

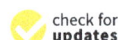

Citation: Abd-Ellah, H.S.; Mudududdla, R.; Carter, G.P.; Baell, J.B. Novel Perspectives on the Design and Development of a Long-Acting Subcutaneous Raltegravir Injection for Treatment of HIV—In Vitro and In Vivo Evaluation. *Pharmaceutics* 2023, 15, 1530. https://doi.org/10.3390/pharmaceutics15051530

Academic Editors: Hamdy Abdelkader and Adel Al-Fatease

Received: 11 April 2023
Revised: 11 May 2023
Accepted: 15 May 2023
Published: 18 May 2023

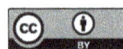

Copyright: © 2023 by the authors. Licensee MDPI, Basel, Switzerland. This article is an open access article distributed under the terms and conditions of the Creative Commons Attribution (CC BY) license (https://creativecommons.org/licenses/by/4.0/).

Abstract: Antiretrovirals (ARVs) are a highly effective therapy for treatment and prevention of HIV infection, when administered as prescribed. However, adherence to lifelong ARV regimens poses a considerable challenge and places HIV patients at risk. Long-acting ARV injections may improve patient adherence as well as maintaining long-term continuous drug exposure, resulting in improved pharmacodynamics. In the present work, we explored the aminoalkoxycarbonyloxymethyl (amino-AOCOM) ether prodrug concept as a potential approach to long-acting ARV injections. As a proof of concept, we synthesised model compounds containing the 4-carboxy-2-methyl Tokyo Green (CTG) fluorophore and assessed their stability under pH and temperature conditions that mimic those found in the subcutaneous (SC) tissue. Among them, probe **21** displayed very slow fluorophore release under SC-like conditions (98% of the fluorophore released over 15 d). Compound **25**, a prodrug of the ARV agent raltegravir (RAL), was subsequently prepared and evaluated using the same conditions. This compound showed an excellent in vitro release profile, with a half-life ($t_{\frac{1}{2}}$) of 19.3 d and 82% of RAL released over 45 d. In mice, **25** extended the half-life of unmodified RAL by 4.2-fold ($t_{\frac{1}{2}}$ = 3.18 h), providing initial proof of concept of the ability of amino-AOCOM prodrugs to extend drug lifetimes in vivo. Although this effect was not as pronounced as seen in vitro—presumably due to enzymatic degradation and rapid clearance of the prodrug in vivo—the present results nevertheless pave the way for development of more metabolically stable prodrugs, to facilitate long-acting delivery of ARVs.

Keywords: HIV; long-acting subcutaneous injection; raltegravir; cyclisation-activated prodrugs

1. Introduction

HIV remains a global health problem. It affects 36.7 million people worldwide, with an additional 2.1 million new cases diagnosed each year, indicating that the AIDS pandemic is far from over [1]. Nevertheless, the introduction of antiretroviral (ARV) treatment and prophylaxis measures has led to remarkable progress in defeating HIV/AIDS infection. These agents have significantly improved treatment efficacy, reduced HIV-related morbidity and mortality, and increased the lifespan of HIV-positive individuals to a level comparable to that of the HIV-negative population [2–4]. However, lifelong compliance with the daily dosing required by ARV regimens remains a great challenge, especially in HIV patients with coexisting mental conditions or drug abuse, or for whom there are multiple medications to be taken daily, complicating the treatment regimen [5,6]. Even short-term non-adherence to ARVs can result in therapeutic failure, as well as promoting development of drug-resistant HIV viral strains that decrease the patient's future treatment opportunities [7].

In fact, only 62% of HIV patients maintain the ≥90% adherence required for optimal viral suppression [8]. Furthermore, despite the high efficacy of pre-exposure prophylaxis (PrEP) in preventing HIV transmission, PrEP compliance ranged from 22–98% in clinical trials [9], also indicating low adherence for a significant number of individuals. In such circumstances, long-acting ARV injections requiring weekly or monthly administration might be an optimal, life-saving alternative to daily oral therapy.

In a 2013 survey, more than 80% of 400 adult patients indicated they would probably try long-acting ARV therapy if the dosage was once a month [10]. In view of this, a number of long-acting injections are currently in phase 2 and phase 3 clinical trials for HIV treatment and prevention. For instance, a phase 2b clinical trial demonstrated that long-acting intramuscular injection of two ARVs (rilpivirine and cabotegravir), administered every 4 or 8 weeks, was as effective as daily oral therapy in maintaining viral suppression over 96 weeks [11]. Two subsequent phase 3 clinical trials on the same drug combination reached equivalent conclusions [12,13]. In 2021, the FDA approved Cabenuva as the first intramuscular long-acting formulation to treat HIV. It is supplied as a packaged kit of two separate long-acting injectable medicines, cabotegravir and rilpivirine, which should be administered once every two months [14,15].

Long-acting injections such as these utilise various approaches to provide sustained therapeutic drug exposure over a period of weeks, or sometimes longer. These include, but are not limited to: incorporation of the active ingredient in either an oil-based solution or a suitable matrix from which the drug is slowly released; using a nanosuspension of drug particles; microsphere encapsulation; implants; and in situ forming depots [16–23]. Each of these approaches has its unique strengths and weaknesses; for example, persistent pain at the injection site that can last for more than three months, low drug loading capacity with subsequently high administration volume, conformational changes, and others. Although many efforts have been directed towards improving the currently available approaches, no reports have yet addressed the potential of chemical transformation methods as a means to develop long-acting injections. Herein, we present our initial work on the amino-alkoxycarbonyloxymethyl (amino-AOCOM) ether moiety as a pH-activated handle to develop long-acting prodrugs for HIV treatment.

Previous work demonstrated that amino-AOCOM prodrugs **1** and **2** (Figure 1) release the parent drug via a pH-dependent intramolecular cyclisation reaction that is completely independent of enzymatic biotransformation [24]. Both prodrugs exhibited enhanced aqueous solubility and oral bioavailability compared with the parent compound [24]. Recently, we applied the same strategy to develop mesalamine prodrugs **3** and **4**—with three- and four-methylene spacers, respectively (Figure 1)—for colonic delivery [25]. In that study, a key finding was that increasing the methylene spacer length to five or six carbons led to pH-sensitive linkers with very slow-release profiles. These were of limited interest for colonic delivery, but could be useful in long-acting injectable formulations. In this paper, we describe our initial efforts to evaluate the utility of those extended handles in such a context. The first part of our study focused on the use of 4-carboxy-2-methyl Tokyo Green (CTG) fluorophore as a model compound, to establish the initial proof of concept. In part two, we applied the same approach to raltegravir (RAL), as a representative ARV drug utilised in the treatment of AIDS. Mechanistically, RAL inhibits the HIV integrase enzyme to block integration of viral DNA into the human genome [26]. The half-life ($t_{\frac{1}{2}}$) of RAL is 7–12 h, allowing for a regimen of two 400 mg doses per day [27]. It also exhibits highly desirable pharmacokinetic properties, such as rapid distribution to the female genital tract and cervicovaginal fluid, as well as greater penetration into the seminal compartment [28–30]. In 2016, a long-acting RAL formulation was developed, involving reconstitution of milled, γ-irradiated drug in a sterile vehicle of water containing poly(ethylene glycol) 3350 (5%), polysorbate 80 (0.2%), and mannitol (5%). Preclinical studies showed that two weeks after a single subcutaneous (SC) injection in BLT mice (7.5 mg) and rhesus macaques (160 mg), the plasma concentration of RAL was comparable to that achieved through the usual oral regimen in humans [28]. Accordingly, it is considered a promising long-acting ARV and prophylactic agent, thereby rationalising its choice in the current study.

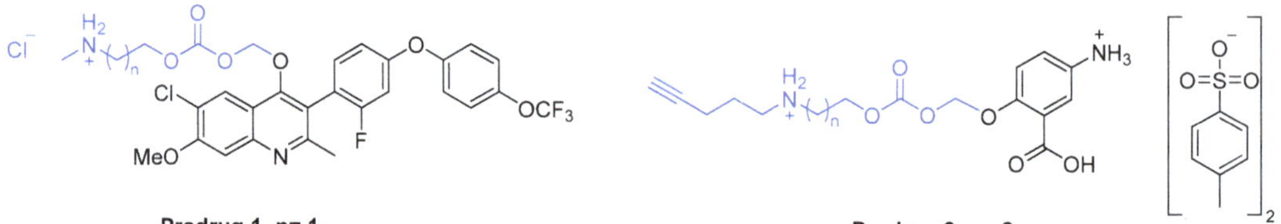

Figure 1. Structure of prodrugs **1–4**.

Prodrug 1, n= 1
Prodrug 2, n = 2
Prodrug 3, n= 2
Prodrug 4, n= 3

2. Materials and Methods

2.1. Synthetic Procedures and Analytical Data

All chemical reagents and solvents were obtained from Combi-Blocks (San Diego, CA, USA), Sigma Aldrich (Burghausen, Germany), and Thermo Fisher Scientific (Waltham, MA, USA), kept in appropriate storage conditions, and used without further purification. Reactions were monitored by thin layer chromatography (TLC) using silica gel 60 F254 coated aluminium plates with 0.25 mm thickness. TLC plates were visualised under UV light at 254 nm or 366 nm, and staining with $KMnO_4$ solution when necessary. The ^1H NMR and ^{13}C NMR spectra were obtained at 400.13 MHz, 100.62 MHz, respectively, on Bruker spectrometer (Bruker Corporation, Billerica, MA, USA), using tetramethylsilane as an internal reference. Chemical shifts were measured in parts per million (ppm) and referenced to an internal standard of residual deuterated solvent: $CDCl_3$ (7.26 ppm for ^1H and 77.16 ppm for ^{13}C), DMSO-d_6 (2.50 ppm for ^1H and 39.52 ppm for ^{13}C), or MeOD (3.31 ppm for ^1H and 49.00 ppm for ^{13}C). Missing or/and overlapping ^{13}C signals were identified using 2D NMR experiments (HSQC and HMBC) and are distinguished with a * symbol. The ESI–MS and HRMS analyses were run on Agilent UHPLC/MS (1260/6120) and Agilent 6224 TOF-MS systems (Agilent Technologies, Santa Clara, CA, USA), respectively. The purity of the final target compounds was determined by analytical HPLC (Agilent 1260 Infinity, Agilent Technologies, Santa Clara, CA, USA) and was >95% in every case.

2.2. In Vitro Release Tests

Probes **14–15** and **20–21** stock solutions were prepared at 1000 µM (1 mM) in a 1:1 mixture of MeCN/water, followed by serial dilution with deionised water to give a 50 µM working concentration. Each experiment was run in triplicate after dilution of 0.5 mL of the stock solution with 0.5 mL of PBS (pH 7.4) or Tris buffer (pH 7.4), giving a final assay concentration of 25 µM for the probes. The samples were incubated at 34 °C to mimic the conditions found in SC tissue. Every day, a 2 µL aliquot of each sample was subjected to HPLC analysis using an Agilent 1260 Infinity instrument, with conditions as follows. Column: Agilent ZORBAX Eclipse Plus C18 Rapid Resolution, 3.5 µm (4.6 × 100 mm), pore size (95 Å); column temperature (35 °C). The mobile phases were solvent A: 0.1% TFA in ultrapure H_2O and solvent B: 0.1% TFA in MeCN. The injection volume was 2 µL and the flow rate was kept at 1.0 mL/min. The analysis was performed using a gradient elution of 5–100% of solvent B in solvent A over 9 min, then maintained for a further 1 min at two wavelengths: 254 nm and 214 nm. The retention times of CTG and probes **14–15** and **20–21** were 4.13, 4.27, 4.93, 5.55, and 5.71 min, respectively. A calibration curve for the free CTG fluorophore was constructed over the concentration range of 10–100 µM at pH 7.4. The data were fit by linear regression to the equation $y = 14.615x - 0.067$, where y is the peak area of the analyte and x is the analyte concentration (µM). The correlation coefficient (R^2) was computed as 0.999, confirming the linearity of used method under the specified measured concentrations.

Likewise, a test solution of prodrug **25** was incubated in 50% PBS at 100 µM final concentration, and analysed using the same HPLC method but with detection at 254 nm only. A higher concentration of **25** was used due to its relatively weaker absorption at 254 nm, compared with CTG. The retention times of RAL and prodrug **25** were 4.47 and 5.55 min, respectively. A calibration curve of RAL was constructed over the range 50–1000 µM. The data were fit by linear regression as before to give the equation y = 5.1961x − 20.064, with a similar goodness of fit ($R^2 \geq 0.999$).

2.3. Pharmacokinetic Study of Prodrug 25

2.3.1. Study Design

The pharmacokinetic profile of prodrug **25** was evaluated in mice, in a study undertaken at WuXi AppTec. Prodrug **25** was dissolved in a sterile vehicle of DMSO/Solutol HS15/water (10:10:80) to give a clear solution with a final concentration of 6 mg/mL. The same procedure was used to prepare a 6 mg/mL solution of RAL as a control. Six male BALB/c mice were used, each weighing 18–25 g and aged between 7–9 weeks (three per group). A single 30 mg/kg dose of prodrug **25** was administered to each animal in the treatment group (subcutaneously, in the thoracic region). Similarly, RAL (30 mg/kg) was administered to each animal in the control group. Blood samples were taken at the time points indicated below, up to the experiment endpoint (96 h).

2.3.2. Blood and Sample Preparation

For each animal, blood samples (30 µL each) were collected from the submandibular or saphenous vein over a period of 96 h, at the following time points: zero/pre-dose; then 0.25, 0.5, 1, 2, 3, 4, 5, 6, 24, 48, and 96 h. All samples were transferred into pre-chilled commercial K2EDTA tubes and placed on wet ice until processing for plasma, which was obtained by centrifugation at 4 °C and 3200× g for 10 min, within 30 min of sampling. The plasma samples were transferred to polypropylene tubes, snap-frozen on dry ice, and kept at −70 ± 10 °C until LC-MS/MS analysis.

2.3.3. Data Analysis

An LC-MS/MS method was developed to measure the concentrations of prodrug **25** and RAL in the biological matrix. Two mobile phases were used: mobile phase A (0.025% NH_4OH and 2 mM NH_4OAc in 95:5 v/v water/MeCN) and mobile phase B (0.025% NH_4OH and 2 mM NH_4OAc in 5:95 v/v water/MeCN). A UPLC method was performed using an LC-MS/MS-BM Triple Quad 6500 plus system with an ACQUITY UPLC BEH C18 1.7 µm column (2.1 × 50 mm) at a flow rate of 0.65 mL/min. The assay time was 2.5 min, and the solvent B composition was as follows: 10–100% (0.2–1.4 min), 30% (1.41–1.7 min), 95% (2.0–2.4 min), and 10% (2.41–2.5 min). The retention times for the prodrug, RAL and the internal standards (tolbutamide and verapamil) were 0.76, 1.04, 0.66, and 0.97 min, respectively. Quantification was performed by monitoring the transition of m/z 835.3 $[M+H]^+$ to 457.2 for prodrug **25**, representing the cyclisation of the linker with the amidic RAL such as in side-product **22**; whereas for RAL, the transition m/z 445.2 $[M+H]^+$ to 361.2 was followed, representing the loss of the 2-methyl-1,3,4-oxadiazole moiety as the main fragmentation pathway. For the internal standards, the m/z transition from 455.2 $[M+H]^+$ to 164.9 was used for verapamil (corresponding to formation of the verapamil fragment $[CH_2CH_2\text{-}(3,4\text{-dimethoxy phenyl})]^+$), and for tolbutamide, the transition of m/z of 271.1 $[M+H]^+$ to 155.1 was used, representing formation of the $[CH_3\text{-Ph-}SO_2]^+$ fragment. The LLOQ was found to be 1 ng/mL for **25** and 0.3 ng/mL for RAL, respectively. The method was linear over the measured standard concentrations for **25** and RAL. The mean plasma concentration was determined for **25** and RAL (as metabolite or control) at each sampling time point. Pharmacokinetic parameters were then calculated by non-compartmental analysis of plasma concentration/time profiles using the Phoenix WinNonlin 6.3 software. The computed parameters were as follows: peak plasma concentration (C_{max}); the time over which the initial concentration is reduced to half ($t_{\frac{1}{2}}$); area under the plasma concentration versus time curve from time zero to 96 h (AUC 0–96 h); and mean residence time from time zero to 96 h (MRT 0–96 h).

2.3.4. Ethics

Animals were obtained from an approved vendor (Beijing Vital River Laboratory Animal Technology Co., Ltd., Beijing, China), and were acclimated for at least 3 d before being placed in the study. Animals were housed with free access to water and food at all times. The study was approved by the WuXi Institutional Animal Care and Use Committee on Animal Experiments, and was performed in an AAALAC-accredited laboratory, complying with PHS policy and national regulations on the administration of laboratory animals.

3. Results and Discussion

3.1. Proposed Release Mechanism

The proposed mechanism of drug release from the designed prodrugs, based on fundamental principles and supported by the related literature, is shown in Figure 2. Here, the prodrugs become less protonated at physiological pH (7.4), rendering the amino group relatively more nucleophilic and causing subsequent intramolecular cyclisation–elimination to release the payload along with side-products **5** (cyclic carbamate) and **6** (formaldehyde), neither of which is toxic at low concentration [24,31]. The length of the methylene spacer dictates the size of the ring formed, and hence, the rate of cyclisation. Prodrug **1** reportedly cyclises rapidly to give a five-membered ring, releasing >90% of the parent compound within 1 h at pH 7.0. In contrast, prodrug **2** cyclises more slowly to form a six-membered ring, releasing >55% of the payload over 5 h at the same pH [24]. Increasing the methylene spacer length to four carbons—such as in prodrug **4**, which we reported recently [25]— hinders the cyclisation further and slows down drug release accordingly (in this case, achieving 92% release of mesalamine over 6 d at pH 6.5).

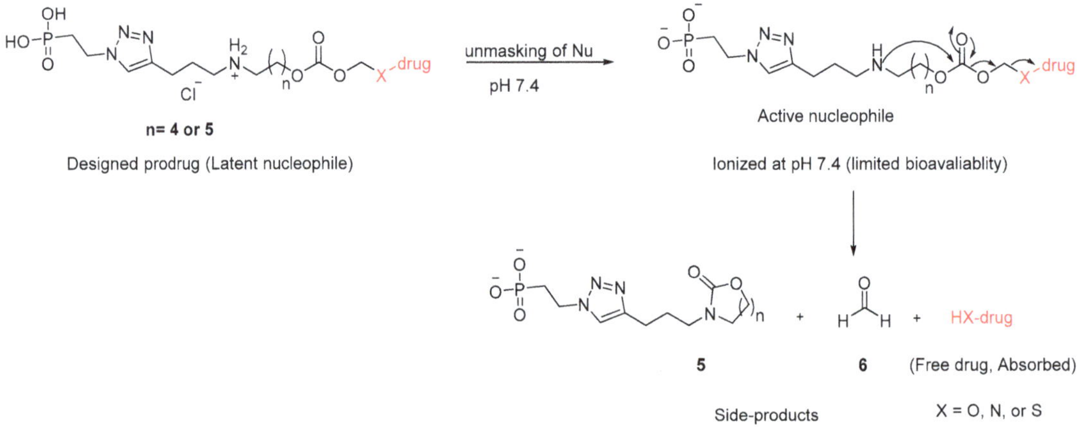

Figure 2. The proposed release mechanism of new cyclization-activated prodrugs for long-acting subcutaneous delivery.

Therefore, in the case of RAL (where long-acting prodrugs are required), we tried extending the methylene spacer to five or six carbons (corresponding to eight- and nine-membered ring cyclisations) in our initial model probes, to obtain the very slow-release kinetics suitable for development of a long-acting SC injection. This goal also necessitates an understanding of the physiology of the SC tissue, also known as the hypodermis, and which is mostly composed of connective tissue, separated primarily by adipose tissues, and to a minor extent by macrophages and fibroblasts. The fibroblasts produce constituents of the extracellular matrix (ECM), including glycosaminoglycans (GAGs), elastin, and collagen [32,33]. In general, a drug after injection reaches the interstitial space of the hypodermis, where absorption occurs mainly according to its molecular size. For instance, smaller molecules (≤16 kDa, as defined in this cited study), are preferentially absorbed through the vascular endothelium of blood capillaries due to their unrestricted permeability, whereas macromolecules (>16 kDa) and small particles are absorbed through the peripheral lymph vessels from the surrounding interstitial space, before entering the systemic circulation [34,35]. However, many other factors can influence the absorption process, rendering it complex and unpredictable. These factors are either physiological (e.g., interaction of the drug with endogenous compounds, lymph flow, or blood), or physicochemical (e.g., hydrophilicity and electrostatic charge) [36]. In the current approach, the prodrug should ideally be retained in the SC tissue, with systemic absorption of only the released payload. In an attempt to decrease the permeability of the prodrug across the vascular endothelium, a phosphonic acid group was introduced via click chemistry using an alkyne group incorporated into the AOCOM structure. Phosphonic acids ionise at physiological pH, resulting here in a highly charged prodrug with presumably poor permeability [37,38]. In support of this hypothesis, phosphonic acid-containing drugs reportedly show impaired diffusion across biological membranes and require endocytosis for cell penetration [37–39]. Nevertheless, given the lack of a reliable in vitro model to predict SC bioavailability, it was difficult to predict whether the phosphonic acid group would play this role in vivo, and we were interested to ascertain whether or not it is useful in such a context.

In addition, due to its anionic nature at physiological pH, this functionality is also reported to increase the water solubility of polymers [38], organic compounds, and ligands for co-ordination chemistry [40]. A phosphonate should therefore improve the aqueous solubility of the current prodrugs, which is a clear requirement for an SC formulation, to avoid any precipitation in vivo that might occlude capillary vessels [41].

3.2. Synthesis

To synthesise probes **14–15** and **20–21**, the AOCOM iodides (**11a–b**) were first constructed as illustrated in Scheme 1. In brief, Boc-protected amino alcohols (**9a–b**) were reacted with chloromethyl chloroformate to give AOCOM chlorides **10a–b**, which were subsequently converted into the corresponding iodides **11a–b** via a Finkelstein reaction as illustrated in Appendix A. *tert*-Butyl-CTG **12** was obtained as described previously [42,43], which was then reacted with **11a–b** in the presence of Cs_2CO_3 to give the desired CTG conjugates **13a–b**. These intermediates (**13a–b**) were deprotected under acidic conditions (aq. HCl) to afford final probes (**14–15**) in good yields (Scheme 1).

To introduce the phosphonic acid moiety, bromophosphonate **16** was used as starting material, and was reacted with NaN_3 in DMSO to give azido ester **17** in high yield (Scheme 2). We noted that in a previous study, the phosphonic acid azide was preferred over the equivalent phosphonate diester for the click reaction, as subsequent dealkylation of the latter (after triazole formation) failed to give the desired product [44]. Therefore, compound **17** was first dealkylated using bromotrimethylsilane followed by methanolysis, to provide azide **18**. Direct coupling of CTG probes **14–15** with **18** was attempted via Cu (I)-catalysed azide/alkyne cycloaddition at room temperature, but the reaction failed and unreacted starting material remained. Further, this was tried at 70 °C using a microwave reactor, however all the starting materials profoundly decomposed, and the free fluorophore was generated. To resolve this issue, an alternative Boc-protected compounds **13a–b** were used to access probes **20–21**, since they are relatively more stable than probes **14–15** at elevated temperatures. Thus, **13a–b** were reacted with azide **18** to give intermediates **19a–b**, which were deprotected under acidic conditions to give the final probes **20–21**, as shown in Scheme 2.

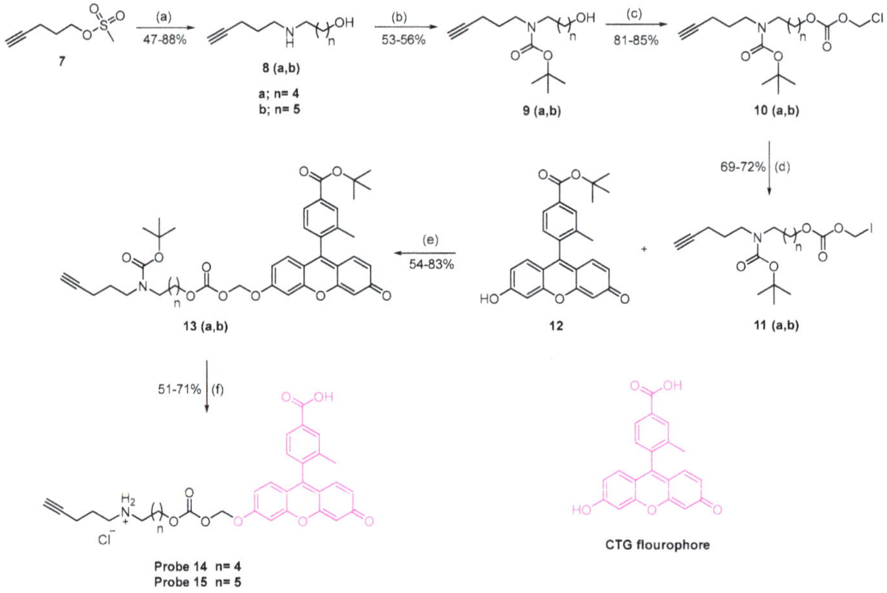

Scheme 1. Synthetic route for probes **14–15**. Reagents and conditions: (a) respective amino alcohol, TEA (cat), DMF, rt 2d; (b) Boc anhydride, NaOH, THF, 16 h; (c) chloromethyl chloroformate, pyridine (cat), DCM 0 °C to rt, 5 h; (d) sodium iodide, acetone, 40 °C, 16 h; (e) Cs_2CO_3, DMF, 0 °C to rt, 4 h; (f) Aqueous HCl (32%), MeCN, 3 h.

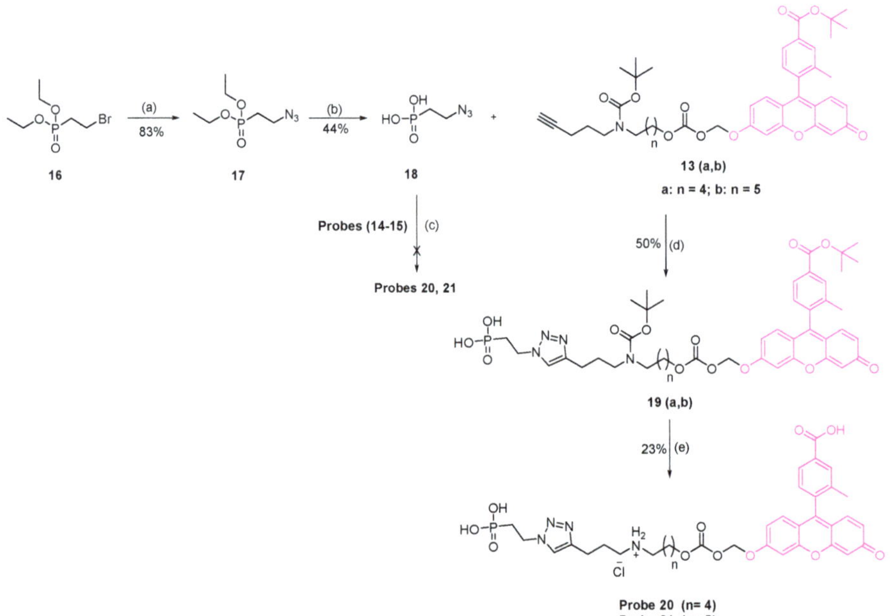

Scheme 2. Synthetic route for probes **20–21**. Reagents and conditions: (a) NaN_3, DMSO, 2 d, rt; (b) (i) trimethylbromosilane, MeCN, 0 °C to rt, 16 h; (ii) CH_3OH/H_2O (1:1), rt, 24 h; (c,d) $CuSO_4$ (20% mol), sodium-L ascorbate (40% mol), $DCM/H_2O/t$-BuOH (1:1:1), μW (100 W), 2 h; (e) Aqueous HCl (32%), MeCN, rt, 2–4 h.

Similarly, RAL was alkylated with AOCOM iodide **11b** using Cs$_2$CO$_3$ (3 equiv.) and DMF as solvent. An unexpected side-product with an m/z of 457.1 [M+H]$^+$ was formed during the reaction, and was identified as **22** based on NMR analysis as shown in Scheme 3, and Figures S31–S33. It was assumed that alkylated product **23** was formed initially but underwent subsequent intramolecular cyclisation via the amidic NH of RAL to give **22**. To avoid this side-reaction, the coupling conditions were optimised with respect to limiting equivalents of Cs$_2$CO$_3$ and reaction time. Using a stoichiometric amount of Cs$_2$CO$_3$ (1 equiv.) and 1 h reaction time resulted in clean reaction conversion to the desired product **23**, without any traces of side-product **22**. Increasing the number of equivalents of Cs$_2$CO$_3$, and/or extending the reaction time promote the base induced cyclisation and side-product formation.

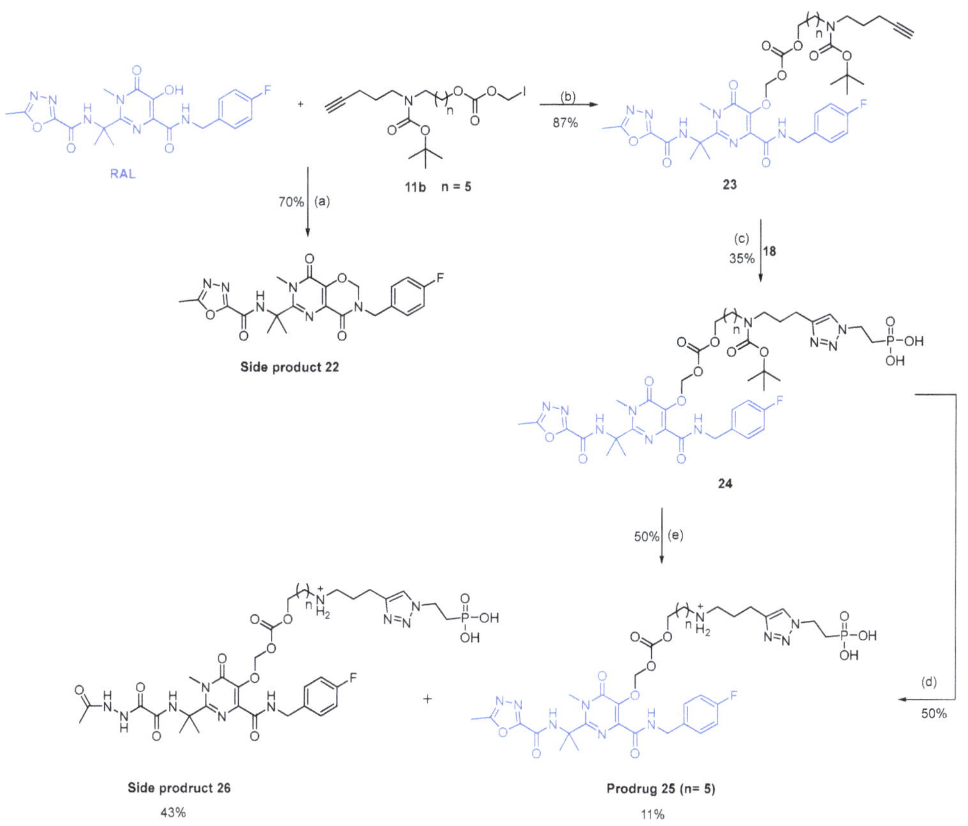

Scheme 3. Synthetic route for prodrug **25**. Reagents and conditions: (a) 3 eq Cs$_2$CO$_3$, DMF, 0 °C to rt, 2 h; (b) 1 eq Cs$_2$CO$_3$, DMF, 0 °C to rt, 1 h. (c) CuSO$_4$ (20% mol), sodium-L-ascorbate (40% mol), DCM/H$_2$O/t-BuOH (1:1:1), μW (100W), 2 h (d) aqueous HCl (32%), MeCN, rt, 3 h; (e) 2 M HCl in Et$_2$O, rt, 4 h.

Next, **23** was reacted with azide **18** to give compound **24**, which was again deprotected under acidic conditions to afford prodrug **25**. Interestingly, the major product formed during this hydrolysis step was identified as **26**, based on its NMR spectra and observed m/z of 853.3 [M+H]$^+$, as demonstrated in Appendix A and shown in Figures S41–S43. This product was believed to arise through hydrolysis of the oxadiazole moiety of **25** in aqueous acidic medium, as shown in Figure 3. A similar tendency for the RAL oxadiazole to hydrolyse has been reported, when it was stirred in a mixture of aqueous KOH and

MeCN [45]. Using 2 M HCl in diethyl ether/MeCN as an alternative to aqueous acid, prodrug **25** was obtained in good yield.

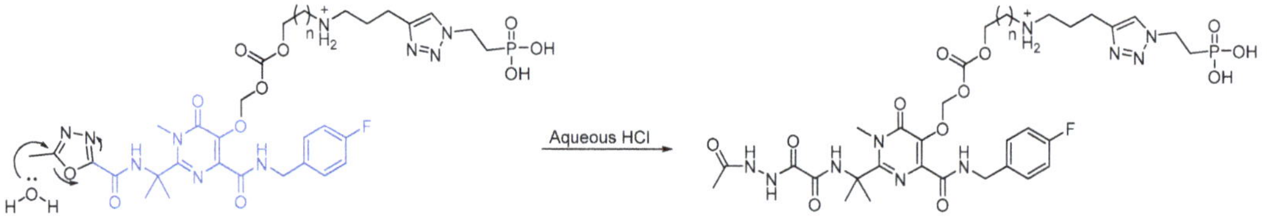

Figure 3. Hydrolysis of prodrug **25** in the presence of aqueous HCl (32%).

3.3. In Vitro Release Study of Probes 14–15 and 20–21

In vitro Release assays for probes **14–15** and **20–21** were conducted using pH and temperature conditions similar to those of SC tissue (pH 7.4 and 34 °C) [46]. Test compounds were dissolved in either MeCN/PBS (1:1, pH 7.4) or MeCN/Tris buffer (1:1, pH 7.4) at 25 µM, then incubated at 34 °C. Aliquots were taken daily and analysed by HPLC and LC-MS until complete fluorophore release was achieved. HPLC was preferred over fluorometric-based assay to study the stability of the synthesised probes because of the bleaching effect that may occur to the fluorophore over the long analysing periods. Photobleaching is the inability of the fluorophore to fluoresce due to the fluorophore instability upon repeated exposure to light over long periods [47]. It can be a particular problem for fluorescence-based assays, thereby rationalising the choice of HPLC in the current work.

The results showed that probe **14**, with a five-methylene spacer, released 36% and 58% of the CTG fluorophore after 1 d and 2 d, respectively, in 50% PBS. Further payload release was slow, reaching 98% after 9 d (Figure 4A). In comparison, probe **15**—with a six-methylene spacer—appeared to be more stable than **14** at every time point. Under the same conditions, it released 29% and 50% of CTG after 1 d and 2 d, respectively, and this value reached 98% after 10 d. Release of CTG from probes **20–21** was then measured to study the influence of the phosphonic acid group on the kinetic profiles. These experiments indicated that CTG release was slower with the phosphonic acid group attached, in both cases. For example, probe **20** gave 25%, 41%, and 98% release of CTG after 1, 2, and 13 d, respectively (Figure 4A). Payload release became much slower with the longer spacer in probe **21**, with 20%, 33%, and 98% of CTG released after 1, 2, and 15 d, respectively, as shown in Figure 4A.

Evaluation of the release kinetics of all CTG probes indicates that they exhibited first-order kinetics. The release rate constants (k_{obs}) and half-lives ($t_{\frac{1}{2}}$) were determined and are shown in Table 1. The results showed that k_{obs} for probe **14**, with a five-methylene spacer, was 0.41 d^{-1}, while it was 0.35 d^{-1} for probe **15**, with a six-methylene spacer; thereby confirming our earlier report that the length of the methylene spacer is a key parameter in the release process. Furthermore, attaching the phosphonic acid group to the AOCOM handles further decreased the reaction rate for reasons that are currently not clear (k_{obs}: 0.41 and 0.35 d^{-1} for **14–15** versus 0.24 and 0.22 d^{-1} for **20–21**, respectively). The half-lives were 1.69, 1.98, 2.88, and 3.15 d for probes **14–15**, and **20–21**, respectively, as summarised in Table 1.

Unexpectedly, the release of CTG from all probes was relatively faster in 50% Tris buffer at the same pH. Furthermore, probes **14–15** and **20–21** gave very similar CTG release rates: 89.2%, 86.2%, 82.5%, and 80.9%, respectively, after 1 d (Figure 4B), indicating a minimal effect of linker length on the release rate. It was assumed that the nucleophilic amino group of Tris had attacked the amino-AOCOM carbonate group to effect CTG release (Scheme 4). This type of reactivity for Tris buffer was first reported in 2016, when an adduct formed by nucleophilic addition to asparagine succinimide-containing proteins was identified (Scheme 4) [48].

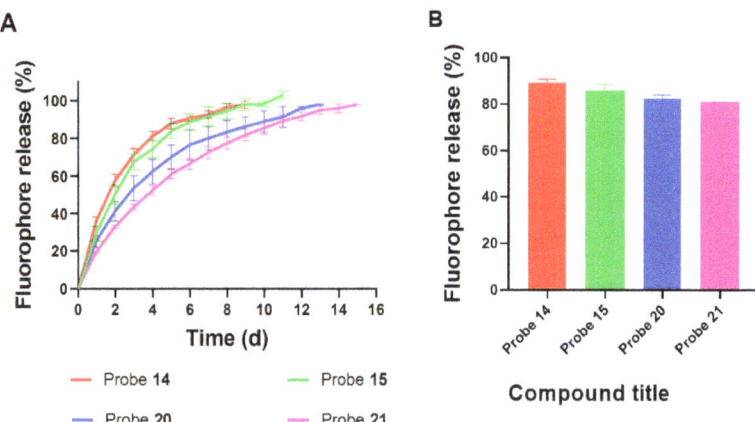

Figure 4. (**A**) The percentage of CTG release with respect to time for 25 µM of CTG probes **14–15** and **20–21** in 50% PBS (pH = 7.4. 34 °C), and (**B**) the percentage of fluorophore release for 25 µM of CTG probes **14–15** and **20–21** in Tris buffer (pH = 7.4. 34 °C) after 1 d. Values were measured in triplicate and error bars represent the standard error of the mean (SEM).

Table 1. Kinetics of release of payload from probes **14–15**, **20–21**, and **25** [a].

Compound	k_{obs} [d^{-1}] [b]	$t_{\frac{1}{2}}$ [d] [c]
14	4.1×10^{-1}	1.69
15	3.5×10^{-1}	1.98
20	2.4×10^{-1}	2.88
21	2.2×10^{-1}	3.15
25	0.36×10^{-1}	19.3

[a] The assay was performed in 50% PBS (pH 7.4) at 37 °C at 25 µM, and 100 µM for CTG probes and prodrug 25, respectively, and the reaction was followed by measuring the peak area change in the substrate using HPLC. [b] Average values of k_{obs} (n = 3), and the error in any measured rate constant is ca. <±0.08. [c] Values of $t_{\frac{1}{2}}$ were calculated from the relationship $0.69/k_{obs}$, with an error being ca. <±0.11.

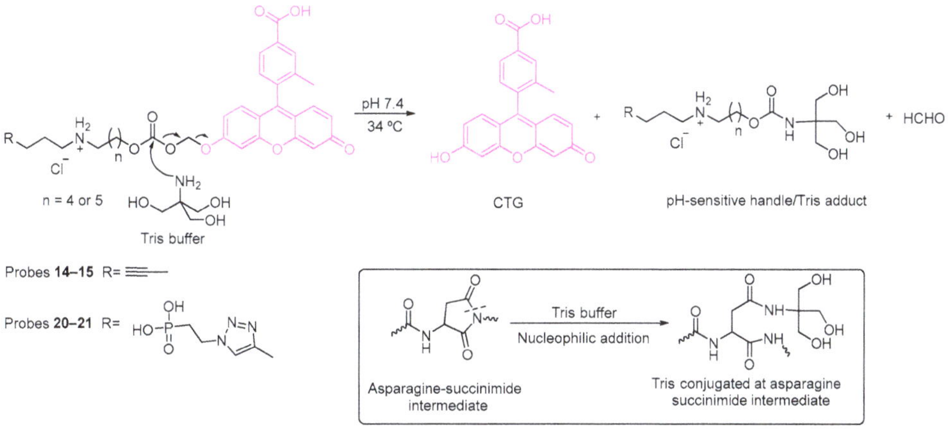

Scheme 4. Proposed mechanism for the reaction of the CTG probes (**14–15**) and (**20–21**) with Tris-HCl buffer and the reported nucleophilic addition of tris buffer to asparagine-succinimide intermediate [46].

Throughout this work, the identity of the fluorophore released from the probes (**14–15** and **20–21**) was confirmed by LC MS analysis in every case. Although the cyclised side product **5** was not separated to confirm the hypothesised mechanism, there are several reasons to believe that the proposed intramolecular cyclisation elimination reaction is the relevant mechanism. The literature reports the cyclisation of similar substrates [24,49–52], and the rate of fluorophore release decreased when the probes were incubated at lower pH (7.0, 5.0), supporting the hypothesis that the amino group plays a crucial role in the release mechanism. Moreover, cyclisation is reported to be slower with increasing methylene spacer length between the amino group and the carbonate group [24,25], and this also matched our results: probe **15**, with a six-methylene spacer, cyclised more slowly than probe **14**, with a five-methylene spacer. Based on the foregoing results, the pH-sensitive amino-AOCOM handle with a six-methylene spacer was chosen to develop the long-acting RAL prodrug (**25**).

3.4. In Vitro Release Study of Prodrug 25

Similarly to the assays above, prodrug **25** (100 µM) was incubated in 50% PBS at 34 °C, and aliquots analysed daily by HPLC and LC-MS until full RAL release was achieved. The results indicated that 8.4% of RAL was released after 1 d, then this value increased slowly to reach 31.5% after 10 d, and finally plateaued at 82.1% after 45 d (Figure 5).

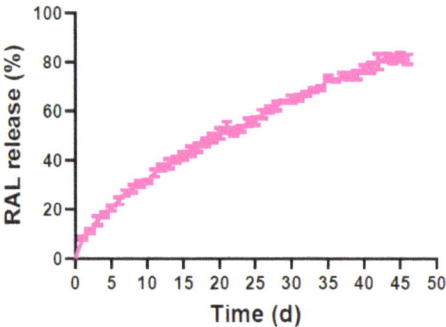

Figure 5. The correlation of RAL was released with respect to time for 100 µM of prodrug **25** when incubated in 50% PBS (pH = 7.4, 34 °C). Values were measured in triplicate and error bars are S.E.M.

Although the identity of the released RAL was confirmed by LC-MS throughout the assay, it also became apparent that payload release was incomplete due to side-product formation as the experiment progressed. Analysis of LC-MS spectra indicated that the side-product formed was due to instability of RAL under the assay conditions, giving rise to **27** as shown in Figure 6. Side-product **27** was produced by hydrolysis of RAL's 2-methyl-1,3,4-oxadiazole moiety, similarly to the formation of side-product **26**. The same result was obtained after incubation of unmodified RAL as a control under identical assay conditions. Oxadiazole hydrolysis can occur under acidic and neutral conditions, and reportedly also in basic media [45], confirming that the observed side-reaction can take place relatively easily and does not need strongly acidic or basic conditions to proceed. In this study, the degree of side-product formation was estimated as 15.2%, accounting for the unreleased RAL from **25**. Furthermore, maximal release of RAL from this prodrug was evidently prolonged compared with that for CTG from probe **21** (45 d versus 15 d).

The release profile of prodrug **25** at pH 7.4 indicates that it exhibited the same release pattern as the CTG probes; i.e., first-order kinetics. However, the reaction rate was significantly slower for probe **21** with the same methylene spacer (k_{obs} values were 0.036 d^{-1} for **25** versus 0.22 d^{-1} for **21**; Table 1). The $t_{\frac{1}{2}}$ of **25** was prolonged accordingly, at 19.3 d compared with 3.15 d for **21**. CTG is more acidic than RAL (pK_a 4.33 versus 6.7) [53], and as illustrated in the literature for similar substrates, the rate of payload release increases with the payload's acidity [52,54], thereby justifying the present findings.

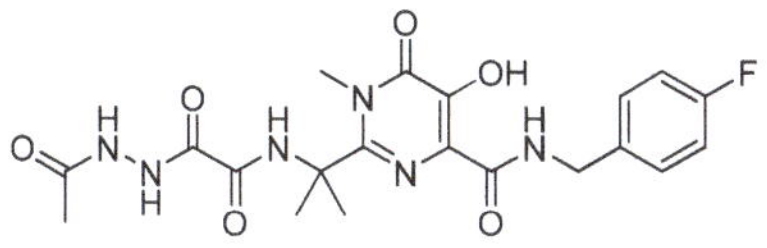

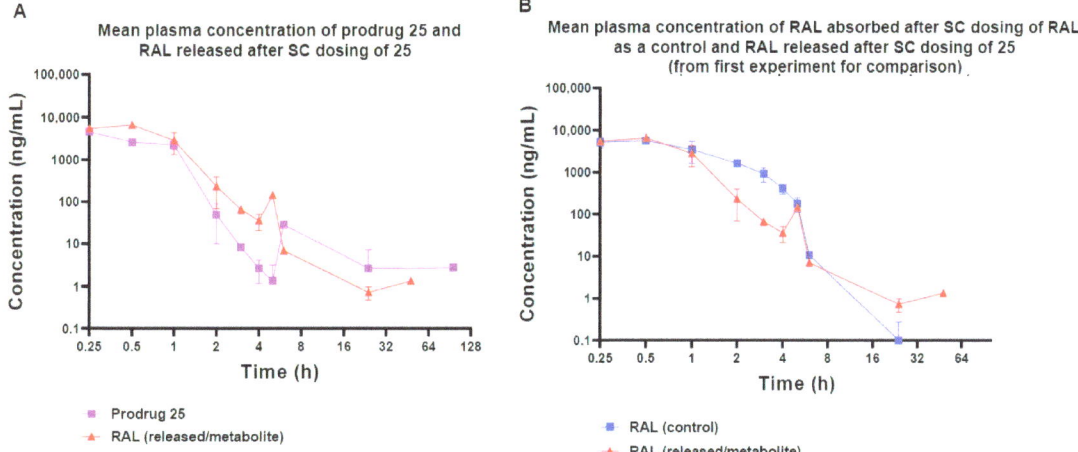

Figure 6. Degradation products of RAL under the assay conditions (50% PBS, pH 7.4, 34 °C).

3.5. Pharmacokinetic Release Profile of 25 in BALB/c Mice

Since in vitro models are not fully predictive of in vivo pharmacokinetics, especially for prodrugs, assessment of these characteristics still relies on in vivo studies [55]. Therefore, the pharmacokinetic profile of prodrug **25** was evaluated in mice. Compound **25** and the control (RAL) were dissolved in DMSO/Solutol HS15/water (10:10:80). For a single SC injection of **25** (30 mg/kg) in BALB/c mice (n = 3), the plasma concentrations of prodrug and released RAL were measured at the following time points: zero/pre-dose; then 0.25, 0.5, 1, 2, 3, 4, 5, 6, 24, 48, and 96 h. The plasma profile (Figure 7) was obtained by plotting the measured concentrations (ng/mL) against time (h). The same analysis was performed for the control group (n = 3), with administration of a single SC dose of RAL (30 mg/kg). The lower limit of quantification (LLOQ) was calculated as 1 ng/mL for **25** and 0.3 ng/mL for RAL. In both cases, the experiment continued until the concentration of the measured compounds had fallen below the LLOQ (96 h).

Figure 7. The pharmacokinetic profiles of a single SC injection of (**A**) prodrug **25** (30 mg/kg) and (**B**) RAL as a control in BALB/c mice. The mean plasma concentrations were measured at predose/zero, then; 0.25, 0.5, 1, 2, 3, 4, 5, 6, 24, 48, and 96 h by LC-MS assays and LLOQ were 1.3 ng/mL and 0.3 ng/mL for **25** and RAL, respectively.

The results indicated rapid absorption of the RAL control, with the maximum plasma concentration (C_{max}) of 6.23 µg/mL reached after 0.33 h (t_{max}), as shown in Table 2. The concentration then declined quickly, with only 10.7 ng/mL remaining after 6 h (Figure 7B), and displaying an observed half-life of 0.76 h. These findings confirmed that RAL is rapidly absorbed and cleared in vivo following SC administration, illustrating the need to extend its half-life for parenteral formulations.

Table 2. Pharmacokinetic parameters for single SC dosing of prodrug **25**, and RAL as control, in male BALB/c mice.

Compound	Dose (mg/kg)	C_{max} (µg/mL) [b]	t_{max} (h) [b]	AUC 0–96 h (µg h/mL) [c]	$t_{\frac{1}{2}}$ (h) [b]
25 [a]	30	4.55	0.25	3.27	0.85
Metabolite (released RAL)	–	6.59	0.42	5.59	3.18
Control (RAL) [a]	30	6.23	0.33	9.89	0.76

[a] Each compound was administered to three males per group. [b] Mean and SD values were calculated based on the data obtained per individual mouse and the error in any measured C_{max}, t_{max}, and $t_{1/2}$ is ca. <±0.32, <±0.14, and <±0.19, respectively. [c] Observed drug exposure (AUC 0–96 h, in µg h/mL) was obtained from the mean plasma concentrations at the different time points, and error in any measured AUC 0–96 h is ca. <±0.61.

Unexpectedly, in case of doing with compound **25**, this prodrug was detected intact in plasma shortly after SC dosing, with the highest concentration (C_{max} = 4.55 µg/mL) found at the t_{max} of 0.25 h (Figure 7A), indicating that the prodrug was rapidly absorbed and was not retained in the SC tissue as designed. Furthermore, **25** was cleared quickly, with a $t_{\frac{1}{2}}$ of 0.85 h. The released payload (RAL) was also measured in plasma, with C_{max} = 6.59 µg/mL and t_{max} = 0.42 h (Table 2). The released drug concentration then declined, with 1.3 ng/mL remaining at 48 h.

The mean exposure to RAL over the analysis period (AUC 0–96 h) was 5.59 µg h/mL for SC administration of prodrug **25**, compared with 9.89 µg h/mL for control administration of the unmodified drug by the same route (i.e., relative bioavailability = 56% of control exposure). This appeared to be related to the slightly extended release of RAL from prodrug **25**, since the $t_{\frac{1}{2}}$ of the released drug was successfully increased (3.18 h versus 0.76 h for the control group; ~4.2 fold). Although these results were not as promising as the earlier in vitro tests ($t_{\frac{1}{2}}$ = 19.3 d), they did provide initial proof of concept that the amino-AOCOM approach can successfully extend the half-life of RAL in vivo. At the same time, the significant difference between the in vitro and in vivo release profiles suggests that the prodrug may be susceptible to enzymatic hydrolysis, thus explaining why a steady plasma concentration of released RAL was not obtained.

In summary, the intention was that prodrug **25** should be retained in SC tissue, where it gradually breaks down through intramolecular cyclisation rather than enzymatic activation to give a slow but steady release of RAL over a long period. Unexpectedly, prodrug **25** was detected in plasma within a very short time-frame after dosing SC and cleared rapidly in vivo and cannot be practically used for the intended application. The significant difference between the in vitro and in vivo release profiles of **25** suggested that the major issue with the current design is the enzymatic instability of the prodrug in SC tissue or in plasma, and thus explaining why a steady plasma concentration of released RAL was not obtained. The other outstanding problem was the inability of the phosphonate to retain the prodrug in the SC tissue as designed. In terms of lack of retention in SC tissue, we thought it possible that electrostatic repulsion might have occurred between the negatively charged ECM and the negatively charged prodrug, leading to rapid absorption and transport of the prodrug via the blood capillaries. Although it may seem counterintuitive that a negatively charged species may be more rapidly absorbed, this assumption is supported by previous work in which negatively charged antibodies had enhanced bioavailability (70%) after SC injection relative to their positively charged counterparts (31%) [56,57], although this cannot be entirely confirmed due to the complexity of the absorption process from the hypodermis.

In order to improve the current design and to put the amino-AOCOM approach into practice, two challenges need to be overcome. Firstly, the instability of prodrug in vivo which could potentially be avoided by incorporating a bulky group into the carbon chain of the linker, as shown in Figure 8. This modification has been reported to lead to more enzymatically stable prodrugs [54]. The second challenge is to find a suitable way to achieve long-acting drug delivery in vivo as an alternative to the phosphonate group. In general, two approaches are mainly used to develop long acting-subcutaneous injection: prolonging SC drug retention (as aimed in the current work by using the phosphonate) and as reported in the literature through direct immobilization [58–60], and hydrogel formation [61,62], or extending the half-life of drugs via extending their blood circulation such as poly(ethylene glycol)ylation (PEGylation) [63]. We had many reasons to prefer PEGylation in future work to achieve our goal. Initially, PEGylation is the most common approach to delay in vivo clearance, by forming a hydration shell around the drug to increase its hydrodynamic radius and slow renal clearance [64]. One previous study demonstrated that PEGylation of an HIV fusion inhibitory peptide (C34) was able to decrease its clearance in vivo after SC administration and extend its half-life by 4.6-fold [65], in line with previous reports [66]. As we previously mentioned, prodrug **25** was able to extend the half-life of RAL by 4.2-fold, which is comparable to the PEGylation case just mentioned. Combining the amino-AOCOM-based approach with PEGylation would represent a novel strategy that could presumably lead synergistic extension of in vivo half-life of the prodrug, compared with either approach alone. However, the effect of PEGylation on the release rate of the drug (via the intramolecular cyclisation mechanism) would be an important parameter to address. Further, the proposed PEGylation approach should also confer protection against enzymatic degradation. It would also be preferable to retain the phosphonic acid functionality, since it improved the aqueous solubility of **25**. In brief, we believe that the high in vivo clearance of the prodrug and enzymatic instability can be decreased by PEGylation. The PEGylated, α-hydroxy, ω-phosphonic acid compound **28** features both phosphonic acid and hydroxy groups, to make it suitable for our intended future work. The hydroxy group can be converted into an azide functionality, as a handle for attachment to the prodrug via click chemistry (Figure 8).

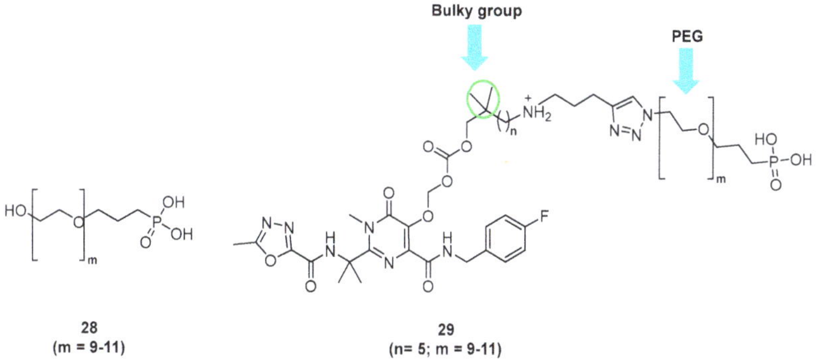

Figure 8. Proposed structure of compound **28** and prodrug **29**.

The potential immunogenicity of the PEG moiety has recently been reported to increase the hydrophobicity of PEG end group [67]. Since compound **28** has a polar phosphonic acid end-group, we believe it should have lower immunogenicity, which we consider to be an extra advantage. Therefore, future efforts will be dedicated towards the synthesis of **29**, enabling us to study the effect of different bulky groups on the enzymatic stability of the prodrug (for example, using in vitro assays performed using isolated blood plasma). Furthermore, we intend to look for reliable in vitro models to study the effect of PEGylation on the prodrug's clearance and correlate the results with subsequent in vivo findings.

4. Conclusions

A series of amino-AOCOM ether prodrugs have been designed and evaluated for long-acting SC delivery. Model compound **21**, with a six-methylene spacer, exhibited very slow-release kinetics in vitro (98% CTG released over 15 d) under pH and temperature conditions chosen to mimic those found in SC tissue. Based on this finding, RAL prodrug **25** was synthesised and evaluated in vitro and in vivo. Compound **25** degraded slowly in vitro to release RAL over 45 d ($t_{\frac{1}{2}}$ = 19.3 d). On SC administration in mice, the plasma half-life of RAL was extended by 4.2-fold for **25** compared with the control drug (3.18 h versus 0.76 h), but this result was not as promising as the earlier in vitro observations. Thus, future optimisation is required to translate the early potential of this approach into long-acting in vivo delivery.

Supplementary Materials: The following supporting information can be downloaded at: https://www.mdpi.com/article/10.3390/pharmaceutics15051530/s1. NMR spectra for intermediates **9a–b**, **10a–b**, **11a**, **13a–b**, and **19a–b**, and final probes **14–15** and **20–21** (Figures S1–S30); NMR spectra of intermediates **23** and **24**, side products **22** and **26** and prodrug **25** (Figures S31–S44).

Author Contributions: The research has been conducted by H.S.A.-E.; under the supervision of J.B.B. as the main supervisor and R.M. and G.P.C. as co-supervisors; The initial draft was written by H.S.A.-E., reviewed and edited by J.B.B. and R.M. All authors have read and agreed to the published version of the manuscript.

Funding: The authors acknowledge the financial support provided by Monash University for the studies presented in this work.

Institutional Review Board Statement: The animal study protocol was approved by Institutional Committee Animal Care and Use Committee, Shanghai Site (IACUC-SH) (protocol code: (A) PK01-001-2019v1.9a and approval date: 16 June 2021).

Informed Consent Statement: Not applicable.

Data Availability Statement: All the data obtained within this work were provided in Supplementary Materials.

Conflicts of Interest: The authors declare no conflict of interest.

Abbreviations

ARVs	Antiretrovirals
Amino-AOCOM	Amino-alkoxycarbonyloxymethyl
CTG	4-Carboxy-2-methyl Tokyo Green
SC	Subcutaneous
RAL	Raltegravir
$t_{\frac{1}{2}}$	Half-life
PrEP	Pre-exposure prophylaxis
ECM	Extracellular matrix
GAGs	Glycosaminoglycans
LLOQ	Lower limit of quantification

Appendix A

Appendix A.1. General Procedure for the Synthesis of Compounds 8(a–b)

Compound **3** (0.02 mol), respective amino alcohol (0.29 mol) and Et$_3$N (0.02 mol) were stirred in DMF at rt for 2d. Then, the reaction mixture was diluted with ethyl acetate and ice-cold water. The organic phase was isolated and dried over MgSO$_4$. The solvent was evaporated, and the crude product was used in the next step without further purification. Compounds **8(a–b)** were identified as follow:

5-(Pent-4-yn-1-ylamino)pentan-1-ol (**8a**). A yellow oil (1.80 g, 47%). ^{1}H NMR (400 MHz, CDCl$_3$): δ 3.65 (t, J = 6.4 Hz, 2H), 2.73 (t, J = 7.0 Hz, 2H), 2.64 (t, J = 7.0 Hz, 2H), 2.26 (td, J = 7.0, 2.7 Hz, 2H), 1.95 (t, J = 2.7 Hz, 1H), 1.77–1.67 (m, 2H), 1.58–1.49 (m, 4H), 1.46–1.37 (m, 2H); ^{13}C NMR (101 MHz, CDCl$_3$): δ 84.1, 68.7, 62.6, 49.8, 48.9, 32.6, 29.8, 28.7, 23.6, 16.5; LR-MS (ESI+) m/z: 170.1 [M+H]$^+$; HRMS m/z (ESI) calcd. for C$_{10}$H$_{19}$NO [M+1]$^+$, 170.1539; found, 170.1544.

6-(Pent-4-yn-1-ylamino)hexan-1-ol (**8b**). A yellow oil (3.65 g, 88%). ^{1}H NMR (400 MHz, CDCl$_3$): δ 3.67–3.62 (m, 2H), 2.77–2.69 (m, 2H), 2.63 (t, J = 6.8 Hz, 2H), 2.26 (td, J = 7.0, 2.7 Hz, 2H), 1.95 (t, J = 2.7 Hz, 1H), 1.77–1.68 (m, 2H), 1.54–1.45 (m, 4H), 1.41 –1.35 (m, 4H); ^{13}C NMR (101 MHz, CDCl$_3$): δ 84.0, 68.8, 62.9, 49.7, 48.7, 32.7, 29.7, 28.4, 27.1, 25.7, 16.5; LR-MS (ESI+) *m/z*: 184.2 [M+H]$^+$; HRMS *m/z* (ESI) calcd. for C$_{11}$H$_{21}$NO [M+H]$^+$, 184.1696; found, 184.1700.

Appendix A.2. General Procedure for the Synthesis of Compounds ***9(a–b)***

Compound **8(a–b)** (2.40 g, 14.80 mmol) was stirred with Boc anhydride (4.60 g, 22.00 mmol) in THF and to this solution, 1 M NaOH (25 mL) was added. Then, the reaction was stirred at rt for 16 h. The product was extracted by Et$_2$O, and the ether layer was washed with H$_2$O, brine, dried over MgSO$_4$, and filtered. The solvent was then evaporated, and the residue was purified using silica gel chromatography (16% EtOAc in pet. spirits).

Tert-butyl (5-hydroxypentyl)(pent-4-yn-1-yl)carbamate (**9a**). A yellow oil (1.10 g, 56%). ^{1}H NMR (400 MHz, CDCl$_3$): δ 3.64 (t, J = 6.5 Hz, 2H), 3.30–3.12 (m, 4H), 2.19 (td, J = 7.0, 2.7 Hz, 2H), 1.96 (t, J = 2.7 Hz, 1H), 1.80–1.68 (m, 2H), 1.64–1.52 (m, 4H), 1.45 (s, 9H), 1.40–1.30 (m, 2H); ^{13}C NMR (101 MHz, CDCl$_3$): δ 155.8, 83.9, 79.5, 68.8, 62.9, 47.1*, 46.3, 32.5, 28.6, 28.1, 27.7*, 23.0, 16.1; LR-MS (ESI+) *m/z*: 292.2 [M+Na]$^+$; HRMS *m/z* (ESI) calcd. for C$_{15}$H$_{27}$NO$_3$ [M+H]$^+$, 270.2064; found, 270.2060.

Tert-butyl (6-hydroxyhexyl)(pent-4-yn-1-yl)carbamate (**9b**). A yellow oil (2.2 g, 53%). ^{1}H NMR (400 MHz, CDCl$_3$): δ 3.66–3.62 (m, 2H), 3.30–3.12 (m, 4H), 2.19 (td, J = 7.1, 2.7 Hz, 2H), 1.96 (t, J = 2.7 Hz, 1H), 1.79–1.71 (m, 2H), 1.61–1.57 (m, 2H), 1.55–1.48 (m, 2H), 1.45 (s, 9H), 1.42–1.36 (m, 2H), 1.34–1.27 (m, 2H); ^{13}C NMR (101 MHz, CDCl$_3$): δ 155.8, 83.9, 79.4, 68.8, 62.9, 47.3*, 46.3, 32.8, 28.6, 28.4, 27.7, 26.6, 25.5, 16.2; LR-MS (ESI+) *m/z*: 306.2 [M+Na]$^+$; HRMS *m/z* (ESI) calcd. for C$_{16}$H$_{29}$NO$_3$ [M+Na]$^+$ 306.2040; found, 306.2043.

Appendix A.3. General Procedure for the Synthesis of Compounds ***10(a–b)***

Chloromethyl chloroformate (2 mmol) was added dropwise to a mixture of compound **9(a–b)** (1 mmol) and pyridine (0.1 mmol) in DCM (25 mL). The reaction was stirred at rt for 2 h. Then, HCl (5 mL, 3 M) was added to quench pyridine and the desired product was extracted from the reaction mixtures using CH$_2$Cl$_2$. The organic layer was washed with NaHCO$_3$, and brine, dried over MgSO$_4$, and concentrated under vacuum. Purification by column chromatography (5% EtOAc in pet. spirits) gave the pure compounds which were characterized as follows:

Tert-butyl (5-(((chloromethoxy)carbonyl)oxy)pentyl)(pent-4-yn-1-yl)carbamate (**10a**). A yellow oil (0.31 g, 85%). ^{1}H NMR (400 MHz, CDCl$_3$): δ 5.73 (s, 2H), 4.22 (t, J = 6.6 Hz, 2H), 3.31–3.12 (m, 4H), 2.19 (td, J = 7.0, 2.6 Hz, 2H), 1.96 (t, J = 2.6 Hz, 1H), 1.80–1.67 (m, 4H), 1.61–1.50 (m, 2H), 1.45 (s, 9H), 1.41–1.30 (m, 2H); ^{13}C NMR (101 MHz, CDCl$_3$): δ 155.7, 153.5, 83.8, 79.5, 72.3, 69.2, 68.9, 47.1, 46.3, 28.6, 28.0 (2C), 27.9*, 23.1, 16.1; LR-MS (ESI+) *m/z*: 384.1 [M+Na]$^+$; HRMS *m/z* (ESI) calcd. for C$_{17}$H$_{28}$ClNO$_5$ [M+Na]$^+$, 384.1548; found, 384.1552.

Tert-butyl (6-(((chloromethoxy)carbonyl)oxy)hexyl)(pent-4-yn-1-yl)carbamate (**10b**). A yellow oil (0.31 g, 82%). ^{1}H NMR (400 MHz, CDCl$_3$): δ 5.73 (s, 2H), 4.22 (t, J = 6.6 Hz, 2H), 3.30–3.10 (m, 4H), 2.19 (td, J = 6.8, 2.5 Hz, 2H), 1.96 (t, J = 2.5 Hz, 1H), 1.78–1.65 (m, 4H), 1.60–1.51 (m, 2H), 1.45 (s, 9H), 1.42–1.35 (m, 2H), 1.34–1.27 (m, 2H); ^{13}C NMR (101 MHz, CDCl$_3$): δ 155.7, 153.6, 83.9, 79.6, 72.3, 69.3, 68.8, 47.4*, 46.4, 28.6, 28.4* (2C), 27.5*, 26.6, 25.6, 16.2; LR-MS (ESI+) *m/z*: 398.2 [M+Na]$^+$; HRMS *m/z* (ESI) calcd. for C$_{18}$H$_{30}$ClNO$_5$ [M+Na]$^+$, 398.1705; found, 398.1710.

Appendix A.4. General Procedure for the Synthesis of Compounds ***11(a–b)***

A mixture of compound **10a** or **10b** (1 mmol) and sodium iodide (3 mmol) was heated in acetone (25 mL) at 45 °C for 16 h. The reaction mixture was filtered and extracted with CHCl$_3$. The chloroform layer was washed with sodium thiosulfate, NaHCO$_3$, and brine, dried over MgSO$_4$, and concentrated under pressure to yield the desired products which were purified by Silica gel chromatography (5% EtOAc in pet spirits) and were identified as follows:

Tert-butyl(5-(((iodomethoxy)carbonyl)oxy)pentyl)(pent-4-yn-1-yl)carbamate (**11a**). A brown oil (0.33 g, 72%). ^{1}H NMR (400 MHz, CDCl$_3$): δ 5.95 (s, 2H), 4.22 (t, *J* = 6.6 Hz, 2H), 3.27–3.12 (m, 4H), 2.20 (td, *J* = 7.2, 2.8 Hz, 2H), 1.96 (t, *J* = 2.6 Hz, 1H), 1.78–1.68 (m, 4H), 1.59–1.52 (m, 2H), 1.45 (s, 9H), 1.41–1.30 (m, 2H); ^{13}C NMR (101 MHz, CDCl$_3$): δ 155.7, 153.3, 83.8, 79.5, 69.2, 68.9, 47.1, 46.3, 34.1, 28.6, 28.4* (2C), 27.5, 23.1, 16.1; LR-MS (ESI+) *m/z*: 354.1 [M+H]$^+$; HRMS *m/z* (ESI) calcd. for C$_{17}$H$_{28}$INO$_5$ [M+Na]$^+$, 476.0904; found, 476.0901.

Tert-butyl(6-(((iodomethoxy)carbonyl)oxy)hexyl)(pent-4-yn-1-yl)carbamate (**11b**). A brown oil (0.32 g, 69%). ^{1}H NMR (400 MHz, CDCl$_3$): δ 5.95 (s, 2H), 4.21 (t, *J* = 6.6 Hz, 2H), 3.29–3.11 (m, 4H), 2.19 (td, *J* = 7.1, 2.6 Hz, 2H), 1.96 (t, *J* = 2.6 Hz, 1H), 1.79–1.65 (m, 4H), 1.52–1.47 (m, 2H), 1.45 (s, 9H), 1.42–1.36 (m, 2H), 1.34–1.27 (m, 2H); ^{13}C NMR (101 MHz, CDCl$_3$): δ 155.7, 153.4, 83.9, 79.4, 69.3, 68.8, 47.3, 46.3, 34.1, 28.6, 28.3(2C)*, 27.5*, 26.5, 25.5, 16.1; LR-MS (ESI+) *m/z*: 490.10 [M+Na]$^+$; HRMS *m/z* (ESI) calcd. for C$_{18}$H$_{30}$INO$_5$ [M+Na]$^+$, 490.1061; found, 490.1066.

Appendix A.5. General Procedure for the Synthesis of CTG-Based Conjugates 13(a–b)

A mixture of cesium carbonate (3.0 mmol) and Boc-protected CTG (1 mmol) was stirred in DMF for 1 h at 0 °C. Then, the respective alkylating agent (2.0 mmol) was added dropwise and the reaction was left to stir for 2–3 h at rt. The reaction was diluted with water and extracted with ethyl acetate, dried over Na$_2$SO$_4$, and concentrated under vacuum. Compounds **13(a–b)** were purified by column chromatography (10:50% EtOAc in pet. Spirits).

Tert-butyl 4-(6-((13,13-dimethyl-3,11-dioxo-10-(pent-4-yn-1-yl)-2,4,12-trioxa-10-azatetra decyl)oxy)-3-oxo-3*H*-xanthen-9-yl)-3-methylbenzoate (**13a**). An orange solid (0.60 g, 83%). ^{1}H NMR (400 MHz, CDCl$_3$): δ 8.04–8.02 (m, 1H), 7.99–7.98 (dd, *J* = 7.6, 0.8 Hz, 1H), 7.22 (d, *J* = 7.9 Hz, 1H), 7.16 (d, *J* = 2.3 Hz, 1H), 6.93 (d, *J* = 8.8 Hz, 1H) 6.89–6.85 (m, 2H), 6.56 (dd, *J* = 9.7, 1.9 Hz, 1H), 6.45 (d, *J* = 1.9 Hz, 1H), 5.84 (s, 2H), 4.20 (t, *J* = 6.6 Hz, 2H), 3.28–3.11 (m, 4H), 2.18 (td, *J* = 7.0, 2.7 Hz, 2H), 2.12 (s, 3H), 1.95 (t, *J* = 2.7 Hz, 1H), 1.77–1.67 (m, 4H), 1.64 (s, 9H), 1.56–1.49 (m, 2H), 1.44 (s, 9H), 1.39–1.30 (m, 2H); ^{13}C NMR (101 MHz, CDCl$_3$): δ 185.9, 165.2, 160.9, 158.6, 155.7, 154.1, 154.0, 147.5, 136.7, 136.6, 133.5, 131.7, 131.0, 130.2, 129.4, 129.3, 127.4, 119.2, 115.6, 114.1, 106.4, 103.4, 87.5, 83.8, 81.8, 79.5, 69.1, 68.9, 47.1, 46.3, 28.6, 28.3, 28.0* (2C), 27.6, 23.1, 19.7, 16.1; LR-MS (ESI+) *m/z*: 728.3 [M+H]$^+$; HRMS *m/z* (ESI) calcd. for C$_{42}$H$_{49}$NO$_{10}$ [M+H]$^+$, 728.3429; found, 728.3435; HPLC: t$_R$ 8.22 min = (>99%).

Tert-butyl4-(6-((14,14-dimethyl-3,12-dioxo-11-(pent-4-yn-1-yl)-2,4,13-trioxa-11azapen tadecyl)oxy)-3-oxo-3*H*-xanthen-9-yl)-3-methylbenzoate (**13b**). An orange solid (0.4 g, 54%). ^{1}H NMR (400 MHz, CDCl$_3$): δ 8.03 (d, *J* = 0.5 Hz, 1H), 8.00 (dd, *J* = 7.9, 1.1 Hz, 1H), 7.24 (d, *J* = 7.9 Hz, 1H), 7.21 (d, *J* = 2.2 Hz, 1H), 7.02 - 6.87 (m, 3H), 6.70–6.60 (m, 2H), 5.86 (s, 2H), 4.20 (t, *J* = 6.6 Hz, 2H), 3.30–3.07 (m, 4H), 2.18 (td, *J* = 7.0, 2.6 Hz, 2H), 2.12 (s, 3H), 1.95 (t, *J* = 2.6 Hz, 1H), 1.78–1.66 (m, 4H), 1.64 (s, 9H), 1.56–1.47 (m, 2H), 1.42 (s, 9H), 1.40–1.24 (m, 4H). ^{13}C NMR (101 MHz, CDCl$_3$): δ 185.8, 165.2, 161.1, 158.7, 155.7, 154.8, 154.0, 147.8, 136.8, 136.6, 133.6, 131.7, 130.9, 130.3, 129.5, 129.4, 127.4, 119.2, 115.7, 114.2, 106.5, 103.5, 87.6, 83.9, 81.8, 79.6, 69.1, 68.8, 47.3, 46.3, 28.6, 28.4, 27.6* (2C), 26.6 (2C), 25.6, 19.7, 16.13; LR-MS (ESI+) *m/z*: 742.4 [M+H]$^+$; HRMS *m/z* (ESI) calcd. for C$_{43}$H$_{51}$NO$_{10}$, [M+Na]$^+$ 764.3405; found, 764.3418; HPLC: t$_R$ 8.35 mins = (>99%).

Appendix A.6. General Procedures for the Synthesis of Probes 14–15

A mixture of the respective CTG conjugates **13(a–b)** (0.36 mmol), and aqueous HCL (0.3 mL, 32%) in acetonitrile or Et$_2$O was stirred for 4–5 h, and the excess HCl and solvent were removed by freeze-drying. The crude products were washed with cyclohexane, and Et$_2$O to yield the pure products which are characterised as follow:

N-(5-(((((9-(4-Carboxy-2-methylphenyl)-3-oxo-3*H*-xanthen-6-yl)oxy)methoxy)carbonyl)oxy) pentyl)pent-4-yn-1-aminium chloride (probe **14**). An orange solid (0.11 g, 51%). ^{1}H NMR (400 MHz, DMSO-d$_6$): δ 8.83 (bs, 2H), 8.07 (m, 1H), 7.99 (d, *J* = 8.0 Hz, 1H), 7.55 (d, *J* = 2.1 Hz, 1H), 7.44 (d, *J* = 8.0 Hz, 1H), 7.19–7.09 (m, 2H), 7.07 (d, *J* = 9.6 Hz, 1H), 6.72 (dd, *J* = 9.6, 1.9 Hz, 1H), 6.66 (d, *J* = 1.9 Hz, 1H), 6.00 (s, 2H), 4.15 (t, *J* = 6.4 Hz, 2H), 2.96–2.79 (m, 5H), 2.27 (td, *J* = 7.0, 2.8 Hz, 2H), 2.08 (s, 3H), 1.85–1.72 (m, 2H), 1.69–1.54 (m, 4H), 1.39–1.27 (m, 2H); ^{13}C NMR (101 MHz, DMSO-d$_6$): δ 181.4, 167.0, 161.9, 158.9, 154.8, 153.4, 152.5, 136.6, 136.1, 132.2, 131.4, 130.3 (2C), 129.7, 128.1, 127.1, 118.1, 115.7, 115.6, 104.4, 103.0, 87.3, 83.6, 72.2, 68.3, 46.6, 45.9, 27.4, 25.0, 24.5, 22.3, 19.2, 15.3; LR-MS (ESI+) *m*/*z*: 572.2 [M+H]$^+$; HRMS *m*/*z* (ESI) calcd. for C$_{33}$H$_{33}$NO$_8$ [M+H]$^+$, 572.2279; found, 572.2283; HPLC: t$_R$ = 5.17 mins. (96%).

6-(((((9-(4-Carboxy-2-methylphenyl)-3-oxo-3*H*-xanthen-6-yl)oxy)methoxy)carbonyl)oxy)-*N*-(pent-4-yn-1-yl)hexan-1-aminium chloride (probe **15**). An orange solid (0.13 g, 71%). ^{1}H NMR (400 MHz, DMSO-d$_6$): δ 8.77 (bs, 2H), 8.07 (s, 1H), 7.99 (dd, *J* = 7.9, 1.0 Hz, 1H), 7.53 (d, *J* = 2.2 Hz, 1H), 7.44 (d, *J* = 7.9 Hz, 1H), 7.15–7.08 (m, 2H), 7.04 (d, *J* = 9.6 Hz, 1H), 6.68 (dd, *J* = 9.6, 2.0 Hz, 1H), 6.60 (d, *J* = 2.0 Hz, 1H), 5.99 (s, 2H), 4.14 (t, *J* = 6.6 Hz, 2H), 2.95–2.87 (m, 5H), 2.27 (td, *J* = 7.1, 2.6 Hz, 2H), 2.08 (s, 3H), 1.83–1.73 (m, 2H), 1.65–1.49 (m, 4H), 1.35–1.23 (m, 4H). ^{13}C NMR (101 MHz, DMSO-d$_6$): δ 182.1, 166.9, 161.5, 158.7, 154.5, 153.4, 151.3 136.5, 136.2, 132.2, 131.3, 131.1, 130.1, 129.6, 128.5, 127.1, 118.1, 115.4, 115.3, 104.6, 103.0, 87.3, 83.1, 72.1, 68.4, 46.7, 45.8, 27.7, 25.5, 25.3, 24.6, 24.5, 19.1, 15.2; HRMS *m*/*z* (ESI) calcd. for C$_{34}$H$_{35}$NO$_8$ [M+H]$^+$, 586.2435; found, 586.2442; HPLC t$_R$ = 5.28 mins (92%).

*Appendix A.7. Procedure for the Synthesis of Diethyl (2-Azidoethyl)Phosphonate (**17**)*

Compound **17** was synthesised as previously described in the literature [68]. ^{1}H NMR (400 MHz, CDCl$_3$): δ 4.12 (m, 4H), 3.54 (dt, *J* = 12.1, 7.8 Hz, 2H), 2.05 (dt, *J* = 15.2, 7.6 Hz, 2H), 1.34 (t, *J* = 7.1 Hz, 6H); ^{13}C NMR (101 MHz, CDCl$_3$): δ 62.1, 62.03, 45.5, 26.9, 25.5, 16.6, 16.5; LR-MS (ESI+) *m*/*z*: 208.1 [M+H]$^+$. Spectroscopic data were matched with those reported in the literature [68].

*Appendix A.8. Preparation of (2-Azidoethyl)Phosphonic Acid (**18**)*

Compound **18** was synthesised as previously described in the literature. ^{1}H NMR (400 MHz, D$_2$O): δ 3.56 (dt, *J* = 13.5, 7.6 Hz, 2H), 2.06 (dt, *J* = 17.9, 7.6 Hz, 2H); ^{13}C NMR (101 MHz, D$_2$O): δ 46.6, 27.3, 26.0; ESI-MS *m*/*z* 152.1 [M+H]$^+$. Spectroscopic data were matched with those reported in the literature [68].

*Appendix A.9. General Procedures to Synthesise Compounds **19(a–b)***

A 10 mL microwave tube was charged with either compound **13a** or **13b** (0.39 mmol) and **18** (0.59 mmol) in a 6 mL mixture of DCM: H$_2$O: *t*BuOH (1:1:1). Then, a mixture of CuSO$_4$ (78 µL, 0.2 equivalents, 1 M) and sodium-L-ascorbate (154 µL, 0.4 equivalents, 1 M) was added and the reaction was heated at 70 °C (100 W) in a microwave reactor for 2 h. When the starting material was completely consumed, the reaction was left to cool. The solvents were removed under vacuum and ethyl acetate was added. The resultant solution was washed with NH$_4$Cl (3 × 5 mL) and the solvent was removed under vacuum. The crude product was purified by flash chromatography (20% MeOH in DCM) to give the title compound which are characterised as follow:

(2-(4-(3-((*tert*-butoxycarbonyl)(5-(((((9-(4-(*tert*-butoxycarbonyl)-2-methylphenyl)-3-oxo-3*H*-xanthen-6-yl)oxy)methoxy)carbonyl)oxy)pentyl)amino)propyl)-1*H*-1,2,3-triazol-1-yl)ethyl)phosphonic acid (**19a**). A brownish-red solid (0.17 g, 50%). ^{1}H NMR (400 MHz, MeOD): δ 8.06 (d, *J* = 1.7 Hz, 1H), 8.01 (dd, *J* = 7.9, 1.7 Hz, 1H), 7.80 (s, 1H), 7.39–7.36 (m, 2H), 7.13–7.04 (m, 3H), 6.62 (dd, *J* = 9.6, 2.0 Hz, 1H), 6.50 (d, *J* = 2.0 Hz, 1H), 5.94 (s, 2H), 4.60–4.54 (m, 2H), 4.20 (t, *J* = 6.4 Hz, 2H), 3.25 –3.15 (m, 4H), 2.65 (t, *J* = 7.6 Hz, 2H), 2.22–2.15 (m, 2H), 2.13 (s, 3H), 1.90 –1.83 (m, 2H), 1.73–1.66 (m, 2H), 1.64 (s, 9H), 1.58–1.49 (m, 2H), 1.40 (s, 9H), 1.36–1.29 (m, 2H); ^{13}C NMR (101 MHz, MeOD) δ 187.7, 172.9, 166.7, 163.3, 161.2, 157.4, 155.9, 155.3, 152.6, 148.4, 138.1, 137.8, 134.7, 132.5, 131.2, 130.6, 130.6,

128.2, 123.0, 119.6, 116.6, 116.0, 106.1, 104.5, 88.6, 82.9, 80.8, 69.8, 47.8 (2C)*, 32.4, 31.1, 29.3 (3C)*, 28.7, 28.4, 24.0, 23.7, 19.6; ESI-MS m/z 879.3 [M+H]$^+$; HRMS m/z (ESI) calcd. for $C_{44}H_{55}N_4O_{13}P$ [M+H]$^+$, 879.3576; found, 879.3593; HPLC t_R = 3.80 min (>99%).

(2-(4-(3-((*tert*-butoxycarbonyl)(6-(((((9-(4-(*tert*-butoxycarbonyl)-2-methylphenyl)-3-oxo-3H-xanthen-6-yl)oxy)methoxy)carbonyl)oxy)hexyl)amino)propyl)-1H-1,2,3-triazol-1-yl) ethyl)phosphonic acid (**19b**). A brownish red solid (0.17 g, 50%).^{1}H NMR (400 MHz, MeOD): δ 8.09 (s, 1H), 8.04 (d, *J* = 7.9 Hz, 1H), 7.84 (s, 1H), 7.44–7.37 (m, 2H), 7.19–7.08 (m, 3H), 6.68 (d, *J* = 9.5 Hz, 1H), 6.58 (s, 1H), 5.97 (s, 2H), 4.62 (bs, 2H), 4.21 (t, *J* = 6.4 Hz, 2H), 3.28–3.14 (m, 4H), 2.74 –2.63 (m, 2H), 2.40–2.24 (m, 2H), 2.15 (s, 3H), 1.93–1.82 (m, 2H), 1.74–1.71 (m, 2H) 1.67 (s, 9H), 1.56–1.49 (m, 2H), 1.43 (s, 9H), 1.42–1.36 (m, 2H), 1.33–1.25 (m, 2H); ^{13}C NMR (101 MHz, MeOD): δ 186.5, 166.5, 163.7, 161.3, 157.3, 156.3, 155.3, 154.0, 143.6, 138.0, 137.6, 134.8, 132.7, 132.5, 131.4, 130.6, 128.2, 123.6, 119.5, 116.8, 116.5, 106.0, 104.4, 88.6, 82.8, 80.8, 69.8, 46.6(2C)*, 30.7, 29.5(2C)*, 28.8, 28.4, 27.4 (2C)*, 26.5 (2C)*, 23.7, 19.7; ESI-MS m/z 893.3 [M+H]$^+$; HRMS m/z (ESI) calcd. for $C_{44}H_{55}N_4O_{13}P$ [M+H]$^+$, 893.3733; found, 893.3733; HPLC: t_R = 3.86 mins (> 97%).

Appendix A.10. Preparation of 5-(((((9-(4-Carboxy-2-Methylphenyl)-3-Oxo-3H-Xanthen-6-yl) Oxy)Methoxy)Carbonyl)Oxy)-N-(3-(1-(2-Phosphonoethyl)-1H-1,2,3-triazol-4-yl)Propyl) Pentan-1-Aminium Chloride (20)

Probe **20** was synthesised according to the general procedure used for the synthesis of probes **14–15** and was purified by revered-phase HPLC and obtained as a brownish-red solid (19 mg, 23%). ^{1}H NMR (400 MHz, MeOD): δ 8.22 (s, 1H), 8.17–8.08 (m, 2H), 7.89 (d, *J* = 2.3 Hz, 1H), 7.68 (d, *J* = 9.3 Hz, 2H), 7.51–7.43 (m, 3H), 7.36 (dd, *J* = 9.3, 2.2 Hz, 1H), 6.12 (s, 2H), 4.73–4.63 (m, 2H), 4.23 (t, *J* = 6.4 Hz, 2H), 3.07–2.93 (m, 4H), 2.87 (t, *J* = 7.2 Hz, 2H), 2.46–2.34 (m, 2H), 2.11 (s, 3H), 2.09–2.03 (m, 2H), 1.79–1.64 (m, 4H), 1.52–1.40 (m, 2H); ^{13}C NMR (101 MHz, MeOD): δ 184.1, 174.8, 168.9, 161.7, 157.6, 155.2, 138.1, 137.4, 134.0, 133.5, 133.0, 132.2, 130.6, 128.5, 127.7, 123.9, 119.5, 118.0, 117.6, 105.2, 104.3, 88.7, 69.5, 58.3, 48.2, 46.4, 29.1, 28.9, 26.8, 23.8, 23.3, 19.7, 18.4; ESI-MS m/z 723.2 [M+H]$^+$; HRMS m/z (ESI) calcd. for $C_{35}H_{39}N_4O_{11}P$ [M+H]$^+$, 723.2426; found, 723.2413; HPLC: t_R = 2.99 mins (>99%).

Appendix A.11. Preparation of 6-(((((9-(4-(Tert-Butoxycarbonyl)-2-Methylphenyl)-3-Oxo-3H-Xanthen-6-yl)Oxy)Methoxy)Carbonyl)Oxy)-N-(3-(1-(2-Phosphonoethyl)-1H-1,2,3-Triazol-4-yl)Propyl)Hexan-1-Aminium Chloride (21)

Probe **21** was synthesised according to the general procedure used for the synthesis of probes **14–15** and was purified by revered-phase HPLC and obtained as a brownish-red solid (20 mg, 23%). ^{1}H NMR (400 MHz, MeOD): δ 8.21 (s, 1H), 8.14 (d, *J* = 8.2 Hz, 1H), 7.86 (s, 1H), 7.66 (d, *J* = 2.5 Hz, 1H), 7.48–7.39 (m, 3H), 7.30 (dd, *J* = 9.2, 2.4 Hz, 1H), 7.04–7.00 (m, 2H), 6.05 (s, 2H), 4.68–4.60 (m, 2H), 4.23 (t, *J* = 6.6 Hz, 2H), 3.07–2.96 (m, 4H), 2.82 (t, *J* = 7.3 Hz, 2H), 2.42–2.31 (m, 2H), 2.14 (s, 3H), 2.09–2.01(m, 2H), 1.77–1.63 (m, 4H), 1.49–1.40 (m, 4H); ^{13}C NMR (101 MHz, MeOD) δ 187.8, 181.0, 168.9, 166.1, 161.9, 158.3, 155.2, 138.1, 137.2, 134.2, 133.8, 133.1, 132.6, 130.6, 128.5, 126.6, 123.9, 119.5, 118.8, 117.9, 104.8, 104.2, 88.6, 69.8, 46.2 (2C), 30.3, 29.3, 27.1, 27.1, 26.8, 26.2, 23.3, 19.7; ESI-MS m/z 737.2 [M+H]$^+$; HRMS m/z (ESI) calcd. for $C_{36}H_{41}N_4O_{11}P$ [M+H]$^+$, 737.2582; found, 737.2581, HPLC: t_R = 3.03 mins (>99%).

Appendix A.12. N-(2-(3-(4-Fluorobenzyl)-7-Methyl-4,8-Dioxo-3,4,7,8-Tetrahydro-2H-Pyrimido[4,5-E][1,3]Oxazin-6-yl)Propan-2-yl)-5-Methyl-1,3,4-Oxadiazole-2-Carboxamide (22)

^{1}H NMR (400 MHz, CDCl$_3$): δ 7.77 (s, 1H), 7.34–7.28 (m, 2H), 7.07–6.99 (m, 2H), 5.24 (s, 2H), 4.71 (s, 2H), 3.67 (s, 3H), 2.62 (s, 3H), 1.93 (s, 6H); ^{13}C NMR (101 MHz, CDCl$_3$): δ 164.0, 161.5, 160.4, 158.2, 154.9, 152.29, 144.7, 131.6, 131.5, 131.3, 129.9, 129.9, 116.2, 116.0, 78.5, 58.9, 47.6, 33.5, 27.4, 11.3; ESI-MS m/z 457.1 [M+H]$^+$; HRMS m/z (ESI) calcd. for $C_{21}H_{21}FN_6O_5$ [M+H]$^+$, 457.163; found, 457.1616; HPLC: t_R = 4.44 mins (>99%) at 254 nm.

Appendix A.13. Preparation of Tert-Butyl(6-(((((4-((4-Fluorobenzyl)Carbamoyl)-1-Methyl-2-(2-(5-Methyl-1,3,4-Oxa-Diazole-2-Carboxamido)Propan-2-yl)-6-Oxo-1,6-Dihydropyrimidin-5yl)Oxy)Methoxy)Carbonyl)Oxy)Hexyl)(Pent-4-yn-1-yl)Carbamate (23)

A mixture of RAL (0.10 g, 0.22 mmole) and cesium carbonate (0.07 g, 0.22 mmole) in DMF (10 mL) was stirred at 0 °C for 1 h. Then, compound 7b (0.21 g, 0.45 mmole) in 5 mL DMF was added dropwise and the resultant mixture was left to stir at rt for 1 h. The crude product was extracted by ethyl acetate and the organic layer was then removed under pressure. The product was purified by flash chromatography (5% MeOH in DCM) and yielded as a white solid (0.15 g, 87%). ^{1}H NMR (400 MHz, CDCl$_3$): δ 8.13 (s, 1H), 7.82 (t, J = 6.1 Hz, 1H), 7.37–7.32 (m, 2H), 7.03–6.98 (m, 2H), 5.88 (s, 2H), 4.56 (d, J = 6.0 Hz, 2H), 4.14 (t, J = 6.7 Hz, 2H), 3.63 (s, 3H), 3.23 (t, J = 7.3 Hz, 2H), 3.14 (bs, 2H), 2.62 (s, 3H), 2.17 (td, J = 7.0, 2.6 Hz, 2H), 1.95 (t, J = 2.6 Hz, 1H), 1.87 (s, 6H), 1.73–1.62 (m, 4H), 1.53–1.46 (m, 2H), 1.43 (s, 9H), 1.39–1.33 (m, 2H), 1.30–1.23 (m, 2H); ^{13}C NMR (101 MHz, CDCl$_3$): δ 166.6, 163.5, 161.9, 161.1, 160.9, 158.7, 155.7, 155.4, 154.7, 152.1, 141.1, 138.7, 134.1, 134.0, 129.7, 129.6, 12.5, 115.7, 115.5, 90.5, 83.9, 79.3, 68.8, 68.6, 58.3, 47.3*, 46.3, 42.8, 33.4, 28.6* (2C), 27.3*, 26.7, 26.6, 25.6, 16.1, 11.3; ESI-MS m/z 782.3 [M − H]$^+$; HRMS m/z (ESI) calcd. for C$_{38}$H$_{50}$FN$_7$O$_{10}$ [M+H]$^+$ 784.3676; found, 784.3695; HPLC: t$_R$ = 6.52 mins (>99%).

Appendix A.14. Preparation of (2-(4-(3-((Tert-Butoxycarbonyl)(6-(((((4-((4-Fluorobenzyl) Carbamoyl)-1-Methyl-2-(2-(5-Methyl-1,3,4-Oxadiazole-2-Carboxamido)Propan-2-yl)-6-Oxo-1,6-Dihydropyrimidin-5-yl)Oxy)Methoxy)Carbonyl)Oxy)Hexyl)Amino)Propyl)-1H-1,2,3-Triazol-1-yl)Ethyl)Phosphonic Acid (24)

Compound **24** was synthesised according to the procedure used for the synthesis of compounds **19 (a–b)**, purified by flash chromatography (20% MeOH in DCM), and obtained as a brownish-red solid (0.17 g, 50%). ^{1}H NMR (400 MHz, MeOD): δ 7.77–7.74 (m, 1H), 7.31–7.28 (m, 2H), 6.99–6.94 (m, 2H), 5.67 (s, 2H), 4.53 (q, J = 9.2 Hz, 2H), 4.44 (s, 2H), 4.01 (t, J = 6.6 Hz, 2H), 3.53 (s, 3H), 3.14 (t, J = 7.4 Hz, 2H), 3.08 (t, J = 7.4 Hz, 2H), 2.58 (t, J = 7.6 Hz, 2H), 2.50 (s, 3H), 2.35–2.21 (m, 2H), 1.84–1.76 (m, 2H), 1.72 (s, 6H), 1.59–1.50 (m, 2H), 1.46–1.38 (m, 2H), 1.33 (bs, 9H), 1.31–1.24 (m, 2H), 1.22–1.14 (m, 2H); ^{13}C NMR (101 MHz, MeOD): δ 167.9, 165.2, 164.7, 162.3, 159.7, 158.8, 157.4, 156.0, 154.7, 148.3*, 142.7, 140.5, 135.7, 130.5, 130.4, 123.8, 116.3, 116.1, 91.4, 80.8, 69.5, 59.6, 47.7*, 47.4*, 46.4*, 43.4, 34.0, 30.2*, 29.6, 29.2 (2C)*, 28.7, 27.4, 27.2, 26.5, 23.5*, 10.8; ESI-MS m/z 935.3 [M+H]$^+$; HRMS m/z (ESI) calcd. for C$_{40}$H$_{56}$FN$_{10}$O$_{13}$P [M+H]$^+$, 935.3823; found, 935.3828; HPLC: t$_R$ = 2.99 mins (>99%).

Appendix A.15. Preparation of 6-(((((4-((4-Fluorobenzyl)Carbamoyl)-1-Methyl-2-(2-(5-Methyl-1,3,4-Oxadiazole-2-Carboxa-Mido)Propan-2-Yl)-6-Oxo-1,6-Dihydropyrimidin-5yl)Oxy)Methoxy)Carbonyl)Oxy)-N-(3-(1-(2-Phosphonoethyl)-1H-1,2,3-Triazol-4-Yl) Propyl)Hexan-1-Aminium Chloride (25)

HCl in diethyl ether (1 mL, 2 M) was added to compound **24** in diethyl ether (5 mL) and the reaction mixture was stirred at rt for 4 h. The excess HCl acid was evaporated by freeze-drying and the obtained solid was purified by reversed-phase chromatography to give the pure product as a white solid (45 mg, 50%). ^{1}H NMR (400 MHz, MeOD): δ 7.87 (s, 1H), 7.44–7.37 (m, 2H), 7.12–7.04 (m, 2H), 5.78 (s, 2H), 4.61 (q, J = 8.3 Hz, 2H), 4.55 (s, 2H), 4.15 (t, J = 6.4 Hz, 2H), 3.65 (s, 3H), 3.08–2.96 (m, 4H), 2.82 (t, J = 7.0 Hz, 2H), 2.62 (s, 3H), 2.26–2.14 (m, 2H), 2.10–2.01 (m, 2H), 1.81 (s, 6H), 1.74–1.64 (m, 4H), 1.49–1.39 (m, 4H); ^{13}C NMR (101 MHz, MeOD): δ 167.9, 165.3, 164.7, 162.3, 159.8, 158.9, 156.0, 154.8, 142.8, 140.5, 135.7, 135.7, 130.5, 130.4, 123.8, 116.3, 116.1, 91.5, 69.4, 59.6, 48.8*, 48.2, 47.5, 43.4, 34.0, 30.6, 29.2*, 27.2, 27.1, 27.0, 26.8, 26.2, 23.3, 10.8; ESI-MS m/z 833.3 [M−H]$^+$; HRMS m/z (ESI) calcd. for C$_{35}$H$_{48}$FN$_{10}$O$_{11}$P [M+H]$^+$ 835.3298, found, 835.3289; HPLC: t$_R$ = 3.07 mins (>99%).

Appendix A.16. (E)-6-(((((4-((4-Fluorobenzyl)Carbamoyl)-2-(2-(2-(2-(1-Hydroxyethylidene) Hydrazineyl)-2-Oxoacetamido)Propan-2-yl)-1-Methyl-6-Oxo-1,6-Dihydropyrimidin-5-yl) Oxy)Methoxy)Carbonyl)Oxy)-N-(3-(1-(2-Phosphonoethyl)-1H-1,2,3-Triazol-4-yl)Propyl) Hexan-1-Aminium Chloride (26)

Compound **26** was produced as by-product during the synthesis of compound **25** using aqueous concentrated HCl (32%). ^{1}H NMR (400 MHz, MeOD) δ 8.78 (t, J = 6.2 Hz, 1H), 7.86 (s, 1H), 7.44–7.36 (m, 2H), 7.11–7.02 (m, 2H), 5.76 (s, 2H), 4.61 (q, J = 9.2 Hz, 2H), 4.54 (d, J = 4.3 Hz, 2H), 4.15 (t, J = 6.4 Hz, 2H), 3.61 (s, 3H), 3.06–2.95 (m, 4H), 2.81 (t, J = 7.2 Hz, 2H), 2.28–2.16 (m, 2H), 2.09–2.03 (m, 2H), 2.02 (s, 3H), 1.78 (s, 6H), 1.74–1.64 (m, 4H), 1.47–1.40 (m, 4H); ^{13}C NMR (101 MHz, MeOD): δ 171.9, 165.3, 164.7, 162.3, 160.2, 160.1, 159.1, 156.0, 142.6, 140.6, 135.7, 135.7, 130.5, 130.4, 123.8, 116.3, 116.1, 91.6, 69.3, 59.0, 48.8*, 48.2, 47.3, 43.4, 34.0, 31.6, 29.3, 27.2, 27.1, 27.0, 26.8, 26.2, 23.3, 20.5; ESI-MS m/z 853.3[M+H]$^+$; HRMS m/z (ESI) calcd. for C$_{35}$H$_{50}$FN$_{10}$O$_{12}$P [M+H]$^+$ 853.3404, found, 853.3423.

References

1. Barnhart, M. Long-acting HIV treatment and prevention: Closer to the threshold. *Glob. Health Sci. Pract.* **2017**, *5*, 182–187. [CrossRef]
2. Walensky, R.P.; Paltiel, A.D.; Losina, E.; Mercincavage, L.M.; Schackman, B.R.; Sax, P.E.; Weinstein, M.C.; Freedberg, K.A. The survival benefits of AIDS treatment in the united states. *J. Infect. Dis.* **2006**, *194*, 11–19. [CrossRef] [PubMed]
3. Blanc, F.X.; Sok, T.; Laureillard, D.; Borand, L.; Rekacewicz, C.; Nerrienet, E.; Madec, Y.; Marcy, O.; Chan, S.; Prak, N.; et al. Earlier versus later start of antiretroviral therapy in HIV-infected adults with tuberculosis. *N. Engl. J. Med.* **2011**, *365*, 1471–1481. [CrossRef] [PubMed]
4. Wada, N.; Jacobson, L.P.; Cohen, M.; French, A.; Phair, J.; Muñoz, A. Cause-specific life expectancies after 35 years of age for human immunodeficiency syndrome-infected and human immunodeficiency syndrome-negative individuals followed simultaneously in long-term cohort studies, 1984–2008. *Am. J. Epidemiololgy* **2013**, *177*, 116–125. [CrossRef] [PubMed]
5. Chesney, M.A. Factors affecting adherence to antiretroviral therapy. *Clin. Infect. Dis.* **2000**, *30* (Suppl. S2), S171–S176. [CrossRef]
6. Gonzalez, J.S.; Batchelder, A.W.; Psaros, C.; Safren, S.A. Depression and HIV/AIDS treatment nonadherence: A review and meta-analysis. *J. Acquiedr Immune Defic. Syndr.* **2011**, *58*, 181–187. [CrossRef]
7. Barnabas, R.V.; Celum, C. Closing the gaps in the HIV care continuum. *PLoS Med.* **2017**, *14*, 1002443. [CrossRef]
8. Ortego, C.; Huedo-Medina, T.B.; Llorca, J.; Sevilla, L.; Santos, P.; Rodríguez, E.; Warren, M.R.; Vejo, J. Adherence to highly active antiretroviral therapy (HAART): A meta-analysis. *AIDS Behavoir* **2011**, *15*, 1381–1396. [CrossRef]
9. Amico, K.R.; Stirratt, M.J. Adherence to preexposure prophylaxis: Current, emerging, and anticipated bases of evidence. *Clin. Infect. Dis.* **2014**, *59* (Suppl. S1), S55–S60. [CrossRef]
10. Williams, J.; Sayles, H.R.; Meza, J.L.; Sayre, P.; Sandkovsky, U.; Gendelman, H.E.; Flexner, C.; Swindells, S. Long-acting parenteral nanoformulated antiretroviral therapy: Interest and attitudes of HIV-infected patients. *Nanomedicine* **2013**, *8*, 1807–1813. [CrossRef]
11. Margolis, D.A.; Gonzalez-Garcia, J.; Stellbrink, H.-J.; Eron, J.J.; Yazdanpanah, Y.; Podzamczer, D.; Lutz, T.; Angel, J.B.; Richmond, G.J.; Clotet, B.; et al. Long-acting intramuscular cabotegravir and rilpivirine in adults with HIV-1 infection (LATTE-2): 96-week results of a randomised, open-label, phase 2b, non-inferiority trial. *Lancet* **2017**, *390*, 1499–1510. [CrossRef]
12. Swindells, S.; Andrade-Villanueva, J.-F.; Richmond, G.J.; Rizzardini, G.; Baumgarten, A.; Masiá, M.; Latiff, G.; Pokrovsky, V.; Bredeek, F.; Smith, G.; et al. Long-Acting Cabotegravir and Rilpivirine for Maintenance of HIV-1 Suppression. *N. Engl. J. Med.* **2020**, *382*, 1112–1123. [CrossRef]
13. Orkin, C.; Arasteh, K.; Górgolas Hernández-Mora, M.; Pokrovsky, V.; Overton, E.T.; Girard, P.-M.; Oka, S.; Walmsley, S.; Bettacchi, C.; Brinson, C.; et al. Long-Acting cabotegravir and rilpivirine after oral induction for HIV-1 infection. *N. Engl. J. Med.* **2020**, *382*, 1124–1135. [CrossRef]
14. Markham, A. Cabotegravir plus rilpivirine: First approval. *Drugs* **2020**, *80*, 915–922. [CrossRef]
15. FDA Approves First Extended-Release, Injectable Drug Regimen for Adults Living with HIV. Available online: https://www.fda.gov/news-events/press-announcements/fda-approves-first-extended-release-injectable-drug-regimen-adults-living-hiv (accessed on 29 November 2022).
16. Harrison, T.S.; Goa, K.L. Long-acting risperidone: A review of its use in schizophrenia. *CNS Drugs* **2004**, *18*, 113–132. [CrossRef]
17. Draper, B.H.; Morroni, C.; Hoffman, M.; Smit, J.; Beksinska, M.; Hapgood, J.; Van der Merwe, L. Depot medroxyprogesterone versus norethisterone oenanthate for long-acting progestogenic contraception. *Cochrane Database Syst. Rev.* **2006**, *19*, Cd005214. [CrossRef]
18. Rabinow, B.E. Nanosuspensions in drug delivery. *Nat. Rev. Drug Discov.* **2004**, *3*, 785–796. [CrossRef]
19. Müller, R.H.; Peters, K. Nanosuspensions for the formulation of poorly soluble drugs: I. Preparation by a size-reduction technique. *Int. J. Pharm.* **1998**, *160*, 229–237. [CrossRef]
20. Paik, J.; Duggan, S.T.; Keam, S.J. Triamcinolone acetonide extended-release: A review in osteoarthritis pain of the knee. *Drugs* **2019**, *79*, 455–462. [CrossRef]

21. Kanwar, N.; Sinha, V.R. In Situ Forming Depot as Sustained-Release Drug Delivery Systems. *Crit. Rev. Ther. Drug Carr. Syst.* **2019**, *36*, 93–136. [CrossRef]
22. Shi, Y.; Lu, A.; Wang, X.; Belhadj, Z.; Wang, J.; Zhang, Q. A review of existing strategies for designing long-acting parenteral formulations: Focus on underlying mechanisms, and future perspectives. *Acta Pharm. Sin. B* **2021**, *11*, 2396–2415. [CrossRef] [PubMed]
23. Benhabbour, S.R.; Kovarova, M.; Jones, C.; Copeland, D.J.; Shrivastava, R.; Swanson, M.D.; Sykes, C.; Ho, P.T.; Cottrell, M.L.; Sridharan, A.; et al. Ultra-long-acting tunable biodegradable and removable controlled release implants for drug delivery. *Nat. Commun.* **2019**, *10*, 4324. [CrossRef] [PubMed]
24. Monastyrskyi, A.; Brockmeyer, F.; LaCrue, A.N.; Zhao, Y.; Maher, S.P.; Maignan, J.R.; Padin-Irizarry, V.; Sakhno, Y.I.; Parvatkar, P.T.; Asakawa, A.H. Aminoalkoxycarbonyloxymethyl ether prodrugs with a pH-triggered release mechanism: A case study improving the solubility, bioavailability, and efficacy of antimalarial 4 (1*H*)-quinolones with single dose cures. *J. Med. Chem.* **2021**, *64*, 6581–6595. [CrossRef] [PubMed]
25. Abd-Ellah, H.S.; Mudududdla, R.; Carter, G.P.; Baell, J.B. Design, development, and optimisation of smart linker chemistry for targeted colonic delivery— in vitro evaluation. *Pharmaceutics* **2023**, *15*, 303. [CrossRef] [PubMed]
26. Croxtall, J.D.; Keam, S.J. Raltegravir: A review of its use in the management of HIV infection in treatment-experienced patients. *Drugs* **2009**, *69*, 1059–1075. [CrossRef]
27. Evering, T.H.; Markowitz, M. Raltegravir: An integrase inhibitor for HIV-1. *Expert Opin. Investig. Drugs* **2008**, *17*, 413–422. [CrossRef]
28. Kovarova, M.; Swanson, M.D.; Sanchez, R.I.; Baker, C.E.; Steve, J.; Spagnuolo, R.A.; Howell, B.J.; Hazuda, D.J.; Garcia, J.V. A long-acting formulation of the integrase inhibitor raltegravir protects humanized BLT mice from repeated high-dose vaginal HIV challenges. *J. Antimicrob. Chemother.* **2016**, *71*, 1586–1596. [CrossRef]
29. Cottrell, M.L.; Patterson, K.B.; Prince, H.M.; Jones, A.; White, N.; Wang, R.; Kashuba, A.D. Effect of HIV infection and menopause status on raltegravir pharmacokinetics in the blood and genital tract. *Antivir. Ther.* **2015**, *20*, 795–803. [CrossRef]
30. Clavel, C.; Peytavin, G.; Tubiana, R.; Soulié, C.; Crenn-Hebert, C.; Heard, I.; Bissuel, F.; Ichou, H.; Ferreira, C.; Katlama, C.; et al. Raltegravir concentrations in the genital tract of HIV-1-infected women treated with a raltegravir-containing regimen (DIVA 01 study). *Antimicrob. Agents Chemother.* **2011**, *55*, 3018–3021. [CrossRef]
31. Heck, H.D.; Casanova-schm1tz, M.; Dodd, P.B.; Schachter, E.N.; Witek, T.J.; Tosun, T. Formaldehyde (CH_2O) concentrations in the blood of humans and Fischer-344 rats exposed to CH_2O under controlled conditions. *Am. Ind. Hyg. Assoc. J.* **1985**, *46*, 1–3. [CrossRef]
32. Arda, O.; Göksügür, N.; Tüzün, Y. Basic histological structure and functions of facial skin. *Clin. Dermatol.* **2014**, *32*, 3–13. [CrossRef] [PubMed]
33. Viola, M.; Sequeira, J.; Seiça, R.; Veiga, F.; Serra, J.; Santos, A.C.; Ribeiro, A.J. Subcutaneous delivery of monoclonal antibodies: How do we get there? *J. Control. Release* **2018**, *286*, 301–314. [CrossRef] [PubMed]
34. Ruiz, M.; Scioli Montoto, S. *Routes of Drug Administration: Dosage, Design, and Pharmacotherapy Success*; Springer: Berlin/Heidelberg, Germany, 2018; pp. 97–133. [CrossRef]
35. Supersaxo, A.; Hein, W.R.; Steffen, H. Effect of molecular weight on the lymphatic absorption of water-soluble compounds following subcutaneous administration. *Pharm. Res. Off. J. Am. Assoc. Pharm. Sci.* **1990**, *7*, 167–169. [CrossRef]
36. Usach, I.; Martinez, R.; Festini, T.; Peris, J.E. Subcutaneous injection of drugs: Literature review of factors influencing pain sensation at the injection site. *Adv. Ther.* **2019**, *36*, 2986–2996. [CrossRef] [PubMed]
37. Hecker, S.J.; Erion, M.D. Prodrugs of phosphates and phosphonates. *J. Med. Chem.* **2008**, *51*, 2328–2345. [CrossRef]
38. Schull, T.L.; Fettinger, J.C.; Knight, D.A. Synthesis and characterization of palladium(ii) and platinum(ii) complexes containing water-soluble hybrid phosphine−phosphonate ligands. *Inorg. Chem.* **1996**, *35*, 6717–6723. [CrossRef]
39. Wiemer, A.J.; Wiemer, D.F. Prodrugs of phosphonates and phosphates: Crossing the membrane barrier. *Top. Curr. Chem.* **2015**, *360*, 115–160. [CrossRef]
40. Jiang, J.; Yang, E.; Reddy, K.R.; Niedzwiedzki, D.M.; Kirmaier, C.; Bocian, D.F.; Holten, D.; Lindsey, J.S. Synthetic bacteriochlorins bearing polar motifs (carboxylate, phosphonate, ammonium and a short PEG). Water-solubilization, bioconjugation, and photophysical properties. *New J. Chem.* **2015**, *39*, 5694–5714. [CrossRef]
41. Bittner, B.; Richter, W.; Schmidt, J. Subcutaneous administration of biotherapeutics: An overview of current challenges and opportunities. *BioDrugs* **2018**, *32*, 425–440. [CrossRef]
42. Mineno, T.; Ueno, T.; Urano, Y.; Kojima, H.; Nagano, T. Creation of superior carboxyfluorescein dyes by blocking donor-excited photoinduced electron transfer. *Org. Lett.* **2006**, *8*, 5963–5966. [CrossRef]
43. Yamagishi, K.; Sawaki, K.; Murata, A.; Takeoka, S. A Cu-free clickable fluorescent probe for intracellular targeting of small biomolecules. *Chem. Commun.* **2015**, *51*, 7879–7882. [CrossRef] [PubMed]
44. Yang, S.H.; Lee, D.J.; Brimble, M.A. Synthesis of an NDPK phosphocarrier domain peptide containing a novel triazolylalanine analogue of phosphohistidine using click chemistry. *Org. Lett.* **2011**, *13*, 5604–5607. [CrossRef] [PubMed]
45. Patil, G.D.; Kshirsagar, S.W.; Shinde, S.B.; Patil, P.S.; Deshpande, M.S.; Chaudhari, A.T.; Sonawane, S.P.; Maikap, G.C.; Gurjar, M.K. Identification, synthesis, and strategy for minimization of potential impurities observed in raltegravir potassium drug substance. *Org. Process Res. Dev.* **2012**, *16*, 1422–1429. [CrossRef]

46. Webb, P. Temperatures of skin, subcutaneous tissue, muscle and core in resting men in cold, comfortable and hot conditions. *Eur. J. Appl. Physiol. Occup. Physiol.* **1992**, *64*, 471–476. [CrossRef] [PubMed]
47. Demchenko, A.P. Photobleaching of organic fluorophores: Quantitative characterization, mechanisms, protection. *Methods Appl. Fluoresc.* **2020**, *8*, 022001. [CrossRef]
48. Kabadi, P.G.; Sankaran, P.K.; Palanivelu, D.V.; Adhikary, L.; Khedkar, A.; Chatterjee, A. Mass spectrometry based mechanistic insights into formation of tris conjugates: Implications on protein biopharmaceutics. *J. Am. Soc. Mass Spectrom.* **2016**, *27*, 1677–1685. [CrossRef]
49. Saari, W.S.; Schwering, J.E.; Lyle, P.A.; Smith, S.J.; Engelhardt, E.L. Cyclization-activated prodrugs. Basic esters of 5-bromo-2'-deoxyuridine. *J. Med. Chem.* **1990**, *33*, 2590–2595. [CrossRef]
50. Thomsen, K.F.; Bundgaard, H. Cyclization-activated phenyl carbamate prodrug forms for protecting phenols against first-pass metabolism. *Int. J. Pharm.* **1993**, *91*, 39–49. [CrossRef]
51. Matsumoto, H.; Sohma, Y.; Kimura, T.; Hayashi, Y.; Kiso, Y. Controlled drug release: New water-soluble prodrugs of an HIV protease inhibitor. *Bioorganic Med. Chem. Lett.* **2001**, *11*, 605–609. [CrossRef]
52. Sharma, I.; Kaminski, G.A. Calculating pKa values for substituted phenols and hydration energies for other compounds with the first-order Fuzzy-Border continuum solvation model. *J. Comput. Chem.* **2012**, *33*, 2388–2399. [CrossRef]
53. Moss, D.M.; Siccardi, M.; Back, D.J.; Owen, A. Predicting intestinal absorption of raltegravir using a population-based ADME simulation. *J. Antimicroibial Chemother.* **2013**, *68*, 1627–1634. [CrossRef]
54. Fredholt, K.; Mørk, N.; Begtrup, M. Hemiesters of aliphatic dicarboxylic acids as cyclization-activated prodrug forms for protecting phenols against first-pass metabolism. *Int. J. Pharm.* **1995**, *123*, 209–216. [CrossRef]
55. Sánchez-Félix, M.; Burke, M.; Chen, H.H.; Patterson, C.; Mittal, S. Predicting bioavailability of monoclonal antibodies after subcutaneous administration: Open innovation challenge. *Adv. Drug Deliv. Rev.* **2020**, *167*, 66–77. [CrossRef]
56. Pitiot, A.; Heuzé-Vourc'h, N.; Sécher, T. Alternative routes of administration for therapeutic antibodies-state of the art. *Antibodies* **2022**, *11*, 56. [CrossRef]
57. Bumbaca Yadav, D.; Sharma, V.K.; Boswell, C.A.; Hotzel, I.; Tesar, D.; Shang, Y.; Ying, Y.; Fischer, S.K.; Grogan, J.L.; Chiang, E.Y.; et al. Evaluating the use of antibody variable region (Fv) charge as a risk assessment tool for predicting typical cynomolgus monkey pharmacokinetics. *J. Biol. Chem.* **2015**, *290*, 29732–29741. [CrossRef]
58. Uhrich, K.E.; Cannizzaro, S.M.; Langer, R.S.; Shakesheff, K.M. Polymeric systems for controlled drug release. *Chem. Rev.* **1999**, *99*, 3181–3198. [CrossRef]
59. Luginbuhl, K.M.; Schaal, J.L.; Umstead, B.; Mastria, E.M.; Li, X.; Banskota, S.; Arnold, S.; Feinglos, M.; D'Alessio, D.; Chilkoti, A. One-week glucose control via zero-order release kinetics from an injectable depot of glucagon-like peptide-1 fused to a thermosensitive biopolymer. *Nat. Biomed. Eng.* **2017**, *1*, 0078. [CrossRef]
60. Lau, J.; Bloch, P.; Schäffer, L.; Pettersson, I.; Spetzler, J.; Kofoed, J.; Madsen, K.; Knudsen, L.B.; McGuire, J.; Steensgaard, D.B.; et al. Discovery of the once-weekly glucagon-like peptide-1 (GLP-1) Analogue semaglutide. *J. Med. Chem.* **2015**, *58*, 7370–7380. [CrossRef]
61. Lee, P.Y.; Cobain, E.; Huard, J.; Huang, L. Thermosensitive hydrogel PEG-PLGA-PEG enhances engraftment of muscle-derived stem cells and promotes healing in diabetic wound. *Mol. Ther.* **2007**, *15*, 1189–1194. [CrossRef]
62. Kuzma, P.; Moo-Young, A.J.; Mora, D.; Quandt, H.; Bardin, C.W.; Schlegel, P.H. Subcutaneous hydrogel reservoir system for controlled drug delivery. *Macromol. Symp.* **1996**, *109*, 15–26. [CrossRef]
63. Zhang, X.; Zhang, S.; Kang, Y.; Huang, K.; Gu, Z.; Wu, J. Advances in long-circulating drug delivery strategy. *Curr. Drug Metab.* **2018**, *19*, 750–758. [CrossRef] [PubMed]
64. Van Witteloostuijn, S.B.; Pedersen, S.L.; Jensen, K.J. Half-life extension of biopharmaceuticals using chemical methods: Alternatives to PEGylation. *ChemMedChem* **2016**, *11*, 2474–2495. [CrossRef] [PubMed]
65. Wang, C.; Cheng, S.; Zhang, Y.; Ding, Y.; Chong, H.; Xing, H.; Jiang, S.; Li, X.; Ma, L. Long-Acting HIV-1 fusion inhibitory peptides and their mechanisms of action. *Viruses* **2019**, *11*, 811. [CrossRef] [PubMed]
66. Cheng, S.; Wang, Y.; Zhang, Z.; Lv, X.; Gao, G.F.; Shao, Y.; Ma, L.; Li, X. Enfuvirtide-PEG conjugate: A potent HIV fusion inhibitor with improved pharmacokinetic properties. *Eur. J. Med. Chem.* **2016**, *121*, 232–237. [CrossRef]
67. Sherman, M.R.; Williams, L.D.; Sobczyk, M.A.; Michaels, S.J.; Saifer, M.G. Role of the methoxy group in immune responses to mPEG-protein conjugates. *Bioconjugate Chem.* **2012**, *23*, 485–499. [CrossRef]
68. Ma, C.; Bian, T.; Yang, S.; Liu, C.; Zhang, T.; Yang, J.; Li, Y.; Li, J.; Yang, R.; Tan, W. Fabrication of versatile cyclodextrin-functionalized upconversion luminescence nanoplatform for biomedical imaging. *Anal. Chem.* **2014**, *86*, 6508–6515. [CrossRef]

Disclaimer/Publisher's Note: The statements, opinions and data contained in all publications are solely those of the individual author(s) and contributor(s) and not of MDPI and/or the editor(s). MDPI and/or the editor(s) disclaim responsibility for any injury to people or property resulting from any ideas, methods, instructions or products referred to in the content.

Article

Hydroxypropyl Methylcellulose Bioadhesive Hydrogels for Topical Application and Sustained Drug Release: The Effect of Polyvinylpyrrolidone on the Physicomechanical Properties of Hydrogel

Patrick Pan [1], Darren Svirskis [1], Geoffrey I. N. Waterhouse [2] and Zimei Wu [1,*]

1 School of Pharmacy, Faculty of Medical and Health Sciences, The University of Auckland, Auckland 1142, New Zealand; t.pan@auckland.ac.nz (P.P.); d.svirskis@auckland.ac.nz (D.S.)
2 School of Chemical Sciences, Faculty of Science, The University of Auckland, Auckland 1142, New Zealand; g.waterhouse@auckland.ac.nz
* Correspondence: z.wu@auckland.ac.nz; Tel.: +64-9-9231709

Abstract: Hydrogels are homogeneous three-dimensional polymeric networks capable of holding large amounts of water and are widely used in topical formulations. Herein, the physicomechanical, rheological, bioadhesive, and drug-release properties of hydrogels containing hydroxypropyl methylcellulose (HPMC) and polyvinylpyrrolidone (PVP) were examined, and the intermolecular interactions between the polymers were explored. A three-level factorial design was used to form HPMC–PVP binary hydrogels. The physicomechanical properties of the binary hydrogels alongside the homopolymeric HPMC hydrogels were characterized using a texture analyzer. Rheological properties of the gels were studied using a cone and plate rheometer. The bioadhesiveness of selected binary hydrogels was tested on porcine skin. Hydrophilic benzophenone-4 was loaded into both homopolymeric and binary gels, and drug-release profiles were investigated over 24 h at 33 °C. Fourier transform infrared spectroscopy (FTIR) was used to understand the inter-molecular drug–gel interactions. Factorial design analysis supported the dominant role of the HPMC in determining the gel properties, rather than the PVP, with the effect of both polymer concentrations being non-linear. The addition of PVP to the HPMC gels improved adhesiveness without significantly affecting other properties such as hardness, shear-thinning feature, and viscosity, thereby improving bioadhesiveness for sustained skin retention without negatively impacting cosmetic acceptability or ease of use. The release of benzophenone-4 in the HPMC hydrogels followed zero-order kinetics, with benzophenone-4 release being significantly retarded by the presence of PVP, likely due to intermolecular interactions between the drug and the PVP polymer, as confirmed by the FTIR. The HPMC–PVP binary hydrogels demonstrate strong bioadhesiveness resulting from the addition of PVP with desirable shear-thinning properties that allow the formulation to have extended skin-retention times. The developed HPMC–PVP binary hydrogel is a promising sustained-release platform for topical drug delivery.

Keywords: hydrogels; factorial design; controlled release; topical delivery; texture analysis; rheology; bioadhesion; intermolecular interactions; hydroxypropyl methylcellulose; polyvinylpyrrolidone

1. Introduction

Topical drug delivery attracts significant attention due to its potential to provide targeted and localized therapy for various dermatological conditions. However, the efficacy of topical formulations can often be compromised by factors such as poor retention on the skin and low drug penetration into the skin, leading to the need for frequent application [1]. The outermost layer of the skin, the stratum corneum, constitutes a strong barrier and makes it difficult for drug molecules to penetrate and cross the skin at clinically relevant rates. An increase in the contact time of topically applied formulation allows for a higher quantity of the active agents to eventually be delivered. In dermatological conditions such as in psoriasis, a controlled-release formulation will allow for the local release of a drug over a prolonged period, reducing the frequency of administration, and improving patient compliance and clinical outcomes. Controlled-release technologies using bioadhesive gels provide a solution to overcome these challenges and improve the effectiveness of topical drug delivery [2–5]. These gel formulations can regulate the release rate of drugs over time. They can be designed to provide sustained drug exposure to the target site, reducing the risk of systemic side effects, and provide flexibility in dosing regimens to match the specific requirements of different dermatological conditions [2–5]. Thus, topical controlled-release gel formulations offer significant advantages and hold great promise in advancing the field of dermatological drug delivery.

Among the various topical controlled-release formulations, hydrogels have been extensively explored as an effective medium for sustained topical drug delivery [2–5]. Hydrogels are homogeneous semisolids which consist of a water-swollen hydrophilic polymer three-dimensional network possessing a high water content [6]. Hydrogels offer numerous benefits as a controlled-release medium, including the ability to quickly dry and form a thin-film that is non-greasy and non-occlusive, whilst also being cosmetically elegant and easy to apply [2,7]. Such systems have been used to locally deliver anti-inflammatories and anesthetics such as borneol, curcumin, and lignocaine during the treatment of skin wounds [3,5,8], where an extended local retention time is desirable. Furthermore, polymers in gels ensure good film formation and stability on the skin, as well as good water and sweat resistance [9].

Various physicomechanical properties (rheological and mechanical properties) of a gel-based topical formulation determine its retention, penetration, and drug-release rates. Viscosity of the gel medium plays an important role in increasing the retention time of the formulation on the skin while prolonging drug release [3,4]. Bioadhesiveness is another important factor to consider when designing topical controlled-delivery formulations where extended skin contact is required for the drug to be delivered to the target site over a period of time [10,11]. The main mechanism of bioadhesion is intermolecular bonding, and, for many materials, it is due to the formation of interfacial hydrogen bonds between the adhesive gel and biological surface [12,13].

With hydrogels, the low polymer and high water content allows for soft, deformable, and flexible networks that can accommodate skin movement [14,15], making them desirable for topical drug delivery. However, the adhesiveness of hydrogels is generally low due to the majority of their volume being composed of polar water molecules that do not actively participate in joining materials [15]. To overcome this, combinations of different hydrogel polymers have been explored to boost hydrogel adhesion [14,16,17], resulting in "binary double network-like gels" or "binary gels". However, the addition of the secondary polymer often causes an increase in gel viscosity or decreases the spreadability of the gel on the skin, necessitating the lowering of polymers concentrations, which in turn can reduce adhesiveness [18].

Hydroxypropyl methylcellulose (HPMC) is a commonly used hydrophilic polymer in controlled-release formulations due to its thickening, gelling, and swelling properties, which can form highly stable, clear, and odorless hydrogels [19]. Cosmetically, HPMC gels provide a thick but non-tacky feel, produce a strong and flexible film upon drying, disperse easily on the skin, have a cooling effect, and are non-comedogenic [20]. The bioadhesive property of HPMC has been attributed to the presence of abundant -OH functional groups in the molecule that can form hydrogen bonds with water and other HPMC molecules [21] (Figure 1A). Additionally, HPMC has a minimal interaction with drugs (other than H-bonding interactions) and has demonstrated the ability to improve bioadhesion and enhance local delivery of drugs through improved retention [22,23]. Polyvinylpyrrolidone (PVP), a hydrophilic synthetic polymer, is commonly used in controlled-drug-delivery systems due to its biocompatibility [24,25]. However, the direct use of pure PVP hydrogels is limited due to their low swelling capacity and poor mechanical properties. Therefore, PVP is often blended with different polymers to improve the physicomechanical properties of the preparations according to the requirements of the application [24,26]. Of note, PVP polymers have excellent adhesive properties due to the abundance of carbonyl groups (Figure 1B) that can establish hydrogen bonds with biological surfaces, making PVP an ideal component in bioadhesive delivery systems [25,27–29]. Furthermore, binary hydrogels can form a strong cross-linked film that can adhere to the skin while maintaining a smooth feel, making them ideal for topical formulations for controlled drug delivery [27,30]. Little information is presently available for HPMC–PVP binary hydrogels; however, the addition of PVP has previously been reported to reduce the tackiness of HPMC solutions, as a result of a net reduction in the hydrogen-bonding network between the HPMC chains which is caused by PVP addition [31]. We hypothesized that the HPMC–PVP system may form hydrogels with a high adhesiveness without significantly impacting other mechanical parameters such as viscosity and spreadability, offering a platform for sustained topical drug delivery.

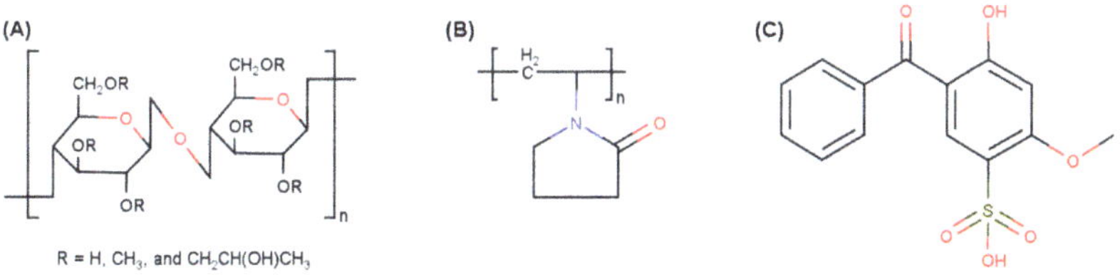

Figure 1. Chemical structures of (**A**) hydroxypropyl methylcellulose (HPMC), (**B**) polyvinylpyrrolidone (PVP), and (**C**) benzophenone-4.

This research aimed to evaluate the effectiveness of using binary HPMC and PVP hydrogels for sustained topical drug delivery. The mechanical properties of the gels were characterized using a texture analyzer and a Brookfield rheometer, and bioadhesiveness was further tested on porcine skin. With the aid of a three-level two-factor (3^2) factorial design, the effects of the addition of PVP on the mechanical parameters of the HPMC-PVP hydrogel's viscosity, bioadhesiveness, and drug-release rates were investigated to determine if an optimal binary gel formulation can produce a topical formulation that is more suited to the sustained release of a drug (benzophenone-4 in this case) into the skin.

2. Materials and Methods

Hydroxypropyl methylcellulose K100 (HPMC), polyvinylpyrrolidone K25 (PVP), benzophenone-4, sodium phosphate dibasic, sodium phosphate monobasic, and dialysis bags from regenerated cellulose membranes with a molecular weight cut-off (MWCO) of 14,000 Da were all purchased from Sigma-Aldrich (Auckland, New Zealand). The HPMC and PVP powders were dried overnight at 60 °C prior to use and were stored in a desiccator. Sodium phosphate dibasic and sodium phosphate monobasic were used to prepare 0.1 M of phosphate buffered saline (PBS), and the final pH was adjusted to 5.5 using hydrochloric acid. Milli-Q water was obtained from a Millipak® 0.22 µm system (Millipore Corporation, Bedford, MA, USA). All other reagents were of analytical grade and purchased from Sigma-Aldrich (Auckland, New Zealand).

Fresh porcine skin (aged 5–6 months) from the flank was obtained from a local abattoir (Auckland Meat Processes, Auckland, New Zealand).

2.1. Preparation of Polymeric Hydrogel Systems

2.1.1. HPMC and PVP Homopolymeric Hydrogels

Homopolymeric gel formulations were prepared using HPMC alone at eight different concentrations (2%, 4%, 6%, 8%, 10%, 12%, 14%, and 16%, w/w) or PVP alone at three different concentrations (3%, 6%, and 9%, w/w). Hydrogels were prepared following a dry-blending method [32]. Briefly, the required amounts of dry HPMC or PVP were weighed and dispersed in half the necessary amounts of PBS (0.1 M, pH 5.5, pre-warmed to 80 °C), followed by vigorous stirring for 10 min to obtain a well-dispersed mixture. Further PBS (at room temperature) was then slowly added to produce the final desired concentration. The mixture was stirred for another 10 min at room temperature, followed by cooling for 10 min in an ice bath. The gels were then sealed and stored at 4 °C for at least 48 h to ensure the complete hydration of the polymers and to allow the escape of the entrapped air bubbles.

2.1.2. HPMC–PVP Binary Hydrogels and Factorial Design Analysis

The dry-blending method was used to prepare the binary gel formulations. Briefly, appropriate amounts of dry HPMC and PVP powders were uniformly mixed before the addition of PBS and mixing well to obtain uniform hydrogels.

A three-level two-factor (3^2) factorial design was used to generate the binary gel formulation (Table 1) and to assess the effect of the polymer concentrations in the HPMC–PVP binary hydrogels on their physicomechanical properties. Based on the properties of the homopolymeric HPMC gels, the concentrations of HPMC (X_1, 4, 8 and 12% w/v) and PVP (X_2; 3, 6, 9% w/v) were considered as independent variables. The response variables Y including adhesiveness and viscosity (at shear rate of 4 s^{-1}) were of interest.

Table 1. Amounts of HPMC (X_1) and PVP (X_2) powders in the binary gels generated by a 3^2 factorial design.

Gel Number	1	2	3	4	5	6	7	8	9
X_1: HMPC (% w/v)	4	4	4	8	8	8	12	12	12
X_2: PVP (% w/v)	3	6	9	3	6	9	3	6	9

2.2. Characterization of Hydrogels

2.2.1. Texture Profile Analysis

The mechanical properties of the homopolymeric and binary hydrogels were investigated using the TA.XT Plus texture analyzer (Stable Micro System, Surrey, UK). A 2 kg loading cell and a cylindrical stainless-steel probe (diameter 25 mm) were used for all measurements. The gel samples (50 g) were placed into glass jars to produce a cylindrical gel mass (diameter 50 mm × 80 mm height) and stored at room temperature for 12 h prior to testing.

During the texture profile analysis, the probe was compressed twice into each gel sample at a defined rate of 1 mm·s^{-1} with a trigger force of 0.001 g, during which the probe would penetrate to a depth of 10 mm into the gel sample. There was a delay period of 15 s between the end of the first and the beginning of the second compression. At least three replicates were performed for each formulation at ambient temperature (21 ± 2 °C) using fresh samples in each case. The data collection and analysis were performed using the Texture Exponent 3.0.5.0 software package provided with the instrument (Stable Micro System, Surrey, UK). The force–time graphs (typically as shown on Figure 2B,C) were recorded for the determination of the mechanical parameters, namely hardness, compressibility, adhesiveness, and cohesiveness [33].

2.2.2. Rheological Characterization

The rheological properties of the gel formulations containing different concentrations of polymers were analyzed using a rotational Brookfield DV-III+ cone and plate rheometer (Brookfield Engineering Laboratories Inc., Middleborough, MA, USA). The rheometer was fitted with a Flat Plate SST ST 40 mm diameter spindle and was operated by the Brookfield Rheocalc operating software version 3.2.47. The sample temperature was controlled at 33 ± 0.1 °C.

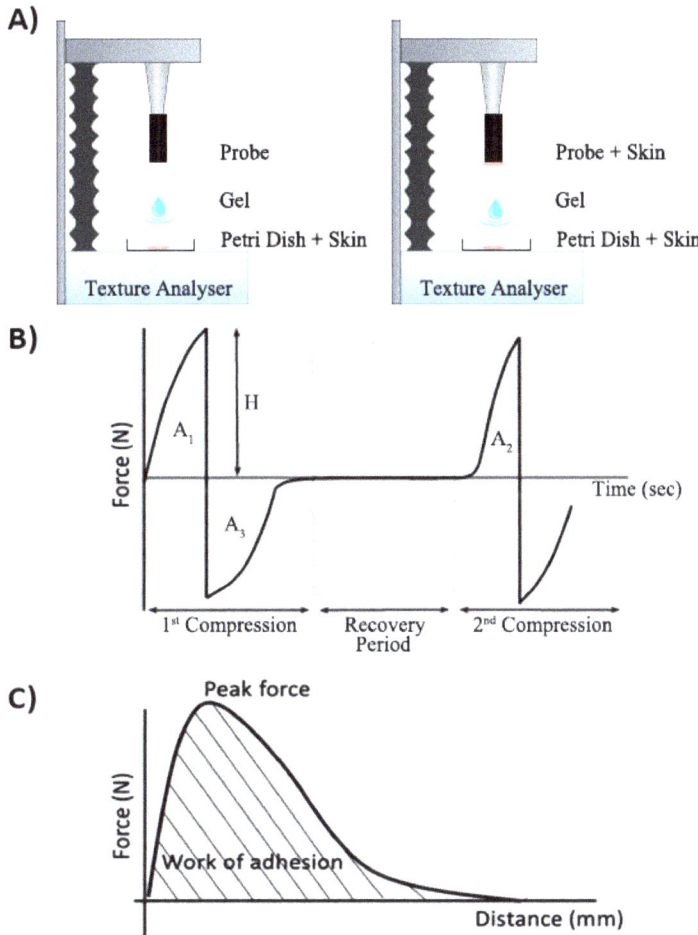

Figure 2. (**A**) Schematic diagram of the TXA setup for bioadhesion testing using a standard setup (**left**) with single skin substrate, or alternative setup (**right**) with gel between two skin substrates. (**B**) Force–time graphical output from texture profile analysis. H = Hardness. A_1 = Compressibility. A_3 = Adhesiveness. A_2/A_1 = Cohesiveness. (**C**) Schematic graph showing the applied peak force and work of adhesion provided by the texture analyzer software (Brookfield Rheocalc version 3.2.47).

For each measurement, 50 µL of gel was carefully pipetted using a large-ended pipette tip, with the tips cut off, to ensure uniform sampling of gel. The sample was applied to the lower chamber of the viscometer avoiding any air bubbles and was allowed to equilibrate for at least 5 min before analysis. The samples were subjected to continuous shear analysis and a logarithmic sweep was performed at shear rates of 4–300 s^{-1}. Each speed was maintained for 30 s to allow for data collection. Three replicates were performed for each formulation, and viscosity curves at shear rates were plotted to understand the flow properties.

2.3. Ex Vivo Bioadhesion Testing

Porcine skin from the flank was used to assess bioadhesiveness of the selected binary hydrogel which contained HPMC 12% and PVP 6% (denoted as H12P6).

2.3.1. Tissue Preparation

The elapsed time from the slaughter of the pig to the removal of the skin was approximately 2 h. The skin sections were stored in normal saline (0.9%) to prevent dehydration during transport to the laboratory for dissection. The damaged or bruised sections were discarded. A scalpel was used to remove the subcutaneous tissue and the remaining full layer of the stratum corneum with epidermis was then cut into either a circular section (diameter of 25 mm) for use as the attached skin, or square sections (30 mm × 30 mm) to be used as the substrate in bioadhesion testing. These length and width measurements reflect the skin in its relaxed state, where the wrinkles and folds were not stretched or flattened. The prepared skin sections were immediately frozen in liquid nitrogen and stored at $-20\ °C$ for no longer than 4 weeks before use.

Porcine skin from the flank, as opposed to the standard porcine ear [34], was used to assess bioadhesion. Evidence has supported that it is an effective in vitro substrate for simulating human skin in terms of histological and physiological properties [35], while also providing the benefit of being able to test using larger sections of skin.

2.3.2. Bioadhesion Analysis

The excised skin sections were thawed overnight at $4\ °C$ and soaked in phosphate-buffered saline (PBS) (0.1 M, pH 5.5) for 10 min. The excess surface moisture was removed by blotting with filter paper after placing a 2 kg weight over the skin for 5 min. Each piece of skin was used only once for each gel preparation.

The bioadhesive force between porcine skin and binary gel was assessed using the TA.XT Plus texture analyzer in Hold-Until-Time mode. To identify differences in bioadhesion results, two setups were used: one testing the steel probe with a single skin substrate, and a second setup testing between two skin sections (Figure 2A).

A total of 1 g of gel was spread homogenously over the entire surface of the substrate skin sections (30 mm × 30 mm), which were secured onto a petri dish with double-sided tape (3M Scotch Mount^{TM}). The circular skin sections were attached using double-sided tape (3M Scotch Mount^{TM}) to the lower end of the cylindrical probe (diameter 25 mm), facing downward and opposing the substrate skin sections.

The upper part of the texture analyzer (with the attached skin) was placed as close as possible to the substrate skin. Contact was avoided between the two skin sheets. In this position, the texture analyzer was lowered to $0.1\ mm·s^{-1}$, which has been shown to give the best discriminative values [36], until contact between the substrate skin and the attached skin was made. The triggering force (by which the contact with the sample was calculated) was 0.01 N. The two skin pieces were in contact for 15 s under a force of 0.5 N. The upper part of the texture analyzer was lifted at a speed of $0.1\ mm·s^{-1}$ until the separation of the two skin sheets occurred.

The tests were conducted at ambient temperature ($21 \pm 2\ °C$) and each experiment was replicated at least three times using a fresh sample of gel. The mucosa was gently cleaned with saline-soaked damp tissue before testing each replicate.

Peak tension can be derived from a force–time graph as the maximum force required to separate the adhesive interface. The area under the force–distance curve during the separation of the hydrogels from the skin surface is regarded as the work of adhesion (Figure 2C).

2.4. Drug Release

The dialysis tubing method [37] was used to investigate the drug release from various gel systems.

Drug-loaded gels were prepared during preparation of the base gel as described above, with the drug pre-added to the PBS phase. The final concentration of benzophenone-4 in each gel was 25 mg/g (2.5%). Drug-loaded gels (2 g) were then packed into 3 mL syringes and loaded into prepared dialysis tubing before sealing with dialysis clips. Care was taken to pack gels tightly, with no air bubbles within the tubing, to form a gel column (diameter 20 mm × 25 mm height), providing a total surface area for diffusion of ~3140 mm^2.

Four formulations (PVP 6%, HPMC 12%, HPMC 13%, H12P6) suspended in PBS and one formulation (HPMC 13% in MeOH) in methanol were tested for drug release by placing the dialysis bags loaded with samples in 50 mL of either PBS or methanol as external media in separate Falcon tubes and suspended in a water bath at 33 °C with oscillation set at 60 rpm. Aliquots (1 mL) from the external media were withdrawn at various time points (0.25, 0.5, 0.75, 1, 2, 3, 4, 5, 6, and 24 h) and immediately replaced with an equivalent volume of PBS or methanol. The drug content in the external media was analyzed directly through a validated high-performance liquid chromatography (HPLC) assay [38].

2.5. Fourier Transform Infrared Spectroscopy

To reveal and identify any intermolecular interactions between functional groups, infrared transmission spectra of pure benzophenone-4 and freeze-dried hydrated gel samples of HPMC, PVP, and HPMC–PVP binary gel mixtures (1:1 weight ratio) with and without benzophenone-4 were obtained using a Fourier transform infrared (FTIR) spectrophotometer (Bruker Alpha Eco-ATR FTIR Spectrometer; OPUS 8.7.41 ALPHA, Mannheim, Germany). The samples were analyzed above a diamond crystal using the ATR mode. The spectra were collected over the wavenumber range 4000 to 400 cm^{-1} at resolution of 4 cm^{-1} to investigate possible interactions between the active functional groups of benzophenone-4 with PVP and HPMC.

The optical spectroscopy software, Spectragryph, Version 1.2.16.1, was used to visualize and manipulate the ATR-FTIR spectra [39]. A baseline correction was applied to all spectra using the standard normal variate approach.

2.6. Stability Studies

The prepared gels (HPMC gels and HPMC–PVP binary gels) were packed into Eppendorf tubes (2 mL) and stability studies were performed in the temperature and relative humidity (RH) conditions stipulated by the International Council for Harmonisation of Technical Requirements for Pharmaceuticals for Human Use. The samples were stored at 4 °C, 25 °C (60% RH), 30 °C (65% RH), and 40 °C (75% RH) for a period of 3 months. The samples were withdrawn at 15-day intervals and evaluated for physical appearance, pH, and viscosity. The drug content was evaluated at 3 months [40].

2.7. Statistical Analysis

All data are expressed as the mean ± standard deviation (SD). A statistical analysis of each parameter of interest was carried out using Student's *t*-test for dependent and independent samples, a one-way analysis of variance (ANOVA) and Tukey's HSD post hoc test. A *p*-value < 0.05 was considered significant. All statistical calculations were performed using the GraphPad Prism for Windows (Version 9, GraphPad Software, La Jolla, CA, USA).

3. Results

3.1. HPMC Homopolymeric Hydrogels

3.1.1. Texture Profile

The hardness, compressibility, and adhesiveness force all showed an exponential relationship to the concentration of HPMC in the homopolymeric HPMC gels (Figure 3A–C). The cohesiveness was largely unaffected by the HPMC concentration (2–16%) (Figure 3D), indicating that the intermolecular forces between the HPMC polymer chains were independent of polymer concentration.

The homopolymeric PVP presented as a free-flowing solution with concentrations of 3%, 6%, and 9%, *w/w*, thus no texture profile analysis could be performed. This was expected, owing to the low swelling capacity of the PVP and thus its inability to establish a viscous hydrogel network [26].

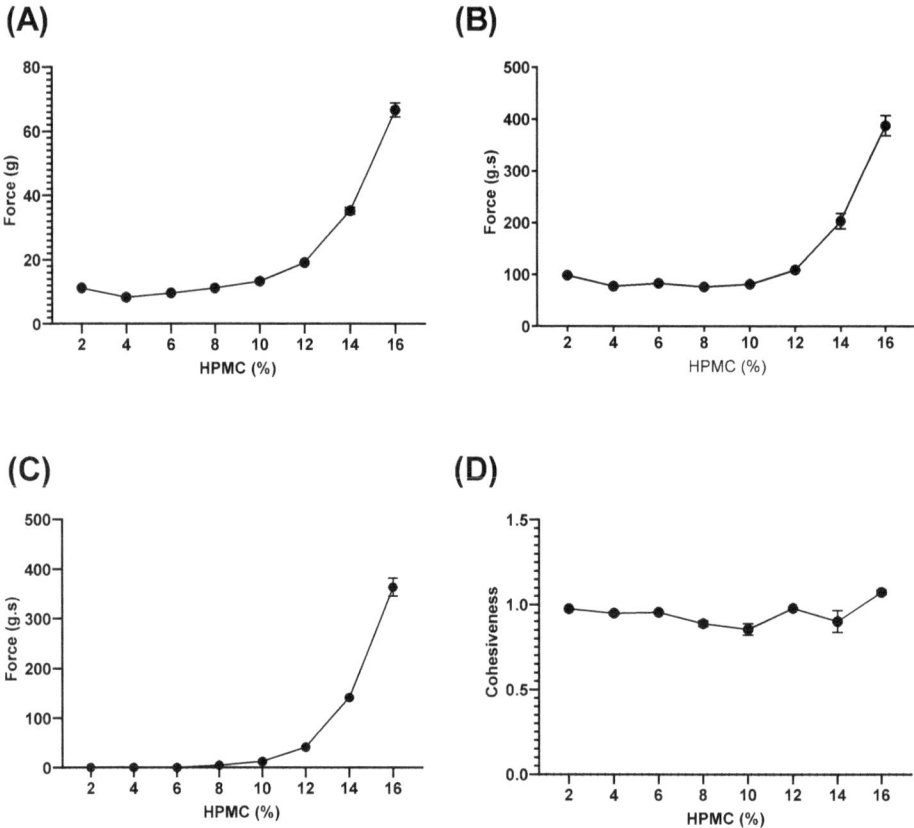

Figure 3. Mechanical properties of homopolymeric HPMC (2–16%) hydrogels obtained with a texture analyzer. (**A**) Hardness; (**B**) Compressibility; (**C**) Adhesiveness; and (**D**) Cohesiveness. Data are mean ± SD (n = 3).

3.1.2. Rheological Properties

The rheological data showed that increasing concentrations of HPMC led to an exponential increase in viscosity, as measured at low shear rate (Figure 4B). The HPMC gels from 2% to 8% exhibited near-Newtonian flow behavior, as evidenced by the almost-linear trend in the rheograms (Figure 4B,C). When the HPMC polymer concentrations increased above 8%, the HPMC hydrogels displayed non-Newtonian (shear-thinning) behavior.

3.2. HPMC–PVP Binary Hydrogel and Factorial Design Analysis

3.2.1. Texture Profile

The adhesiveness of the resulting binary gels increased as a function of the concentration of both polymers. The addition of PVP at 0, 3, 6, or 9% (w/w) to the HPMC gels (4–12%, w/w) increased adhesiveness (Figure 5C) while having a minimal impact on hardness and compressibility (Figure 5A,B). For example, the homopolymeric gel HPMC 12% (H12P0) had an adhesiveness of 40.96 ± 0.37 g·s. The addition of PVP 6% (H12P6) to create a binary gel increased the adhesiveness to 253.64 ± 11.87 g·s, representing a 6.19-fold increase (Figure 5E). At higher concentrations of PVP 9% (H12P9), a higher adhesiveness of 405.08 ± 13.17 g·s was achieved. However, hardness and compressibility, undesirable properties for a topical formulation, also increased significantly for H12P9.

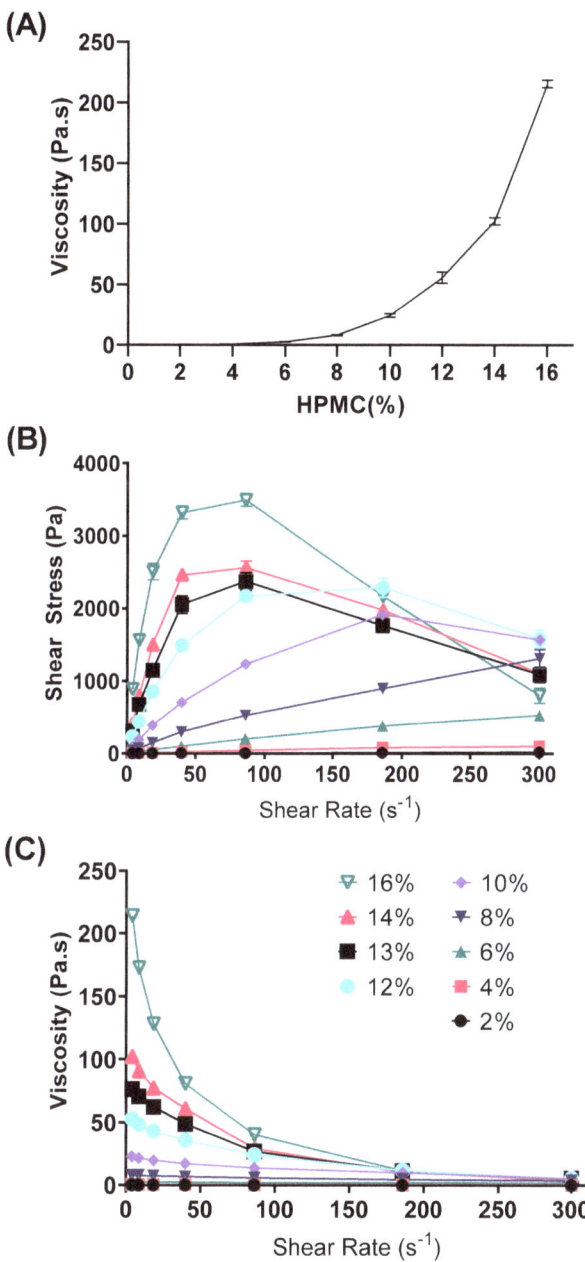

Figure 4. Rheological properties of gels containing HPMC 2–16%: (**A**) Viscosity curve at shear rate = 4 s^{-1}, and rheograms of (**B**) shear stress vs. shear rate and (**C**) viscosity vs. shear rate. Data are mean ± SD (n = 3).

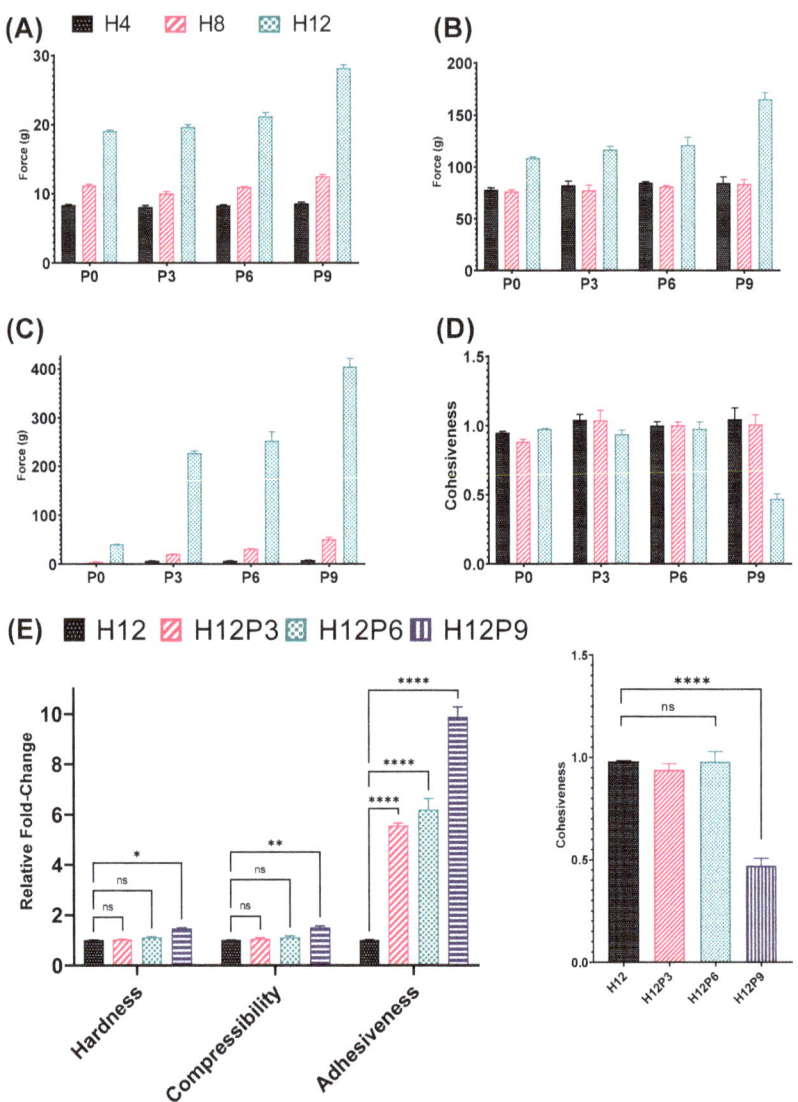

Figure 5. Physicomechanical properties of mono- or binary gels containing HPMC and PVP at various concentrations. (**A**) Hardness; (**B**) Compressibility; (**C**) Adhesiveness; and (**D**) Cohesiveness. Comparisons were made for the following: (**E**) hardness, compressibility, adhesiveness, and cohesiveness. The data show that the addition of PVP only increased the adhesiveness remarkably as a function of PVP concentration. Data are mean ± SD (n = 3). *: $p < 0.05$; **: $p < 0.01$; **** $p < 0.0001$; ns = non-significant difference.

The binary H12P9 formulation exhibited a sharp decrease in the cohesiveness of the gel (Figure 5E), indicating a compromised structure of the polymer network. Thus, this binary gel formulation was excluded from further studies. The results suggested that the H12P6 gel formulation was the most appropriate for further studies examining drug release due to its high adhesiveness, along with acceptable hardness, compressibility, and cohesiveness.

3.2.2. Rheological Properties

Stronger shear-thinning properties were observed with increasing polymer concentrations in the hydrogels (Figure 6A). Increasing the concentration of PVP in the HPMC–PVP binary hydrogels lead to an increase in viscosity, together with more profound shear-thinning properties. The viscosity for all gels dropped to similar levels when the shear rate was increased to 200 s^{-1} (Figure 6B). Interestingly, despite the increase of PVP to 9% for H12P9, there was a slight decrease in the viscosity along with a significant reduction in its' peak shear stress (at shear rate = 86 s^{-1}), which was lower than both H12P3's and H12P6's (Figure 6A). This is aligned with a reduction in the cohesiveness for the same formulation which was seen in the texture analyzer tests, and it further reinforces the finding that the structure of the polymer network in the binary hydrogels was compromised at high PVP concentrations.

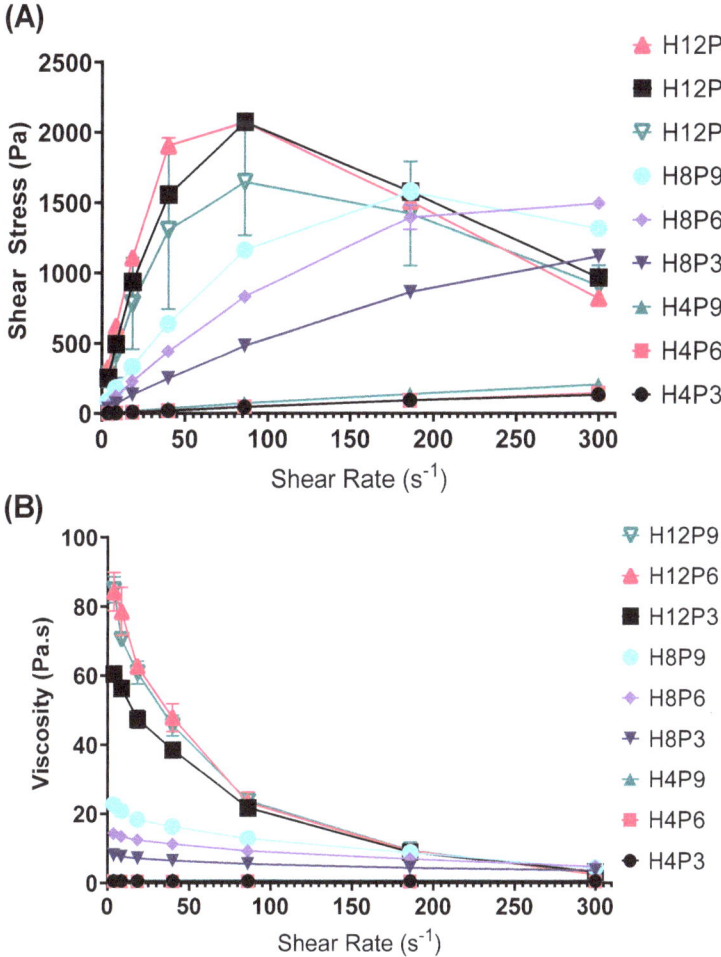

Figure 6. Plots of (**A**) shear stress vs. shear rate and (**B**) viscosity vs. shear rate for HPMC–PVP binary gel formulations. Data are means ± SD (n = 3).

At modest shear rates of 300 s^{-1}, all formulations achieved a very low viscosity value, which makes them suitable for easy application onto the skin.

3.2.3. Factorial Design Analysis

The two-dimensional contour, surface, and interaction plots for adhesiveness and viscosity are shown in (Figure 7). The plots clearly demonstrated that neither adhesiveness nor viscosity increased proportionally to the HPMC concentration in the binary gels. The results also revealed that the increase in adhesiveness and viscosity caused by increasing the PVP concentration from 3% to 6% was only apparent at high concentrations of HPMC (12%). However, further increasing the PVP to 9% increased adhesiveness but not the viscosity.

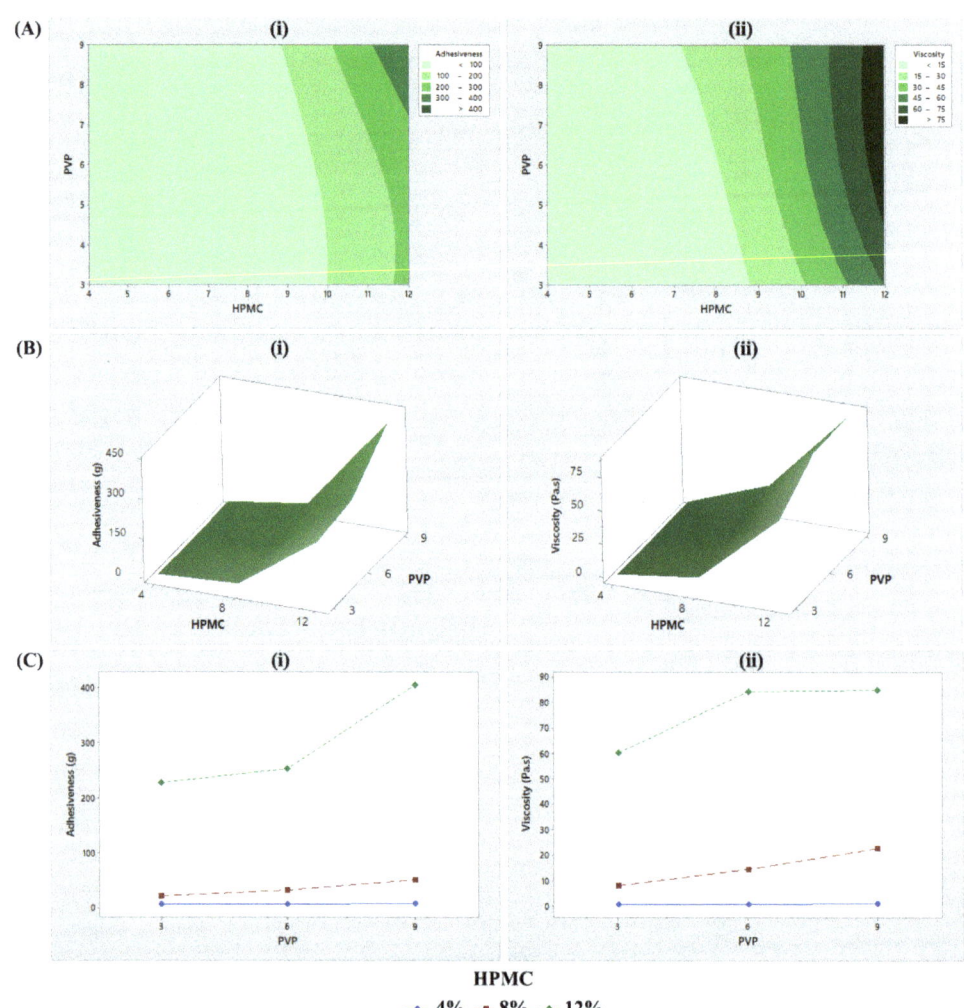

Figure 7. The 3^2 factorial design analysis using Minitab. (**A**) Two-dimensional contour plot, (**B**) three-dimensional surface plot, (**C**) interaction plot, for adhesiveness (**i**) and viscosity (**ii**).

3.3. Ex Vivo Bioadhesiveness

Figure 8 shows bioadhesion results for the binary gel formulation H12P6. This formulation showed the highest adhesiveness, yet an appropriate viscosity for topical application. Significant differences were observed in the peak force and work of adhesion between the two setups used (either single or double skin substrates), but not adhesiveness.

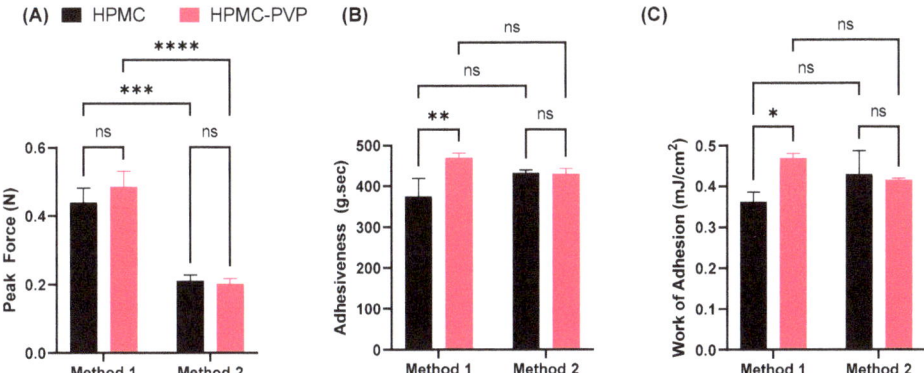

Figure 8. Bioadhesion results for the H12P6 binary gel for either a single (method one) or double (method two) skin substrate setups. (**A**) peak force; (**B**) adhesiveness; and (**C**) work of adhesion. Data are mean ± SD (n = 3). *: $p < 0.05$; **: $p < 0.01$; ***: $p < 0.001$; ****: $p < 0.0001$; ns = non-significant difference.

A significantly large drop in the peak force for both the homopolymeric and binary gels was observed between the single surface skin setup and the double skin setup, possibly attributable to the larger volume of skin that was displaced to reach the specified contact force of 0.5 N. This was also accompanied by a small but non-significant decrease in the adhesiveness and work of adhesion in the double substrate skin setup.

Compared with homopolymeric 12% HPMC gel, the hardness remained the same in the binary gel with addition of 6% PVP. However, a significant increase in the adhesiveness and work of adhesion were observed in the binary gel ($p < 0.01$, $p < 0.05$) using method one. No differences between the two gel formulations were observed using method two.

3.4. Drug-Release Profiles

The cumulative drug release of benzophenone-4 from different gel formulations, including a free drug solution as a control, is illustrated in Figure 9. Release from the drug solution was complete within 3 h, indicating that the dialysis tubing did not impact drug release and that sink conditions were present throughout. Even though it possessed a low viscosity, the homopolymeric PVP 6% impeded the diffusion of benzophenone-4 out of the gel matrix into the external media. The cumulative release amount of benzophenone-4 (Q_t) was linearly dependent on the square root of the time (t), implying that the release kinetics followed a Higuchi model ($R^2 = 0.959$). In contrast, all HPMC gels demonstrated zero-order release kinetics in the first 6 h ($R^2 > 0.983$ to 0.989). The release rate from the 13% HPMC gel was 7.2% (of total dose) h^{-1}, which increased to 8.9% h^{-1} as the HPMC polymer concentration was reduced to 12%, with the increased release being attributed to the reduced viscosity (52.8 Pa·s for 12% HPMC gel vs. 76.4 Pa·s of 13% HPMC gel; at shear rate of 4 s^{-1}, as shown in Figure 4C). No significant difference in drug release was observed between the PBS and methanol (MeOH) as the external media, indicating that the differences in solubility of benzophenone-4 in the external media did not impact drug release and that sink conditions were present throughout. For all HPMC gels, the drug-release rate after 6 h became slower. Of note, no benzophenone-4 was detected in the external media for the binary H12P6 formulation over 24 h, indicating that the rate of drug release was very low and that the total amount of drug released below the limit of detection (LOD) of 1.08 μg/mL (0.11% of total dose).

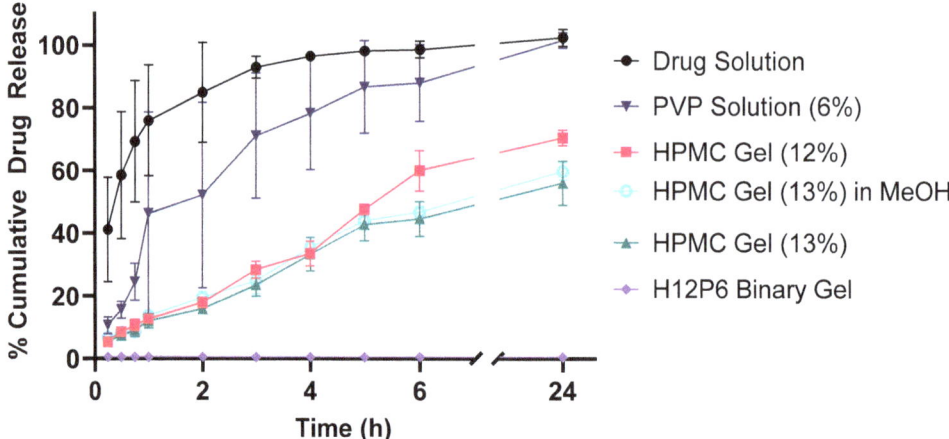

Figure 9. Cumulative drug release of benzophenone-4 over 24 h at 33 °C from formulation samples in dialysis bags. Drug release from the binary gel (H12P6) remained undetected throughout and is graphically represented as the limit of detection. All gel formulations contained 2.5% w/w of benzophenone-4. Data are mean ± SD (n = 3).

3.5. Fourier Transform Infrared Spectroscopy

The FTIR spectra for the various samples are shown in Figure 10. The benzophenone-4 (BNZ4) showed characteristic peaks around 1061 cm^{-1} and 599 cm^{-1} due to S=O and S-O stretching modes, respectively, in the sulfonic acid (-SO$_3$H) group of BNZ4, as well as further peaks in the 1600–1000 cm^{-1} region due to C=O, aromatic C=C, and C-O stretching. The FTIR spectrum of HPMC was dominated by an intense feature at 1049 cm^{-1} due to C-O stretching, along with further peaks at 3395 cm^{-1} and 1373 cm^{-1} due to O-H stretching and C-O-H bending vibrations of hydroxyl groups, respectively. Similar peaks were reported by other groups for HPMC [41]. The PVP showed an intense absorption band at 1654 cm^{-1}, which could readily be assigned to an amide C=O stretching mode [42]. The spectrum for the freeze-dried gel comprising HPMC–PVP (1:1 weight ratio) showed no shift in the characteristic peaks of each polymer, suggesting that no strong intermolecular interactions occur between the two polymers in the dry state. In the PVP + BNZ4 and HPMC–PVP + BNZ4 spectra, the S=O stretching modes for BNZ4 were observed at 1074 cm^{-1} (cf. 1061 cm^{-1} for pristine BNZ4). The same shift was not seen in HPMC + BNZ4, as this peak was obscured by the intense C-O stretching mode of HPMC which occurs at a similar frequency to the S=O stretch of BNZ4. In the low frequency region, HPMC + BNZ4, PVP + BNZ4, and HPMC–PVP + BNZ4 all showed a sharp peak around 605-607 cm^{-1} (assigned to a S-O stretching mode of the -SO$_3$H or -SO$_3^-$ groups), which again was at higher frequencies compared to the same mode for BNZ4 (599 cm^{-1}). Results imply that the BNZ4 interacted with the PVP and through the sulfonate functional group.

3.6. Stability Studies

All gel and binary gel formulations were found to be stable over a 3-month period. No significant changes in physical appearance, pH, viscosity, or drug content were observed.

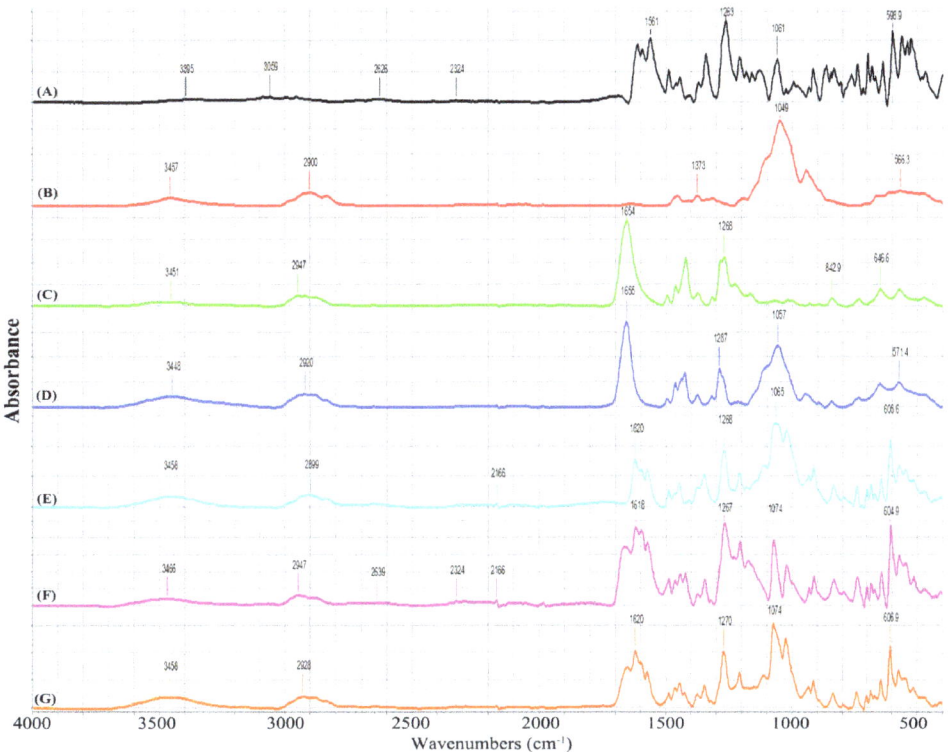

Figure 10. FTIR Spectra for (**A**) benzophenone-4, (**B**) HPMC, (**C**) PVP, (**D**) HPMC–PVP, (**E**) HPMC + BNZ4, (**F**) PVP + BNZ4, and (**G**) HPMC–PVP + BNZ4 freeze-dried gels.

4. Discussion

Hydrogels are an increasingly popular choice in topical applications, particularly in the controlled delivery of drugs through the skin. However, their low adhesiveness can limit their efficacy, and attempts to increase adhesion can negatively impact other properties such as hardness, compressibility, and viscosity. This study aimed to investigate the use of HPMC and PVP binary hydrogels to improve the adhesion of gel-based drug delivery formulations without compromising other texture properties. The results of the study demonstrated that binary hydrogels prepared using HPMC and PVP can improve adhesiveness without significantly impacting other mechanical properties. Other studies that also utilized a binary mixture of polymers, such as HPMC and polycarbophil, have demonstrated similar results in improving bioadhesive properties [43].

The ability to improve adhesiveness without significantly affecting other properties allows for the formulation of highly adhesive topical products to increase the retention time of the drug on the skin for controlled drug delivery, while not negatively affecting the cosmetic acceptability of the gel. A binary formulation (H12P6) was selected for studies on drug release and ex vivo bioadhesiveness, as it exhibited the highest adhesiveness without compromising other mechanical properties. HPMC 12% was used as a reference. Further increasing the PVP concentration from 6% to 9% caused a large reduction in the cohesiveness of the binary gel, indicating a compromised structural integrity of the polymer matrix. This is similar to findings in the literature, where it is suggested that PVP may interact with HPMC chains in the aqueous medium and consequently reduce the extent of HPMC–HPMC bonding [31]. Our results show that no change in gel cohesiveness occurred up to 6% PVP, suggesting that significant intermolecular bond interference only occurs above a critical concentration threshold where there are sufficient PVP molecules to obstruct HPMC–HPMC bonding interactions.

In addition to their texture properties, the rheological properties of binary hydrogels were also investigated. The study found that binary hydrogels exhibit pseudoplastic behavior (shear-thinning), which is desirable for topical products as it ensures uniform distribution on the skin and ease of application or good spreadability [43]. At modest amounts of shear stress (300 s^{-1}), the viscosity of all formulations was extremely low (<10 Pa·s), suggesting that the formulations would be easy to apply in practical settings. The shear stress on application of topicals was in excess of 10^4 s^{-1} [44].

This study also identified the ability of the H12P6 binary gel to "lock" in hydrophilic drugs, with benzophenone-4 remaining below the LOD of the analytical method after 24 h in drug-release studies. This demonstrates that the drug cannot access the matrix surface through the wetted pore network into the external media (PBS or methanol). In contrast, the HMPC homopolymeric hydrogels provided a sustained release with a nearly zero-order kinetic profile. Drug-release kinetics from hydrophilic matrices depend on several processes including the swelling of the polymer, water penetration through the matrix, dissolution of the drug, transport of the drug through the swollen matrix, and erosion of the matrix itself [45,46]. The most commonly used mathematical models to study cumulative drug-release behavior in hydrogels include zero- and first-order kinetic models, Higuchi, Peppas, and Hixon–Crowell models [46]. However, none are suitable for modelling the low drug release from the H12P6 binary gel, as it does not seem to be significantly influenced by the physical properties, such as viscosity, of the gel. This indicates that the binary gel lacks a highly structured matrix due to the low degree of polymer swelling and factors such as drug diffusion, mesh size, and erosion would then not be limiting factors to drug release [46]. Percolation theory is also unsuitable for explaining the drug release of the binary gel owing to the extremely low porosity and lack of connectivity and permeability [45,47,48], indicating that more complex processes such as drug–matrix interactions are influencing the release of the drug. Alternatively, one more explanation for the slow release could be due to the shear-thinning properties that made the gels in the dialysis bags extremely viscous at static conditions, thus impeding drug diffusion and erosion of the gel.

It was reported that the addition of PIP impairs the intermolecular binding of the HPMC polymer chains, thus leading to a reduction in viscosity [31]. Indeed, as shown in Figures 4A and 6B, the addition of PVP to the HPMC gels slightly increased the viscosity, particularly when shear rate was low. The 3^2 factorial design (Figure 7) also confirms the relatively smaller impact of the PVP on these properties compared with that of the HPMC. A similar complex is seen in polyvinylpyrrolidone-iodine [49]. The PVP polymer arranges itself such that a proton is fixed via a short hydrogen bond between two carbonyl groups of two adjacent pyrrolidone rings, forming a positive charge where a negatively charged molecule, such as a triiodide anion, can be bound ionically (Figure 11A) [49]. Benzopohenone-4 may interact with this positively charged area and become retained in the polymer matrix rather than releasing freely to the external media. In the PBS buffer used in this study, the sulfonic acid group ($-SO_3H$) of benzophenone-4 would be deprotonated and exist as the sulfonate ion ($-SO_3^-$). The blue-shift in the S=O and O-S-O peaks of benzopohenone-4 after interactions with the polymers may have been the result of deprotonation of the sulfonic acid group. This would create the possibility of electrostatic interaction between benzophenone-4 and a hydrogen atom between two carbonyl groups of the PVP polymer (Figure 11B). Such electrostatic interactions might account for the very strong binding of benzopohenone-4 in the H12P6 binary gel that led to the slow release.

Finally, this study highlights the lack of a standardized method for measuring the work of adhesion of hydrogels to skin substrates. The results showed that the peak force, adhesiveness, and work of adhesion values used to assess bioadhesion differed substantially depending on whether one or two skin substrates were used. When testing bioadhesion parameters using a double skin substrate setup, a large reduction in the peak force was seen, alongside non-significant decreases in the adhesiveness and work of adhesion. This contrasts with the expected increase due to the larger surface area. The results suggest that an increased deformation occurs between the two layers of skin (as opposed to a single layer of skin and a hard probe surface), making it more difficult for the probe to reach the specified force. A second layer of skin also introduces a small increase in the amount of moisture present between the substrate, which will also reduce the bioadhesion parameters [11]. The disparity between the testing methods is also seen when comparing the homopolymeric HPMC gel to the binary gel, where adhesiveness and work of adhesion have significant differences when tested using a single-skin substrate (method one). These data strongly suggest that the addition of 6% PVP to the homopolymeric HPMC gel only favorably increases the bioadhesiveness, but does not affect the other mechanical properties.

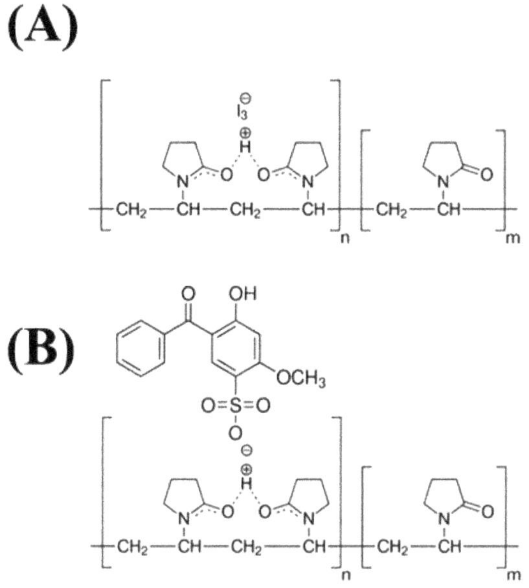

Figure 11. (**A**) Electrostatic adsorption of triiodide by PVP. (**B**) Possible electrostatic adsorption of benzophenone-4 by PVP which retarded the drug release from the gel.

These differences between the two formulations are not apparent when tested using the two-skin layer method (method two). However, compared with method two, method one is closer to the clinical setting.

There are currently no standardized methods for testing bioadhesiveness [10,11], and results vary significantly depending on different experimental setups. This finding emphasizes the need for a standardized method and testing setup for measuring bioadhesion parameters. Presently, it is hard to extrapolate results produced by different research groups under different settings.

Overall, this study contributes to the understanding of the properties and potential applications of binary hydrogels in topical products. The findings demonstrate the versatility and potential of binary hydrogels to improve adhesion, rheological properties, and drug delivery. Potential future directions in developing controlled-release gels should investigate using multiple polymers in gels and their ability to modulate the properties for their applications. This study highlights the ability of a binary gel to modify drug-release properties using parameters outside the classical models, notably, by affecting intermolecular binding. However, further research is needed to better understand and optimize the properties of binary hydrogels for specific applications.

5. Conclusions

The findings in this article demonstrate that the addition of PVP to HPMC to form binary gels provides an effective means of modifying the adhesive properties of the gel without significantly affecting other mechanical properties. This allows for a highly adhesive topical formulation that can still be applied on the skin comfortably while providing the controlled-release of drug over extended periods of time, which is highly desirable in many applications, such as the delivery of anti-inflammatories and chemotherapeutic agents for the treatment of skin conditions such as psoriasis and skin cancers. Furthermore, we demonstrate that binary hydrogels possess favorable pseudoplastic rheological properties that make them well-suited for topical applications. Our study also highlights the ability of binary hydrogels to enhance drug retention for sustained and controlled drug release. Finally, our findings reveal the importance of standardizing the methodology and setup for evaluating bioadhesion parameters. Overall, this research sheds light on the potential of PVP-HPMC binary hydrogels with low viscosity but high bioadhesiveness as a promising platform for sustained drug release in topical applications. When different drug molecules are incorporated, which may have different interactions with the polymers, further studies are needed to optimize the formulation.

Author Contributions: Conceptualization, Z.W.; Methodology, P.P.; Formal analysis, P.P. and Z.W.; Investigation, P.P.; Writing—original draft, P.P.; Writing—review & editing, D.S., G.I.N.W. and Z.W.; Visualization, P.P.; Supervision, D.S., G.I.N.W. and Z.W. All authors have read and agreed to the published version of the manuscript.

Funding: This research received no external funding.

Institutional Review Board Statement: Not applicable.

Informed Consent Statement: Not applicable.

Data Availability Statement: Data is contained within the article. The data presented in this publication are available upon reasonable request from the corresponding authors.

Acknowledgments: The authors wish to acknowledge Patrick Pan's University Doctoral Scholarship from the University of Auckland.

Conflicts of Interest: The authors declare no conflict of interest.

References

1. Guo, J.; Jee, S. Strategies to Develop a Suitable Formulation for Inflammatory Skin Disease Treatment. *Int. J. Mol. Sci.* **2021**, *22*, 6078. [CrossRef] [PubMed]
2. Kathe, K.; Kathpalia, H. Film forming systems for topical and transdermal drug delivery. *Asian J. Pharm. Sci.* **2017**, *12*, 487–497. [CrossRef] [PubMed]
3. Dantas, M.G.; Reis, S.A.; Damasceno, C.M.; Rolim, L.A.; Rolim-Neto, P.J.; Carvalho, F.O.; Quintans-Junior, L.J.; Almeida, J.R. Development and Evaluation of Stability of a Gel Formulation Containing the Monoterpene Borneol. *Sci. World J.* **2016**, *2016*, 7394685. [CrossRef] [PubMed]
4. Binder, L.; Mazál, J.; Petz, R.; Klang, V.; Valenta, C. The role of viscosity on skin penetration from cellulose ether-based hydrogels. *Ski. Res. Technol.* **2019**, *25*, 725. [CrossRef]
5. Nawaz, A.; Farid, A.; Safdar, M.; Latif, M.S.; Ghazanfar, S.; Akhtar, N.; Al Jaouni, S.K.; Selim, S.; Khan, M.W. Formulation Development and Ex-Vivo Permeability of Curcumin Hydrogels under the Influence of Natural Chemical Enhancers. *Gels* **2022**, *8*, 384. [CrossRef]
6. Djekic, L.; Martinović, M.; Dobričić, V.; Čalija, B.; Medarević, Đ.; Primorac, M. Comparison of the Effect of Bioadhesive Polymers on Stability and Drug Release Kinetics of Biocompatible Hydrogels for Topical Application of Ibuprofen. *J. Pharm. Sci.* **2019**, *108*, 1326–1333. [CrossRef]
7. Barnes, T.M.; Mijaljica, D.; Townley, J.P.; Spada, F.; Harrison, I.P. Vehicles for Drug Delivery and Cosmetic Moisturizers: Review and Comparison. *Pharmaceutics* **2021**, *13*, 2012. [CrossRef]
8. Bhubhanil, S.; Talodthaisong, C.; Khongkow, M.; Namdee, K.; Wongchitrat, P.; Yingmema, W.; Hutchison, J.A.; Lapmanee, S.; Kulchat, S. Enhanced wound healing properties of guar gum/curcumin-stabilized silver nanoparticle hydrogels. *Sci. Rep.* **2021**, *11*, 21836. [CrossRef]
9. Puccetti, G.; Fares, H. A new approach for evaluating the water resistance of sunscreens on consumers: Tap water vs. salt water vs. chlorine water. *Int. J. Cosmet. Sci.* **2014**, *36*, 284–290. [CrossRef]

10. Woertz, C.; Preis, M.; Breitkreutz, J.; Kleinebudde, P. Assessment of test methods evaluating mucoadhesive polymers and dosage forms: An overview. *Eur. J. Pharm. Biopharm.* **2013**, *85*, 843–853. [CrossRef]
11. Amorós-Galicia, L.; Nardi-Ricart, A.; Verdugo-González, C.; Arroyo-García, C.M.; García-Montoya, E.; Pérez-Lozano, P.; Suñé-Negre, J.M.; Suñé-Pou, M. Development of a Standardized Method for Measuring Bioadhesion and Mucoadhesion That Is Applicable to Various Pharmaceutical Dosage Forms. *Pharmaceutics* **2022**, *14*, 1995. [CrossRef] [PubMed]
12. Mehdizadeh, M.; Yang, J. Design Strategies and Applications of Tissue Bioadhesives. *Macromol. Biosci.* **2013**, *13*, 271–288. [CrossRef]
13. Uma, K. Bioadhesives for clinical applications—A mini review. *Mater. Adv.* **2023**, *4*, 2062–2069.
14. Brambilla, E.; Locarno, S.; Gallo, S.; Orsini, F.; Pini, C.; Farronato, M.; Thomaz, D.V.; Lenardi, C.; Piazzoni, M.; Tartaglia, G. Poloxamer-Based Hydrogel as Drug Delivery System: How Polymeric Excipients Influence the Chemical-Physical Properties. *Polymers* **2022**, *14*, 3624. [CrossRef] [PubMed]
15. Bovone, G.; Dudaryeva, O.Y.; Marco-Dufort, B.; Tibbitt, M.W. Engineering Hydrogel Adhesion for Biomedical Applications via Chemical Design of the Junction. *ACS Biomater. Sci. Eng.* **2021**, *7*, 4048–4076. [CrossRef] [PubMed]
16. Annabi, N.; Yue, K.; Tamayol, A.; Khademhosseini, A. Elastic sealants for surgical applications. *Eur. J. Pharm. Biopharm.* **2015**, *95 Pt A*, 27–39. [CrossRef]
17. Yang, N.; Huang, Y.; Hou, J.; Zhang, Y.; Tian, L.; Chen, Z.; Jin, Z.; Shen, Y.; Guo, S. Rheological behaviors and texture properties of semi-interpenetrating networks of hydroxypropyl methylcellulose and gellan. *Food Hydrocoll.* **2022**, *122*, 107097. [CrossRef]
18. Shin, S.; Kim, J.; Oh, I. Mucoadhesive and Physicochemical Characterization of Carbopol-Poloxamer Gels Containing Triamcinolone Acetonide. *Drug Dev. Ind. Pharm.* **2000**, *26*, 307–312. [CrossRef]
19. Ghorpade, V.S.; Yadav, A.V.; Dias, R.J. Citric acid crosslinked cyclodextrin/hydroxypropylmethylcellulose hydrogel films for hydrophobic drug delivery. *Int. J. Biol. Macromol.* **2016**, *93 Pt A*, 75–86. [CrossRef]
20. Noval, N.; Rosyifa, R.; Annisa, A. Effect of HPMC Concentration Variation as Gelling Agent on Physical Stability of Formulation Gel Ethanol Extract Bundung Plants (Actinuscirpus Grossus). In Proceedings of the First National Seminar Universitas Sari Mulia, NS-UNISM 2019, Banjarmasin, South Kalimantan, Indonesia, 23 November 2019.
21. Rasool, B.K.; Mohammed, A.A.; Salem, Y.Y. The Optimization of a Dimenhydrinate Transdermal Patch Formulation Based on the Quantitative Analysis of In Vitro Release Data by DDSolver through Skin Penetration Studies. *Sci. Pharm.* **2021**, *89*, 33. [CrossRef]
22. Vrbanac, H.; Trontelj, J.; Kalčič, Š.; Legen, I. Mechanistic study of model drug release from HPMC matrices in fed gastric media. *J. Drug Deliv. Sci. Technol.* **2020**, *60*, 102034. [CrossRef]
23. Kolawole, O.M.; Cook, M.T. In situ gelling drug delivery systems for topical drug delivery. *Eur. J. Pharm. Biopharm.* **2023**, *184*, 36–49. [CrossRef] [PubMed]
24. Luo, Y.; Hong, Y.; Shen, L.; Wu, F.; Lin, X. Multifunctional Role of Polyvinylpyrrolidone in Pharmaceutical Formulations. *AAPS PharmSciTech* **2021**, *22*, 34. [CrossRef]
25. Kurakula, M.; Rao, G.S.N.K. Pharmaceutical assessment of polyvinylpyrrolidone (PVP): As excipient from conventional to controlled delivery systems with a spotlight on COVID-19 inhibition. *J. Drug Deliv. Sci. Technol.* **2020**, *60*, 102046. [CrossRef] [PubMed]
26. Roy, N.; Saha, N. PVP-based hydrogels: Synthesis, properties and applications. In *Hydrogels: Synthesis, Characterization and Applications*; Wiley: Hoboken, NJ, USA, 2012; pp. 1703–1710.
27. Franco, P.; De Marco, I. The Use of Poly(N-vinyl pyrrolidone) in the Delivery of Drugs: A Review. *Polymers* **2020**, *12*, 1114. [CrossRef]
28. Aung, N.N.; Ngawhirunpat, T.; Rojanarata, T.; Patrojanasophon, P.; Opanasopit, P.; Pamornpathomkul, B. Enhancement of transdermal delivery of resveratrol using Eudragit and polyvinyl pyrrolidone-based dissolving microneedle patches. *J. Drug Deliv. Sci. Technol.* **2021**, *61*, 102284. [CrossRef]
29. Suksaeree, J.; Siripornpinyo, P.; Chaiprasit, S. Formulation, Characterization, and In Vitro Evaluation of Transdermal Patches for Inhibiting Crystallization of Mefenamic Acid. *J. Drug Deliv.* **2017**, *2017*, 7358042. [CrossRef]
30. Suvandee, W.; Teeranachaideekul, V.; Jeenduang, N.; Nooeaid, P.; Makarasen, A.; Chuenchom, L.; Techasakul, S.; Dechtrirat, D. One-Pot and Green Preparation of *Phyllanthus emblica* Extract/Silver Nanoparticles/Polyvinylpyrrolidone Spray-On Dressing. *Polymers* **2022**, *14*, 2205. [CrossRef]
31. Chan, L.W.; Wong, T.W.; Chua, P.C.; York, P.; Heng, P.W.S. Anti-tack Action of Polyvinylpyrrolidone on Hydroxypropylmethylcellulose Solution. *Chem. Pharm. Bull.* **2003**, *51*, 107–112. [CrossRef]
32. Lodge, T.P.; Maxwell, A.L.; Lott, J.R.; Schmidt, P.W.; McAllister, J.W.; Morozova, S.; Bates, F.S.; Li, Y.; Sammler, R.L. Gelation, Phase Separation, and Fibril Formation in Aqueous Hydroxypropylmethylcellulose Solutions. *Biomacromolecules* **2018**, *19*, 816–824. [CrossRef]
33. Jones, D.S.; Woolfson, D.A.; Brown, A.F. Textural Analysis and Flow Rheometry of Novel, Bioadhesive Antimicrobial Oral Gels. *Pharm. Res.* **1997**, *14*, 450–457. [CrossRef] [PubMed]
34. Dick, I.P.; Scott, R.C. Pig ear skin as an in-vitro model for human skin permeability. *J. Pharm. Pharmacol.* **1992**, *44*, 640–645. [CrossRef] [PubMed]
35. Khiao In, M.; Richardson, K.C.; Loewa, A.; Hedtrich, S.; Kaessmeyer, S.; Plendl, J. Histological and functional comparisons of four anatomical regions of porcine skin with human abdominal skin. *Anat. Histol. Embryol.* **2019**, *48*, 207–217. [CrossRef] [PubMed]
36. Hägerström, H.; Edsman, K. Interpretation of mucoadhesive properties of polymer gel preparations using a tensile strength method. *J. Pharm. Pharmacol.* **2001**, *53*, 1589–1599. [CrossRef] [PubMed]

37. Sigma-Aldrich. Product Information: Dialysis Tubing, Cellulose Membrane. 2014. Available online: https://www.sigmaaldrich.com/deepweb/assets/sigmaaldrich/product/documents/396/669/d9402pis.pdf (accessed on 6 April 2023).
38. Pan, P.; Svirskis, D.; Waterhouse, G.I.N.; Wu, Z. A simple and reliable isocratic high performance chromatographic assay for the simultaneous determination of hydrophilic benzophenone-4 and lipophilic octocrylene in sunscreens. *Int. J. Cosmet. Sci.* **2023**, *45*, 512–523. [CrossRef]
39. Menges, F. Spectragryph—Optical Spectroscopy Software, Version 1.2.16.1. 2022. Available online: https://www.effemm2.de/spectragryph/ (accessed on 20 June 2023).
40. Center for Drug Evaluation and Research. Q1A(R2) Stability Testing of New Drug Substances and Products. 2020. Available online: https://www.fda.gov/regulatory-information/search-fda-guidance-documents/q1ar2-stability-testing-new-drug-substances-and-products (accessed on 19 April 2023).
41. Furqan, M.; Iqbal, F.; Tulain, R. Microwave radiation induced synthesis of hydroxypropyl methylcellulose-graft-(polyvinylalcohal-co-acrylic acid) polymeric network and its in vitro evaluation. *Acta Pol. Pharm.* **2017**, *74*, 527–541.
42. Rahma, A.; Munir, M.M.; Khairurrijal, K.; Prasetyo, A. Intermolecular Interactions and the Release Pattern of Electrospun Curcumin-Polyvinyl(pyrrolidone). *Fiber* **2016**, *39*, 163–173. [CrossRef]
43. Carvalho, F.C.; Calixto, G.; Hatakeyama, I.N.; Luz, G.M.; Gremião, M.P.D.; Chorilli, M. Rheological, mechanical, and bioadhesive behavior of hydrogels to optimize skin delivery systems. *Drug Dev. Ind. Pharm.* **2013**, *39*, 1750–1757. [CrossRef]
44. Mitsui, T.; Morosawa, K.; Otake, C. Estimation of the rate of shear encountered in topical application of cosmetics. *J. Texture Stud.* **1971**, *2*, 339–347. [CrossRef]
45. Caraballo, I. Factors affecting drug release from hydroxypropyl methylcellulose matrix systems in the light of classical and percolation theories. *Expert Opin. Drug Deliv.* **2010**, *7*, 1291–1301. [CrossRef]
46. Vigata, M.; Meinert, C.; Hutmacher, D.W.; Bock, N. Hydrogels as Drug Delivery Systems: A Review of Current Characterization and Evaluation Techniques. *Pharmaceutics* **2020**, *12*, 1188. [CrossRef] [PubMed]
47. Binglin, H.; Tongwen, X. Mechanism of sustained drug release in diffusion-controlled polymer matrix-application of percolation theory. *Int. J. Pharm.* **1998**, *170*, 139–149.
48. Huang, X.; Yang, D.; Kang, Z. Impact of pore distribution characteristics on percolation threshold based on site percolation theory. *Phys. A Stat. Mech. Its Appl.* **2021**, *570*, 125800. [CrossRef]
49. Schenck, H.U.; Simak, P.; Haedicke, E. Structure of polyvinylpyrrolidone-iodine (povidone-iodine). *J. Pharm. Sci.* **1979**, *68*, 1505–1509. [CrossRef]

Disclaimer/Publisher's Note: The statements, opinions and data contained in all publications are solely those of the individual author(s) and contributor(s) and not of MDPI and/or the editor(s). MDPI and/or the editor(s) disclaim responsibility for any injury to people or property resulting from any ideas, methods, instructions or products referred to in the content.

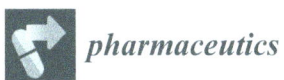

Article

Maillard Reaction Crosslinked Alginate-Albumin Scaffolds for Enhanced Fenofibrate Delivery to the Retina: A Promising Strategy to Treat RPE-Related Dysfunction

Maria Abedin Zadeh [1,2,*], Raid G. Alany [1,3], Leila Satarian [4], Amin Shavandi [5], Mohamed Abdullah Almousa [6], Steve Brocchini [2] and Mouhamad Khoder [1,*]

1. Drug Discovery, Delivery and Patient Care (DDDPC) Theme, School of Life Sciences, Pharmacy and Chemistry, Kingston University London, Kingston Upon Thames KT1 2EE, UK; r.alany@kingston.ac.uk
2. UCL School of Pharmacy, University College London, London WC1N 1AX, UK; s.brocchini@ucl.ac.uk
3. School of Pharmacy, The University of Auckland, Auckland 1010, New Zealand
4. Department of Stem Cells and Developmental Biology, Cell Science Research Center, Royan Institute for Stem Cell Biology and Technology, ACECR, Tehran 1665659911, Iran; l.satarian@royan-rc.ac.ir
5. 3BIO-BioMatter, École Polytechnique de Bruxelles, Université Libre de Bruxelles (ULB), Avenue F.D. Roosevelt, 50-CP 165/61, 1050 Brussels, Belgium; amin.shavandi@ulb.be
6. Duba General Hospital, Saudi Ministry of Health, Duba 49313, Saudi Arabia; maalmousa@gov.sa
* Correspondence: k1824129@kingston.ac.uk (M.A.Z.); m.khoder@kingston.ac.uk (M.K.)

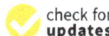

Citation: Abedin Zadeh, M.; Alany, R.G.; Satarian, L.; Shavandi, A.; Abdullah Almousa, M.; Brocchini, S.; Khoder, M. Maillard Reaction Crosslinked Alginate-Albumin Scaffolds for Enhanced Fenofibrate Delivery to the Retina: A Promising Strategy to Treat RPE-Related Dysfunction. *Pharmaceutics* **2023**, *15*, 1330. https://doi.org/10.3390/pharmaceutics15051330

Academic Editor: Monica M. Jablonski

Received: 6 March 2023
Revised: 13 April 2023
Accepted: 20 April 2023
Published: 24 April 2023

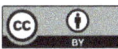

Copyright: © 2023 by the authors. Licensee MDPI, Basel, Switzerland. This article is an open access article distributed under the terms and conditions of the Creative Commons Attribution (CC BY) license (https://creativecommons.org/licenses/by/4.0/).

Abstract: There are limited treatments currently available for retinal diseases such as age-related macular degeneration (AMD). Cell-based therapy holds great promise in treating these degenerative diseases. Three-dimensional (3D) polymeric scaffolds have gained attention for tissue restoration by mimicking the native extracellular matrix (ECM). The scaffolds can deliver therapeutic agents to the retina, potentially overcoming current treatment limitations and minimizing secondary complications. In the present study, 3D scaffolds made up of alginate and bovine serum albumin (BSA) containing fenofibrate (FNB) were prepared by freeze-drying technique. The incorporation of BSA enhanced the scaffold porosity due to its foamability, and the Maillard reaction increased crosslinking degree between ALG with BSA resulting in a robust scaffold with thicker pore walls with a compression modulus of 13.08 KPa suitable for retinal regeneration. Compared with ALG and ALG-BSA physical mixture scaffolds, ALG-BSA conjugated scaffolds had higher FNB loading capacity, slower release of FNB in the simulated vitreous humour and less swelling in water and buffers, and better cell viability and distribution when tested with ARPE-19 cells. These results suggest that ALG-BSA MR conjugate scaffolds may be a promising option for implantable scaffolds for drug delivery and retinal disease treatment.

Keywords: alginate; BSA; Maillard reaction; age-related-macular degeneration; drug release; fenofibrate; retinal cells

1. Introduction

Retinal pigment epithelium (RPE) is a monolayer of nonregenerative cells that is vital for the retinal functional integrity and vision cycle. Located between the neural retina and choroid, RPE plays an essential role in transporting nutrients and waste products, absorbing stray light, phagocytosing shed photoreceptor membranes and secreting growth factors [1]. Ageing, diabetes, and smoking are important factors leading to RPE dysfunction and subsequent retinal degeneration diseases such as age-related macular degeneration (AMD) and Diabetic Retinopathies (DR) which are major causes of visual impairment and vision loss [2]. Globally, the number of AMD cases increases rapidly and is expected to reach about 288 million by 2040 [3].

The intravitreal injection of steroids and anti-vascular endothelial growth factor (anti-VEGF) remains preferred over other conventional treatments, such as laser and photodynamic therapy, for retinal disease management [2,4], especially in the early stages of the disease. However, the main drawback of the intravitreal treatment is the need for repetitive injections due to the poor ocular bioavailability of drugs after topical administration [5]. Fenofibrate (FNB) is a fibric acid derivative used to treat abnormal blood lipid levels. FNB acts as a prodrug that is rapidly hydrolysed in vivo to form its active fenofibric acid metabolite. FNB came into medical use in mid-1970s and was first marketed in the United States in 1988 (Tricor®, Abbott Laboratories) [6]. FNB showed promising therapeutic effects in clinical trials for the management of retinal diseases such as DR and neovascular AMD [7]. When compared with anti-VEGF, FNB is advantageous given its low-cost, fewer side effects, and neuroprotective activity [7,8]. However, the use of FNB for dysfunctional RPE treatment is challenging due to its very hydrophobic nature (log P = 5.24) and poor water solubility. RPE transplantation was introduced as an alternative and effective way to replace damaged RPE cells with healthy ones [9]. However, the implementation of this approach is hindered by the shortage of tissue donors, heavy surgical intervention, and risks of serious post-surgical infections and transplanted cell rejection [1].

Recently, implantable polymeric scaffolds capable of providing structural support for retinal cell growth and proliferation have gained considerable attention for retinal regenerative treatment [10]. The same scaffolds can be used to locally deliver active therapeutics, such as growth factors and active pharmaceutical ingredients, at the damaged retinal sites to enhance cell growth and reduce side effects [11]. Ideally, scaffolds should display physicochemical and biological properties that mimic those of native tissues. This includes good biocompatibility, controllable biodegradability, high porosity and drug loading capacity, and sufficient mechanical stability during and post-implantation [1]. The fundamental features of scaffolds are dependent on the nature of the comprising polymers and composition, crosslinker types (either chemical or physical), and methods of fabrication [1,12]. Due to their safety, biodegradability, chemical versatility, low cost, and processability, naturally occurring polymers, such as sodium alginate (ALG), have been explored to fabricate scaffolds for tissue regenerative applications [1,13]. In the presence of divalent cations, such as calcium, ALG solution forms gel via ionotropic crosslinking, resulting in a 3D hydrogel structure [14]. This unique feature was successfully and widely used to produce ALG scaffolds for different pharmaceutical and biomedical applications [15–17]. However, the hydrophilic nature of ALG leads to fast swelling and poor mechanical properties, hence an uncontrollable drug release behaviour [15]. A promising approach to improve ALG scaffold's performance is to modulate the crosslinking density between ALG chains using chemical crosslinking alongside ionotropic crosslinking [18]. However, chemical crosslinking requires reagents and solvents that often have toxic side effects [19].

Maillard reaction is a natural non-enzymatic process during which covalent bonds are formed between carbonyl groups of reducing sugar and the free amino groups of amino acids, peptides, and proteins [20]. This reaction is spontaneous, thus does not necessitate the use of any toxic chemicals or organic solvents [21]. Furthermore, Maillard reaction products possess antioxidant, anti-inflammatory, and radical scavenging properties which are beneficial for tissue regeneration and development [22,23]. Bovine serum albumin (BSA) is a naturally occurring biocompatible protein that plays a structural support role in cell proliferation and growth and has recently gained considerable attention in the development of scaffolds for tissue repair and regenerative medicine [24,25]. In a previous study, we showed that when ALG is conjugated with BSA via Maillard reaction, the beads produced using the ALG-BSA Maillard product possessed superior water resistance, viscosity, foamability, and capability to control the drug release compared with that of pristine ALG [20].

ALG reinforced by the Maillard reaction has not been previously used to fabricate scaffolds for ocular applications. The aim of this study is to design and develop FNB-loaded scaffolds based on ALG-BSA Maillard conjugate, which can provide a suitable environment for RPE cells to grow, migrate, and produce their own extracellular matrix (ECM). The use of these scaffolds as FNB delivery system is assessed. Morphological and mechanical characteristics as well as the porosity of obtained scaffolds are investigated and the scaffolds swelling, drug loading capacity, and drug release profile are established. Finally, biological investigations are performed to assess the scaffold's biodegradability and biocompatibility with seeded ARPE-19 cells (a spontaneously arising retinal pigment epithelium (RPE) cell line) on ALG-based scaffolds.

2. Materials and Methods

2.1. Materials

ALG (medium molecular weight: 120,000–200,000 g/mol; M/G ratio: 0.8), BSA, FNB, calcium chloride ($CaCl_2$), sodium chloride (NaCl), sodium lauryl sulfate (SLS), phosphate-buffered saline (PBS), 2-(4-(2-hydroxyethyl)-1-piperazinyl) ethane sulphonic acid (HEPES), potassium bromide (KBr), sodium citrate, and acetonitrile (I) were all purchased from Sigma-Aldrich chemicals (Dorset, UK). For the in vitro cell study, ARPE-19 cells, a spontaneously immortalised human RPE cell line, were obtained from ATCC (Manassas, VA, USA). Dulbecco's Modified Eagle Medium: F12 (DMEM/F12), fetal bovine serum (FBS), penicillin/streptomycin, trypan blue and trypsin/ethylenediaminetetraacetic, DAPI (4′,6-diamidino-2-phenylindole), calcein-AM, propidium iodide (PI) were purchased from Gibco (Invitrogen, CA, USA). The MTS assay kit was provided by Promega (Madison, WI, USA). Milli-Q distilled deionised (DI) water was used for all experiments.

2.2. Fabrication of the Scaffolds

Scaffolds were fabricated by a freeze-drying method [26]. Briefly, to prepare ALG solution (1.5% w/v), 0.75 g of ALG was gradually added and dissolved in 50 mL of DI water. For ALG-BSA scaffolds, of BSA (0.25 g) was added to the obtained ALG solution to make ALG-BSA solution. The ALG and a blended mixture of ALG-BSA solutions were separately poured into a well of 96-well culture plate (150 μL per well), and frozen overnight before being freeze-dried (VirTis Benchtop Pro, SP scientific, Winchester, UK) for 48 h. Obtained freeze-dried scaffolds were then crosslinked with calcium by immersion into a 2% (w/v) $CaCl_2$ solution for 30 min. Crosslinked scaffolds were then freeze-dried for another 48 h to remove the solvent completely. For drug-loaded scaffolds, FNB was added and mixed with the obtained ALG and ALG-BSA solution at a concentration of 0.2% (w/v). For MR-ALG-BSA scaffolds, obtained ALG and ALG-BSA scaffolds were placed into a desiccator containing an oversaturated KBr solution to control the relative humidity at 79% and incubated for 24 h at 60 °C in an oven (Binder, Germany).

2.3. Morphological Characterisation

Scanning electron microscopy (SEM) was used to examine the microstructural properties of the scaffolds. Prior to imaging, specimens' surface was coated with a conductive layer of sputtered gold, and the electron microscope (Zeiss Evo50, Oxford instrument, Abingdon-on-Thames, UK) was operated at an accelerating voltage of 30 kV under low-vacuum mode. SEM images were employed to determine the average pore size and porosity of scaffolds. At least twelve pores were randomly selected from each scaffold SEM image and analysed using ImageJ software (V 1.8.0), and pore size data were presented as mean ± standard deviation.

2.4. Mechanical Properties Testing

Mechanical properties of the dry and rehydrated scaffolds were investigated using a texture analyser (Santam, STM-29, Tehran, Iran) with a 1 N load cell at a crosshead speed of 1 mm/min. To simulate the composition of the vitreous humour, scaffold rehydration was performed in HEPES buffer (pH = 7.4 at 37 °C) containing 132 mM NaCl, mimicking the pH and the electrocyte concentration of the vitreous humour [27]. During the experiment, the rehydrated scaffolds remained immersed in the buffer. The compressive stress–strain curves were generated following the methods reported by Wan et al. [28]. The Young's modulus was calculated as the slope of the stress–strain curve at 10% strain.

2.5. Swelling and Degradation Studies

The scaffolds swelling behaviour were evaluated in DI water, PBS, and HEPES-NaCl buffer. Briefly, the scaffold was weighed and placed separately in 10 mL of each medium at 37 ± 0.5 °C. At specific intervals, the scaffold was removed from the swelling medium, and the excess medium was carefully removed with filter paper and weighed. The swelling ratio was calculated using the following equation [29]:

$$swelling\ ratio(\%) = \left[\frac{Ws - Wi}{Wi}\right] \times 100\% \qquad (1)$$

where W_i is the initial weight of the scaffold, and W_s is the weight of swollen scaffold.

The biodegradability of scaffolds was assessed by immersion in DMEM/10% FBS culture medium at 37 ± 0.5 °C to provide conditions similar to those of the cell culture studies. Scaffolds were then incubated in a shaker incubator (ThermoFisher Scientific, Swindon, UK) that was operated at 100 rpm. On days 1, 3, 7, and 14, scaffolds were removed from the medium, frozen, and freeze-dried for 48 h, and the weight loss of scaffolds was calculated using the following equation:

$$Degradation(\%) = \left[\frac{Wd - Wr}{Wd}\right] \times 100 \qquad (2)$$

where W_d is the initial weight of the scaffold and W_r is the weight of the degraded scaffold.

2.6. Drug Loading and Release Studies

To investigate the loading capacity and release of FNB, the saturation solubility of FNB was first determined in HEPES-NaCl buffer solution (pH 7.4) with and without SLS (25 mM). Briefly, an excess amount of FNB (10 mg) was added to the (10 mL) HEPES-NaCl buffer and shaken at the speed of 100 rpm at 37 °C for 48 h. Samples were then centrifuged for 15 min and filtered through a polytetrafluoroethylene (PTFE) syringe-driven filter (average pore size = 0.45 µm). The FNB solubility was determined using HPLC. An Agilent Infinity II HPLC system (Agilent, Waldbronn, Germany) was employed. The flow rate was adjusted at 1 mL/min, and the injection volume was 10 µL. Chromatographic separation was achieved at room temperature using a C18 column (4.6mm × 150 mm, C18, 5 µm) (Phenomenex SphereClone), and a UV detector was set at a (λmax) 286 nm. The mobile phase consisted of 90:10 v/v acetonitrile/HPLC grade water [30,31].

2.6.1. Loading Capacity Study

To determine the loading capacity of drug-loaded formulations, one scaffold was dispersed in 1 mL of a 55 mM sodium citrate solution at 37 °C, resulting in the full release of FNB. The resulting suspension was filtered and diluted with 9 mL of HEPES-NaCl buffer, which contained SLS at a concentration of 25 mM. The FNB content was then measured using HPLC, and the loading capacity was calculated using the following equation [32]:

$$Loading\ capacity\ (\%) = \left[\frac{L}{Lt}\right] \times 100 \qquad (3)$$

where L and L_t are the measured and theoretical amounts of fenofibrate loaded in the scaffold, respectively.

2.6.2. Drug Release Study

The FNB-loaded scaffolds were soaked separately in 10 mL of HEPES-NaCl buffer containing SLS (25 mM) and placed in a shaking incubator at 100 rpm and 37 °C. At specific time intervals (1, 2, 4, 6, and 8 h, and then 2, 3, 4, and 6 days), 500 µL of samples were withdrawn from the release medium and replaced with fresh release medium to keep the initial volume constant. The amount of FNB released was determined using the HPLC.

2.7. Biological Investigations

2.7.1. Cell Culture and Seeding on Scaffolds

ARPE-19 cells were expanded and maintained in a typical RPE medium containing DMEM supplemented with 10% foetal bovine serum (FBS) and 1% penicillin-streptomycin solution. Cells were used between passages 31 and 41 for the experiments. At 80–90% confluency, cells were subcultured using 0.05 trypsin-EDTA. The collected cells were centrifuged at 1500 rpm for 5 min and resuspended in a new medium.

Prior to the cell seeding process, scaffolds were sterilised by immersion in ethanol (70%) for 20 min. The scaffolds were then soaked in the cell culture medium for 30 min and transferred into a well of 48 well-plates. ARPE-19 cells were then counted with a haemocytometer by using the standard trypan blue method and cells in suspension (5×10^4 cells/mL) were seeded on top of the scaffold surface. After 2 h of incubation, fresh culture medium (500 µL) was added to each well of the cell culture well-plate and kept in standard conditions at 95% humidity, 5% CO_2, and 37 °C. The medium was changed every other day intervals during the experiments.

2.7.2. MTS-Based Cytotoxicity Assay

To determine the viability of the ARPE-19 cells, MTS assay was performed [33]. Briefly, after the incubation of the cell-seeded scaffolds for 1, 3, 7, and 14 days, the media was removed, and the scaffolds were rinsed with PBS. MTS solution (1:5 dilution in culture medium) was added to the seeded scaffolds and placed in a dark room for 3 h at 37 °C and 5% CO_2. The optical density of each sample was measured at 490 nm using a UV spectrophotometer microplate reader (FlexStation3 Multi-Mode, Molecular Devices, San Jose, CA, USA). The negative controls were cell culture medium without cells.

2.7.3. Analysis of ARPE-19 Cells-Scaffold Interactions

To visualise the presence of ARPE-19 cells in the scaffolds, the DAPI staining method was used. The cells were first seeded onto each scaffold following the same procedure described above. At day 14, scaffolds were washed twice with PBS before being stained with 200 µL of DAPI solution. Cells-seeded scaffolds were then incubated for 15 min in a dark room at 37 °C. The samples were washed with PBS three times to remove excess DAPI. To assess cell-scaffold interaction, ARPE-19 cells within scaffolds were stained with a LIVE/DEAD staining solution on day 14 of cell seeding. For this purpose, stock solutions of calcein-AM (3 µM) and PI (2.5 µM) were separately prepared, diluted in PBS, and kept at 4 °C. Immediately before use, a working LIVE/DEAD staining solution was prepared by mixing 100µL of calcein-AM and 100 µL PI. Each scaffold was washed with PBS and stained with the LIVE/DEAD solution. After 15 min of incubation at 37 °C in dark, samples were immediately observed under a confocal microscope (Zeiss, Jena, Germany) to evaluate viable and damaged cells. Samples were excited with 498 nm and with 540 nm laser wavelengths and the emitted fluorescence was detected at 515 nm and 615 nm for calcein-AM and PI detections, respectively [34]. Viable cells were illustrated in green fluorescence by calcein-AM and dead cells were illustrated in red by PI. The control was the blank scaffolds without cells.

2.7.4. Distribution of Cells on the Scaffolds

The distribution of ARPE-19 grown on scaffolds was examined using scanning electron microscopy (Vega, Tescan, Czech Republic). On day 14 of cell seeding, scaffolds were rinsed with PBS and washed with double-deionised water. Scaffolds were then frozen in liquid nitrogen and freeze-dried for 48 h. Gold was sputtered on the scaffolds with fixed cells to form a 15 nm thick layer on the surface with a deposition rate of 1 Å/s, and SEM images were captured.

2.8. Statistical Analysis

All experiments were performed at least in triplicate, and results were reported as mean ± standard deviation (SD). Statistical significance was determined using one-way analysis of variance (ANOVA) with post-hoc Tukey's HSD test. p-values < 0.05 indicated statistical significance.

3. Results & Discussion

3.1. Scaffolds Structural Morphology

Maillard reaction is an established method that involves the covalent bonding between the amino group (NH_2) of a protein and the carbonyl group (C=O) of reducing sugars [20]. The conjugation of ALG with BSA via Maillard reaction is therefore expected to add a chemical crosslinking in the polymeric scaffolds, in addition to the ionotropic crosslinking between ALG carboxylic acid and Ca^{+2} [35]. Maillard reaction can also generate other types of chemical bonds, such as those between amino acids and the various reactive intermediates produced during the reaction. Briefly, in the early stage, the reducing sugar reacts with the NH_2 groups of the protein to form a Schiff base. This reaction is reversible and can lead to the formation of Amadori products in the intermediate stage. In the intermediate stage, the Amadori products undergo further reactions, resulting in the formation of advanced glycation end products (AGEs). These products are highly reactive and can react with other proteins, lipids, and nucleic acids, leading to the formation of crosslinks. The intermediate stage can also produce reactive carbonyl compounds, such as 3-deoxyglucosone and glyoxal, which can react with the amino groups of proteins to form covalent crosslinks. In the final stage of the Maillard reaction, melanoidins are formed which are brown pigments responsible for the colour of many food products. In this study, the colour of scaffolds subjected to the Maillard reaction changed from white to brownish (Figure 1b), indicating the formation of ALG-BSA melanoidins [36]. Schematic illustrations of non-treated and treated scaffolds are shown in Figure 1a.

Figure 1b illustrates that all scaffolds possessed porous structures of micro-sized pores, with enhanced porosity observed upon the incorporation of BSA. ImageJ software analysis showed that while the average pore size of ALG scaffolds was 53.16 ± 18.04 µm, this significantly increased in the presence of BSA to 110.8 ± 23.9 µm and 107 ± 21.4 µm in ALG-BSA and MR-ALG-BSA scaffolds, respectively. Notably, a previous study reported that an optimal pore diameter to support retinal cells ranged between 100–200 µm [37]. The porosity of ALG scaffolds was initially 39% and has increased after the incorporation of BSA to 51% and 56% for ALG-BSA and MR-ALG-BSA scaffolds, respectively. BSA is known for its foaming capacity [38], leading to the formation of bubbles during the preparation of the scaffold solutions. Upon freeze-drying, air bubbles that acted as porogen turned into pores that increased pores size diameter and porosity in BSA-containing scaffolds [24,39]. Larger pore size obtained after the incorporation of BSA in the scaffold is expected to facilitate the exchange of nutrients and waste products with the surrounding environment and provide a more favourable structure for cell growth compared to ALG scaffolds [40,41]. Furthermore, the MR-ALG-BSA scaffolds exhibited a thicker pore wall with a measurement of 13.33 ± 2.74 µm, which was significantly higher compared to the pore wall thicknesses of ALG and ALG-BSA scaffolds (5.9 ± 1.85 µm and 4.3 ± 1.21 µm, respectively). This higher thickness of MR scaffold pores walls might potentially increase the overall mechanical properties of the scaffolds, as thicker walls can provide better support and resistance to deformation [42].

3.2. Mechanical Properties of the Scaffolds

The mechanical properties of fabricated scaffolds were evaluated in dry and rehydrated conditions in HEPES-NaCl. The PBS was not used for rehydration to avoid destabilisation of the Ca-ALG structure [43]. Figure 1c–f shows the compressive stress–strain curves and Young's modulus of dried and rehydrated scaffolds, respectively. Both the incorporation of BSA in the scaffolds' formulation and Millard reaction significantly affected the compressive strength of the scaffolds. For non-treated ALG-BSA samples (i.e., did not go through MR reaction), the compressive strength was lower than that of pure ALG scaffold (841.58 KPa and 691.18 KPa respectively). On the other hand, conjugating BSA with ALG reversed its impact, leading to an increase in the compressive strength and young's modulus to 3913.79 KPa and 465.11 KPa, respectively.

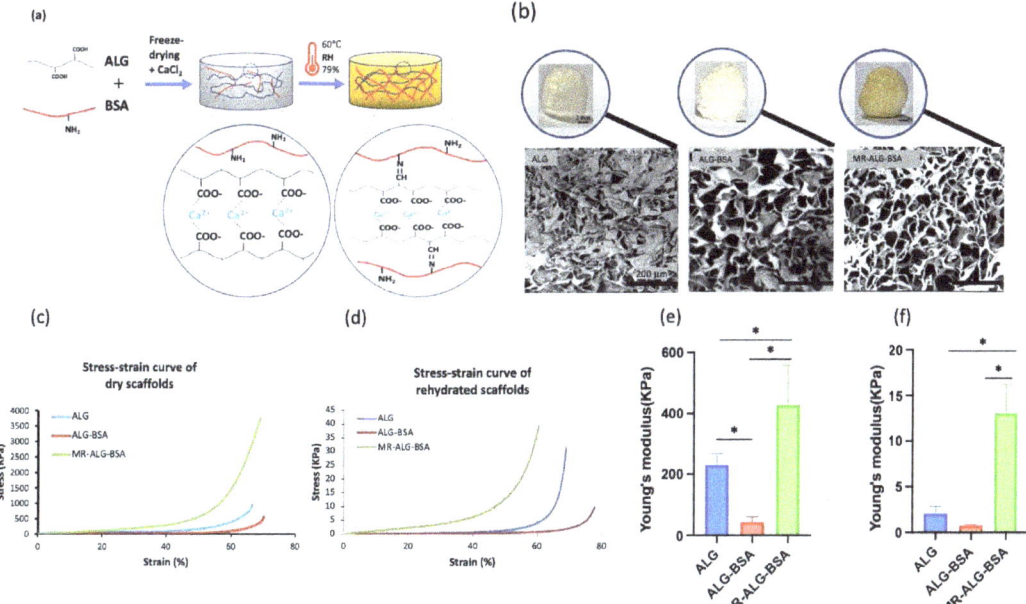

Figure 1. Characteristics of the ALG-based scaffolds; (**a**) schematic illustration of non-treated and MR ALG-based scaffolds, (**b**) the visual (scale bars 1 mm) and SEM (scale bars 200 µm) appearance of ALG, ALG-BSA and MR-ALG-BSA, (**c**) the compressive stress–strain curves of dried and (**d**) rehydrated scaffolds, (**e**) Young's moduli of dried and (**f**) rehydrated scaffolds ($n = 3$). (* denotes a significant difference, $p < 0.05$).

The Maillard reaction results in the formation of covalent bonds between the ALG carboxyl groups and the BSA amino groups, leading to a higher molecular weight product and increased crosslinking [44]. Our results indicated a stiffer structure of MR scaffolds compared to the non-treated ALG-BSA samples. Furthermore, the mechanical strength of scaffolds is influenced by porosity, with larger pore sizes having a negative impact, while thicker pore walls, resulting in smaller pore sizes, improve the strength [41,42].

Since scaffolds are rehydrated before implantation, further investigation was performed on rehydrated scaffolds. Due to water absorption and weakening bonds within the scaffolds structure [45], the Young's modulus of rehydrated pure ALG scaffolds decreased to 2.07 KPa, as shown in Figure 1f. This result is in agreement with the compressive modulus value of about 3 KPa reported by Wan et al. [28] for ALG scaffolds.

As per dry scaffolds, rehydrated MR-ALG-BSA scaffolds displayed the highest Young's modulus at 13.08 KPa. Since scaffolds act as a temporary support that must withstand mechanical stress until the tissues are regenerated, MR-ALG-BSA scaffolds are promising, exhibiting substantially enhanced mechanical performance in both dry and wet conditions. It is worth mentioning that the compressive modulus of MR-ALG-BSA (13.08 KPa) falls within the range of the compressive modulus of a healthy retina, which has been reported to be between 10–20 KPa [46,47]. Thus, the MR-ALG-BSA scaffolds are expected to provide an advantageous environment for retinal cell survival, differentiation and phenotypic maintenance.

3.3. Scaffolds Swelling, Biodegradation, and Drug Release Studies

- Swelling Studies

The swelling behaviour of scaffolds is a determinant factor that affects mechanical properties upon rehydration, drug release, biodegradation, and cellular activities. While excessive swelling might lead to the collapse of scaffolds and uncontrolled release of drugs, failing to swell could prevent drug release [48]. Similarly, adequate swelling is indispensable for cell migration and the transfer of cell nutrients and metabolites in and out of the matrix. Furthermore, swelling expands the pores and maximises the scaffold's surface area, allowing for more room for cells to grow [49].

Swelling studies were performed in three different media: water, PBS, and HEPES-NaCl buffer solutions. Up to six hours, blank and FNB-loaded scaffolds showed identical swelling behaviours in all media.

Considering their mechanical properties, the physical addition of BSA (i.e., BSA-ALG scaffold) led to a significant increase in swelling ratio in all media. However, when BSA was conjugated with ALG (i.e., MR-ALG-BSA scaffolds), the swelling ratio significantly dropped ($p > 0.05$). A similar impact of the Maillard reaction on the swelling capacity of alginate gels was previously reported [50]. All scaffolds exhibited a swelling rate that was approximately five-times higher in buffered solutions (PBS and HEPES) compared to water (Figure 2a–c). ALG scaffolds absorb water and undergo swelling due to the abundance of hydrophilic groups such as hydroxyl and carboxyl [51,52]. In buffered solutions, the ionisation of carboxylic groups causes electrical repulsion, which leads to further swelling.

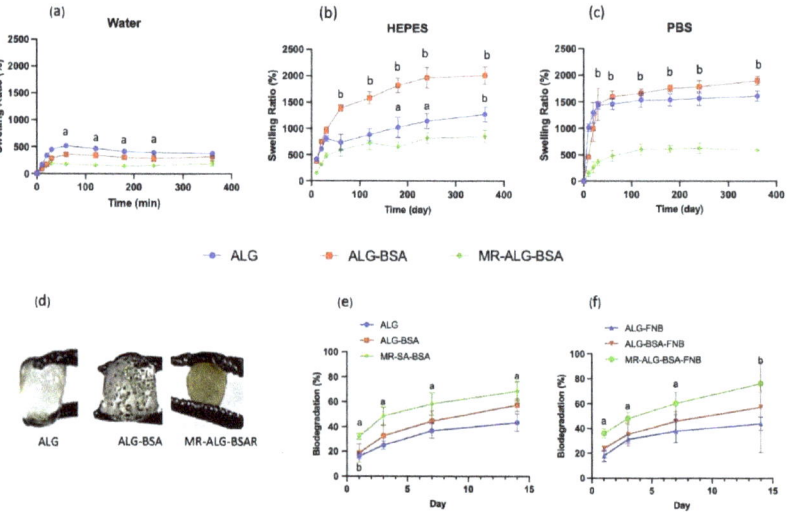

Figure 2. Swelling profiles of ALG, ALG-BSA and MR-ALG-BSA scaffolds in (**a**) water, (**b**) HEPES and (**c**) PBS. (**d**) The visual appearance of scaffolds after rehydration overnight in HEPES-NaCl buffer. The degradation profiles of (**e**) dried and (**f**) rehydrated scaffolds after 1, 3, 7 and 14 days in cell culture medium. (a: $p < 0.01$, b: $p < 0.001$ significant difference between MR scaffold and the other scaffolds) ($n = 3$).

The rate and degree of hydrogel network swelling can be influenced by other factors such as crosslinking density and porosity. In addition, external factors such as the pH, composition and ionic strength of the swelling medium can also affect the extent of swelling behaviour [53]. Contrary to water, PBS and HEPE solutions have the capacity to maintain a stable pH at around 7 [54] which leads to full ionisation of ALG-free carboxylic acid groups (pKa = 4–5). This repulsion amongst the negatively charged carboxylic acid groups causes increased polymer swelling. Buffered media also contain monovalent cations such as Na^+ and K^+ that could penetrate the scaffold matrix and displace the Ca^{2+}. Since monovalent cations cannot crosslink alginate, the matrix structure relaxes and swells. The Maillard reaction converts ALG carboxylic acid groups into an amide group preventing their ionisation and reducing the overall swelling of the scaffolds. Upon extending the swelling study to 48 h, FNB-loaded scaffolds incubated in the PBS buffer fully disintegrated. However, the scaffolds incubated in water and HEPES buffer did not swell any further and maintained their integrity for up to 72 h. A similar destabilising impact of PBS buffer on Ca-ALG structures was reported [14,43,55], which was attributed to the chelating effect that phosphate ions can have on Ca^{2+} and the subsequent formation of a calcium phosphate precipitate. Figure 2d displays the visual appearance of the swollen scaffolds in the HEPES-NaCl solution after 24 h.

- Biodegradation

To investigate the stability of prepared scaffolds in a cell culture medium, the biodegradation of scaffolds was assessed for 14 days. Scaffolds biodegradation is essential for tissue regeneration; in vivo cell activities, such as distance and signal transduction within the matrix, must be maintained until the cells produce their own EMC [1]. Furthermore, scaffolds biodegradation products are eliminated by the eyes, i.e., there is no need to remove them later on. Figure 2e,f shows the degradation profiles of blank and FNB-loaded scaffolds in a cell culture medium over 14 days. Although there was a gradual loss of mass in all scaffolds as incubation time increased, they remained intact for a period of 14 days. The degradability of scaffolds could be explained by the loss of crosslinking Ca^{+2} due to exchange with non-crosslinking monovalent cations (Na^+) that are present in cell culture medium. The incorporation of BSA in scaffold formulation resulted in a faster and higher degradation rate than those of ALG scaffolds, suggesting the dissolution and release of BSA. Compared with ALG and ALG-BSA, MR-ALG-BSA scaffolds (blank and loaded with FNB) showed the highest mass loss of about 25–40% in 24 h and about 60–80% (respectively) after 14 days of incubation in the cell culture medium. This could be due to the uncontrolled nature of the Maillard reaction, leading to the production of intermediate compounds such as Amadori products, that could result in such discrepancy [20,56].

During the degradation process, the scaffolds with larger pores and higher surface area to volume ratio (i.e., ALG-BSA and MR-ALG-BSA scaffolds) became further loose as the surrounding aqueous solution came in contact with the internal network structure. This was expected to correlate with the swelling behaviour in buffered media. However, the MR-ALG-BSA scaffolds showed the lowest swelling ratio with the highest degradation rate. A high degradation rate of BSA-containing scaffolds can be advantageous in providing a better environment to generate ECM and promote cell–cell and cell–scaffold interactions. However, the optimal degradation rate, matching the rate of retinal tissue regeneration, is yet to be identified [1].

- Drug Loading and In-Vitro Release Studies:

To avoid any PBS buffer interference with the drug release, FNB release studies were conducted using HEPES buffer. FNB is a lipophilic compound (Log P = 5.24) that is non-ionisable and insoluble in water [57]. To perform the release studies, the solubility of FNB was first established in the release medium (i.e., HEPES buffer) which was found to be practically insoluble (1.35 ± 0.003 µg/L). To allow the free release of FNB into the surrounding medium, SLS (0.025 M) was added to the HEPES buffer. SLS forms micelles that solubilise the hydrophobic drug such as the FNB. The apparent solubility of FNB in the presence of SLS increased to 105 ± 0.02 µg/L. The scaffold loading capacity was measured by fully dissolving drug-loaded scaffolds in sodium citrate solution, allowing the full release of FNB. The effectiveness of sodium citrate as a chelating agent for the dissolution of Ca-ALG scaffolds has been reported in the literature [58,59]. The dissolution process occurred through ion exchange, where the Na$^+$ ions in sodium citrate were replaced with the chelated Ca^{2+} ions in the ALG-based scaffolds, leading to the loss of crosslinking and the dissolution of the formulated scaffold [60].

Figure 3a shows the FNB loading capacity of scaffolds. ALG, ALG-BSA, and MR-ALG-BSA scaffolds' loading capacities were 39 ± 2.45%, 88 ± 1.90%, and 82 ± 6.28%, respectively. Previous studies have reported that the highly hydrophilic nature of alginate makes loading a significant amount of hydrophobic drugs rather challenging [61,62]. Interestingly, BSA molecules can bind hydrophobic molecules leading to the formation of soluble complexes, which could explain the enhanced FNB loading capacity of BSA-containing scaffolds [63].

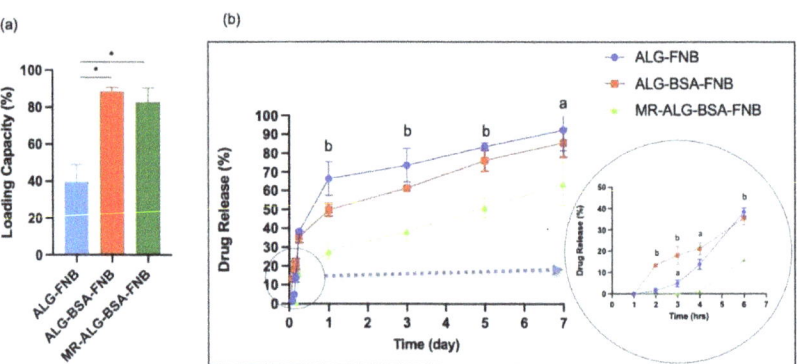

Figure 3. (a) drug loading capacity, (b) FNB release profiles from ALG, ALG-BSA and MR-ALG-BSA scaffolds in HEPES. (*: $p < 0.05$. a: $p < 0.01$, b: $p < 0.001$ significant difference between MR scaffold and the other scaffolds) ($n = 3$).

The release profiles of FNB from the ALG, ALG-BSA and MR-BSA-ALG scaffolds are presented in Figure 3b. All scaffolds revealed 1st order release kinetics where the rate of release decreases over time. Both ALG and ALG-BSA scaffolds exhibited initial burst release with approximately 40% of loaded FNB released in the first 6 h and almost 90% released in 6 days. Interestingly, MR-ALG-BSA scaffolds displayed significantly slower release with no release in the first 4 h, about 25% released at 6 h, and almost 60% release within 6 days. The drug release data correlated with the reduced swelling of MR-ALG-BSA scaffolds, which is plausible given that ALG-based systems typically operate through a swelling/diffusion-controlled release mechanism. Khoder et al. also observed similar findings, where ALG-BSA Maillard product beads demonstrated more sustained release than physically mixed ALG-BSA beads in a simulated intestinal medium. This was attributed to the higher molecular weight of the ALG-BSA conjugate, enhanced viscosity, and reduced swelling of the system [20].

3.4. In Vitro Biological Investigation with ARPE-19 Cells

- Viability of the ARPE-19 cells within scaffolds

The biocompatibility of ALG scaffolds in retinal regenerative medicine was investigated by culturing ARPE-19 cells on them. This cell line is commonly used for eye research applications due to its convenience and consistency for cell culture studies [64]. MTS assay was used to evaluate the viability of ARPE-19 cells in direct contact with the fabricated scaffolds.

Figure 4 shows the MTS absorbance values at 490 nm of all scaffolds, which are directly proportional to cell viability. All ARPE-19 cells seeded scaffolds showed MTS absorbance values from day 1, which gradually increased over incubation time, indicating the biocompatibility of scaffolds and ARPE-19 cells viability. Our results showed that the cell viability on the ALG scaffold gradually increased through the entire incubation period. Compared with blank ALG scaffolds, both blank ALG-BSA and MR-ALG-BSA scaffolds demonstrated significantly higher ARPE-19 cell viability, notably after day 7, which might be attributed to their larger pore diameter.

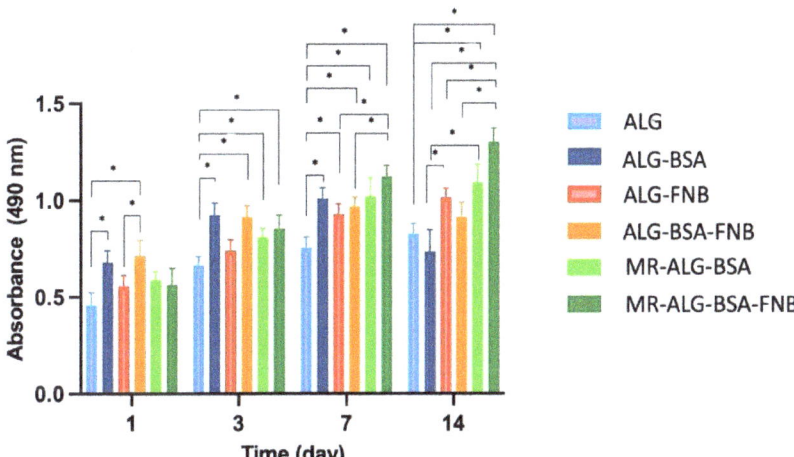

Figure 4. The ARPE-19 cell viability determined by the MTS assay after 1, 3, 7, and 14 days of seeding them seeded on ALG, ALG-BSA, and MR-ALG-BSA scaffolds ($n = 4$). (* denotes a significant difference, $p < 0.05$).

For FNB-loaded scaffolds, an initial significant rise in ARPE-19 cell viability was observed after day one for both ALG-FNB and ALG-BSA-FNB scaffolds. The cell viability on MR-ALG-BSA-FNB consistently increased during the entire cell culture period. This could be due to the anti-inflammatory properties of FNB [65]. It was previously reported that FNB protected retinal cell survival by reducing oxidative stress and inflammation, which was attributed to its PPARα role, decreasing the level of inflammatory mediators, including TNF-α, IL-6, and MCP-1 [66].

The viability of cells on the FNB-loaded MR-ALG-BSA scaffold was significantly higher than the other groups on day 14, which might be explained by the consistent sustained release of FNB from MR-ALG-BSA scaffolds over the tested period. Furthermore, ALG and ALG-BSA scaffolds could be depleted from FNB due to the burst and faster FNB release, as opposed to MR scaffolds, hence could not sustain its beneficial effect until day 14.

- In vitro cell–scaffold interaction studies

In regenerative medicine, the interaction of cells with scaffolds is critical to enhancing the secretion and deposition of ECM, which actively facilitates and regulates cellular activities [12]. Cells–scaffold interaction and cell distribution within scaffolds were studied by staining ARPE-19 cells on the scaffolds with fluorescence staining, including DAPI, calcein-AM, and PI. The DAPI staining forms fluorescent blue products upon binding to DNA in the nucleus [67]. Calcein-AM penetrates the cells and stains the cytoplasm of living cells. Once inside the cells, intracellular esterase enzymatically cleaves acetomethoxy derivative to produce a fluorescent green product. The intensity of green fluorescence is directly proportional to the number of viable cells with intact cell membranes [68]. On the other hand, cells with damaged membranes cannot emit green fluorescence. PI is a non-permeant dye which can penetrate the membrane of damaged cells and produce red fluoresce in dead cells [69].

The confocal fluorescence microscopy images of stained cells in scaffolds (in the depth of 200 µm) after day 14 are presented in Figure 5a. To better understand cell deposition inside scaffolds, the 3D images were reconstructed. The DAPI showed more cells interacting with BSA-containing scaffolds than with ALG scaffolds. Cells seeded on ALG and ALG-FNB scaffolds showed minimal calcein-AM fluorescence, while more PI fluorescence was observed, indicating that cells could not expand nor distribute homogeneously within the scaffold's matrix. In good agreement with the MTS assay, BSA-containing scaffolds showed more intense calcein-AM fluorescence, and reduction in the PI one, suggesting better cell–scaffold interactions and more viable cells within the scaffolds. This could be explained by the larger pore that the incorporation of BSA produced in the scaffolds, allowing deeper cell deposition and better transport of nutrients and oxygen. In addition, larger pores would be occluded later than smaller pores during progressive cell growth, and the presence of open spaces could keep the movement of oxygen and nutrients supply throughout the matrix [70].

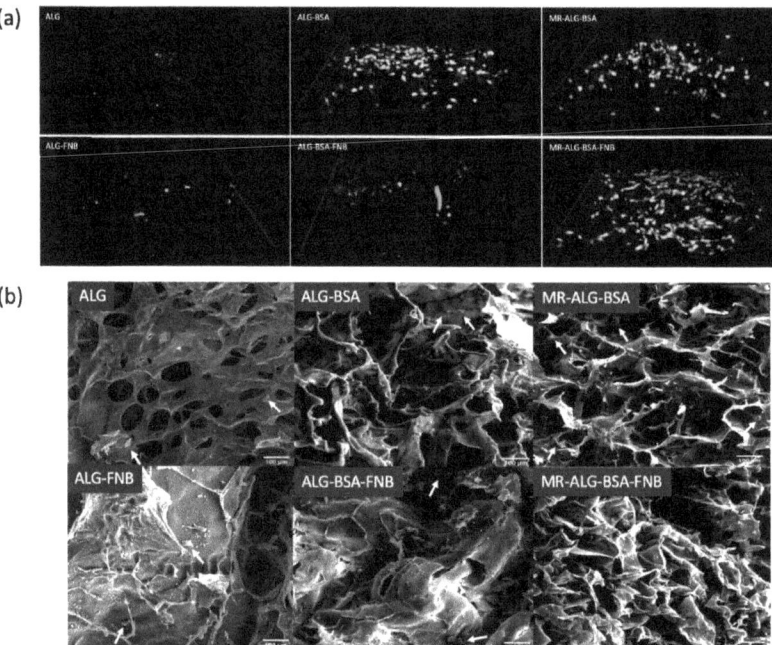

Figure 5. AREP-19 cells seeded on ALG-based scaffolds. (**a**) 3D reconstruction of confocal microscope images of seeded ARPE-19 cells on scaffolds with fluorescence staining after 14 days: DAPI (blue) calcein-AM (green) PI (red) in the depth of 200 µm of scaffolds (scale bar: 100 µm).; y = 1200 µm, x = 1200 µm, thickness = 200 µm, (**b**) SEM images of cells distributed on the ALG-based scaffolds; (Scale bar: 100 µm). White arrows indicate the presence of ARPRE-19 cells.

The capacity of cells to homogenously distribute Inside the scaffold structure is essential to regenerate damaged tissue, as regions devoid of cells might lead to defective tissue structure in regenerated organs [71]. While ALG scaffolds showed a limited deep distribution of cells, a considerably deeper distribution of cells inside BSA-containing scaffolds could be observed. This might indicate the capacity of cells to spread out and populate a deeper scaffold matrix in the presence of BSA. The enhanced porosity associated with the incorporation of BSA in scaffolds formulation might help reduce cell aggregation at scaffolds surfaces which is essential for new tissue formation. In addition, SEM images of seeded cells on scaffolds, shown in Figure 5b, further demonstrated more cells present at the surface of ALG-BSA, MR-ALG-BSA, and MR-ALG-BSA-FNB scaffolds in comparison with ALG and ALG-FNB ones, providing a more favourable environment for cells.

4. Conclusions

This work was undertaken to design and develop different types of ALG-based scaffolds and evaluate their potential use for retinal regenerative and drug delivery applications. The potential role of BSA as a porogenic to enhance the porosity of ALG scaffolds was demonstrated. Furthermore, the incorporation of BSA in ALG scaffold increased their loading capacity toward a hydrophobic drug. On the other hand, the conjugation of BSA with ALG via the Maillard reaction improved the mechanical stability of scaffolds, which is essential for implantation at the back of the eye. It allowed a favourable swelling and sustained release of loaded FNB. In vitro biological investigations demonstrated the biodegradability and biocompatibility of BSA-containing ALG scaffolds, highlighting a significant enhancement of ARPE-19 cell viability distribution within the scaffolds when scaffolds were subjected to the Maillard reaction. Taken together, our results demonstrate that scaffolds made of ALG-BSA Maillard reaction products have a promising role for retinal tissue regenerative application and as an ocular drug delivery system.

Author Contributions: Conceptualisation, M.K. and R.G.A.; methodology, M.K., R.G.A., S.B. and M.A.Z.; formal analysis, M.K., R.G.A., M.A.Z., L.S., A.S. and S.B.; investigation, M.A.Z.; writing—original draft preparation, M.A.Z.; writing—review and editing, M.K., R.G.A., M.A.Z., M.A.A., A.S., L.S. and S.B.; visualization, M.K., R.G.A. and M.A.Z.; supervision, M.K., R.G.A. and S.B. All authors have read and agreed to the published version of the manuscript.

Funding: This research received no external funding.

Institutional Review Board Statement: Not applicable.

Informed Consent Statement: Not applicable.

Data Availability Statement: All data relevant to the publication are included.

Conflicts of Interest: The authors declare no conflict of interest.

References

1. Abedin Zadeh, M.; Khoder, M.; Al-Kinani, A.A.; Younes, H.M.; Alany, R.G. Retinal Cell Regeneration Using Tissue Engineered Polymeric Scaffolds. *Drug Discov. Today* **2019**, *24*, 1669–1678. [CrossRef]
2. Ou, K.; Li, Y.; Liu, L.; Li, H.; Cox, K.; Wu, J.; Liu, J.; Dick, A. Recent Developments of Neuroprotective Agents for Degenerative Retinal Disorders. *Neural Regen. Res.* **2022**, *17*, 1919. [CrossRef]
3. Wong, W.L.; Su, X.; Li, X.; Cheung, C.M.G.; Klein, R.; Cheng, C.-Y.; Wong, T.Y. Global Prevalence of Age-Related Macular Degeneration and Disease Burden Projection for 2020 and 2040: A Systematic Review and Meta-Analysis. *Lancet Glob. Health* **2014**, *2*, e106–e116. [CrossRef]
4. Wallsh, J.O.; Gallemore, R.P. Anti-VEGF-Resistant Retinal Diseases: A Review of the Latest Treatment Options. *Cells* **2021**, *10*, 1049. [CrossRef]
5. Bisht, R.; Mandal, A.; Jaiswal, J.K.; Rupenthal, I.D. Nanocarrier Mediated Retinal Drug Delivery: Overcoming Ocular Barriers to Treat Posterior Eye Diseases. *WIREs Nanomed. Nanobiotechnol.* **2018**, *10*, e1473. [CrossRef]
6. Guay, D.R.P. Update on Fenofibrate. *Cardiovasc. Drug Rev.* **2006**, *20*, 281–302. [CrossRef]
7. Qiu, F.; Meng, T.; Chen, Q.; Zhou, K.; Shao, Y.; Matlock, G.; Ma, X.; Wu, W.; Du, Y.; Wang, X.; et al. Fenofibrate-Loaded Biodegradable Nanoparticles for the Treatment of Experimental Diabetic Retinopathy and Neovascular Age-Related Macular Degeneration. *Mol. Pharm.* **2019**, *16*, 1958–1970. [CrossRef]
8. Bogdanov, P.; Hernández, C.; Corraliza, L.; Carvalho, A.R.; Simó, R. Effect of Fenofibrate on Retinal Neurodegeneration in an Experimental Model of Type 2 Diabetes. *Acta Diabetol.* **2015**, *52*, 113–122. [CrossRef]
9. Tezel, T.H.; Del Priore, L.V.; Berger, A.S.; Kaplan, H.J. Adult Retinal Pigment Epithelial Transplantation in Exudative Age-Related Macular Degeneration. *Am. J. Ophthalmol.* **2007**, *143*, 584–595.e2. [CrossRef]
10. Kim, H.M.; Woo, S.J. Ocular Drug Delivery to the Retina: Current Innovations and Future Perspectives. *Pharmaceutics* **2021**, *13*, 108. [CrossRef]
11. Garg, T.; Singh, O.; Arora, S.; Murthy, R.S.R. Scaffold: A Novel Carrier for Cell and Drug Delivery. *Crit. Rev. Ther. Drug Carr. Syst.* **2012**, *29*, 1–63. [CrossRef]
12. Chan, B.P.; Leong, K.W. Scaffolding in Tissue Engineering: General Approaches and Tissue-Specific Considerations. *Eur. Spine J.* **2008**, *17* (Suppl. S4), 467–479. [CrossRef]
13. White, C.E.; Olabisi, R.M. Scaffolds for Retinal Pigment Epithelial Cell Transplantation in Age-Related Macular Degeneration. *J. Tissue Eng.* **2017**, *8*, 204173141772084. [CrossRef]

14. Al Dalaty, A.; Karam, A.; Najlah, M.; Alany, R.G.; Khoder, M. Effect of Non-Cross-Linked Calcium on Characteristics, Swelling Behaviour, Drug Release and Mucoadhesiveness of Calcium Alginate Beads. *Carbohydr. Polym.* **2016**, *140*, 163–170. [CrossRef]
15. Lee, K.Y.; Mooney, D.J. Alginate: Properties and Biomedical Applications. *Prog. Polym. Sci.* **2012**, *37*, 106–126. [CrossRef]
16. Nayak, A.K.; Mohanta, B.C.; Hasnain, M.S.; Hoda, M.N.; Tripathi, G. Alginate-Based Scaffolds for Drug Delivery in Tissue Engineering. In *Alginates in Drug Delivery*; Academic Press: Cambridge, MA, USA, 2020; pp. 359–386. [CrossRef]
17. Sun, J.; Tan, H. Alginate-Based Biomaterials for Regenerative Medicine Applications. *Materials* **2013**, *6*, 1285–1309. [CrossRef]
18. Oryan, A.; Kamali, A.; Moshiri, A.; Baharvand, H.; Daemi, H. Chemical Crosslinking of Biopolymeric Scaffolds: Current Knowledge and Future Directions of Crosslinked Engineered Bone Scaffolds. *Int. J. Biol. Macromol.* **2018**, *107*, 678–688. [CrossRef]
19. Niknejad, H.; Mahmoudzadeh, R. Comparison of Different Crosslinking Methods for Preparation of Docetaxel-Loaded Albumin Nanoparticles. *Iran. J. Pharm. Res.* **2015**, *14*, 385–394.
20. Khoder, M.; Gbormoi, H.K.; Ryan, A.; Karam, A.; Alany, R.G. Potential Use of the Maillard Reaction for Pharmaceutical Applications: Gastric and Intestinal Controlled Release Alginate-Albumin Beads. *Pharmaceutics* **2019**, *11*, 83. [CrossRef]
21. Lee, Y.-Y.; Tang, T.-K.; Phuah, E.-T.; Alitheen, N.B.M.; Tan, C.-P.; Lai, O.-M. New Functionalities of Maillard Reaction Products as Emulsifiers and Encapsulating Agents, and the Processing Parameters: A Brief Review. *J. Sci. Food Agric.* **2017**, *97*, 1379–1385. [CrossRef]
22. Morales, F.J.; Jiménez-Pérez, S. Free Radical Scavenging Capacity of Maillard Reaction Products as Related to Colour and Fluorescence. *Food Chem.* **2001**, *72*, 119–125. [CrossRef]
23. Chen, X.-M.; Kitts, D.D. Antioxidant and Anti-Inflammatory Activities of Maillard Reaction Products Isolated from Sugar–Amino Acid Model Systems. *J. Agric. Food Chem.* **2011**, *59*, 11294–11303. [CrossRef] [PubMed]
24. Prasopdee, T.; Sinthuvanich, C.; Chollakup, R.; Uttayarat, P.; Smitthipong, W. The Albumin/Starch Scaffold and Its Biocompatibility with Living Cells. *Mater. Today Commun.* **2021**, *27*, 102164. [CrossRef]
25. Yuan, H.; Zheng, X.; Liu, W.; Zhang, H.; Shao, J.; Yao, J.; Mao, C.; Hui, J.; Fan, D. A Novel Bovine Serum Albumin and Sodium Alginate Hydrogel Scaffold Doped with Hydroxyapatite Nanowires for Cartilage Defects Repair. *Colloids Surf. B Biointerfaces* **2020**, *192*, 111041. [CrossRef] [PubMed]
26. Fereshteh, Z. Freeze-Drying Technologies for 3D Scaffold Engineering. In *Functional 3D Tissue Engineering Scaffolds: Materials, Technologies, and Applications*; Elsevier: Amsterdam, The Netherlands, 2018; pp. 151–174. [CrossRef]
27. Li, C. Electrolyte Quantification in Aqueous and Vitreous Humor of Common Preclinical Species. *ARVO Annu. Meet. Abstr.* **2019**, *60*, 3421.
28. Wan, L.Q.; Jiang, J.; Arnold, D.E.; Guo, X.E.; Lu, H.H.; Mow, V.C. Calcium Concentration Effects on the Mechanical and Biochemical Properties of Chondrocyte-Alginate Constructs. *Cell Mol. Bioeng.* **2008**, *1*, 93–102. [CrossRef]
29. Sangkert, S.; Kamolmatyakul, S.; Gelinsky, M.; Meesane, J. 3D Printed Scaffolds of Alginate/Polyvinylalcohol with Silk Fibroin Based on Mimicked Extracellular Matrix for Bone Tissue Engineering in Maxillofacial Surgery. *Mater. Today Commun.* **2021**, *26*, 102140. [CrossRef]
30. Lacroix, P.M.; Dawson, B.A.; Sears, R.W.; Black, D.B.; Cyr, T.D.; Ethier, J.C. Fenofibrate Raw Materials: HPLC Methods for Assay and Purity and an NMR Method for Purity. *J. Pharm. Biomed. Anal.* **1998**, *18*, 383–402. [CrossRef]
31. Jain, D.; Jain, N.; Raghuwanshi, R. Development and Validation of RP-HPLC Method for Simultaneous Estimation of Atorvastatin Calcium and Fenofibrate in Tablet Dosage Forms. *Indian J. Pharm. Sci.* **2008**, *70*, 263. [CrossRef]
32. Shaqour, B.; Reigada, I.; Górecka, Ż.; Choińska, E.; Verleije, B.; Beyers, K.; Święszkowski, W.; Fallarero, A.; Cos, P. 3D-Printed Drug Delivery Systems: The Effects of Drug Incorporation Methods on Their Release and Antibacterial Efficiency. *Materials* **2020**, *13*, 3364. [CrossRef]
33. Wong, F.S.Y.; Tsang, K.K.; Chu, A.M.W.; Chan, B.P.; Yao, K.M.; Lo, A.C.Y. Injectable Cell-Encapsulating Composite Alginate-Collagen Platform with Inducible Termination Switch for Safer Ocular Drug Delivery. *Biomaterials* **2019**, *201*, 53–67. [CrossRef] [PubMed]
34. Chen, C.-Y.; Ke, C.-J.; Yen, K.-C.; Hsieh, H.-C.; Sun, J.-S.; Lin, F.-H. 3D Porous Calcium-Alginate Scaffolds Cell Culture System Improved Human Osteoblast Cell Clusters for Cell Therapy. *Theranostics* **2015**, *5*, 643–655. [CrossRef] [PubMed]
35. Ardiles, C.S.; Rodríguez, C.C. Theoretical Study for Determining the Type of Interactions between a GG Block of an Alginate Chain with Metals Cu^{2+}, Mn^{2+}, Ca^{2+} and Mg^{2+}. *Arab. J. Chem.* **2021**, *14*, 103325. [CrossRef]
36. Liu, F.; Ma, C.; Gao, Y.; McClements, D.J. Food-Grade Covalent Complexes and Their Application as Nutraceutical Delivery Systems: A Review. *Compr. Rev. Food Sci. Food Saf.* **2017**, *16*, 76–95. [CrossRef]
37. Lavik, E.B.; Klassen, H.; Warfvinge, K.; Langer, R.; Young, M.J. Fabrication of Degradable Polymer Scaffolds to Direct the Integration and Differentiation of Retinal Progenitors. *Biomaterials* **2005**, *26*, 3187–3196. [CrossRef] [PubMed]
38. Al-Hakkak, J.; Al-Hakkak, F. Functional Egg White–Pectin Conjugates Prepared by Controlled Maillard Reaction. *J. Food Eng.* **2010**, *100*, 152–159. [CrossRef]
39. Ekemen, Z.; Ahmad, Z.; Stride, E.; Kaplan, D.; Edirisinghe, M. Electrohydrodynamic Bubbling: An Alternative Route to Fabricate Porous Structures of Silk Fibroin Based Materials. *Biomacromolecules* **2013**, *14*, 1412–1422. [CrossRef]
40. Loh, Q.L.; Choong, C. Three-Dimensional Scaffolds for Tissue Engineering Applications: Role of Porosity and Pore Size. *Tissue Eng. Part B Rev.* **2013**, *19*, 485–502. [CrossRef]

41. Stachewicz, U.; Szewczyk, P.K.; Kruk, A.; Barber, A.H.; Czyrska-Filemonowicz, A. Pore Shape and Size Dependence on Cell Growth into Electrospun Fiber Scaffolds for Tissue Engineering: 2D and 3D Analyses Using SEM and FIB-SEM Tomography. *Mater. Sci. Eng. C* **2019**, *95*, 397–408. [CrossRef]
42. Prasadh, S.; Wong, R.C.W. Unraveling the Mechanical Strength of Biomaterials Used as a Bone Scaffold in Oral and Maxillofacial Defects. *Oral Sci. Int.* **2018**, *15*, 48–55. [CrossRef]
43. Khoder, M.; Tsapis, N.; Huguet, H.; Besnard, M.; Gueutin, C.; Fattal, E. Removal of Ciprofloxacin in Simulated Digestive Media by Activated Charcoal Entrapped within Zinc-Pectinate Beads. *Int. J. Pharm.* **2009**, *379*, 251–259. [CrossRef] [PubMed]
44. Etxabide, A.; Ribeiro, R.D.C.; Guerrero, P.; Ferreira, A.M.; Stafford, G.P.; Dalgarno, K.; de la Caba, K.; Gentile, P. Lactose-Crosslinked Fish Gelatin-Based Porous Scaffolds Embedded with Tetrahydrocurcumin for Cartilage Regeneration. *Int. J. Biol. Macromol.* **2018**, *117*, 199–208. [CrossRef]
45. Varley, M.C.; Neelakantan, S.; Clyne, T.W.; Dean, J.; Brooks, R.A.; Markaki, A.E. Cell Structure, Stiffness and Permeability of Freeze-Dried Collagen Scaffolds in Dry and Hydrated States. *Acta Biomater.* **2016**, *33*, 166–175. [CrossRef]
46. Wendland, R.J.; Jiao, C.; Russell, S.R.; Han, I.C.; Wiley, L.A.; Tucker, B.A.; Sohn, E.H.; Worthington, K.S. The Effect of Retinal Scaffold Modulus on Performance during Surgical Handling. *Exp. Eye Res.* **2021**, *207*, 108566. [CrossRef]
47. Worthington, K.S.; Wiley, L.A.; Bartlett, A.M.; Stone, E.M.; Mullins, R.F.; Salem, A.K.; Guymon, C.A.; Tucker, B.A. Mechanical Properties of Murine and Porcine Ocular Tissues in Compression. *Exp. Eye Res.* **2014**, *121*, 194–199. [CrossRef] [PubMed]
48. Li, J.; Mooney, D.J. Designing Hydrogels for Controlled Drug Delivery. *Nat. Rev. Mater.* **2016**, *1*, 16071. [CrossRef]
49. Gentile, P.; Mattioli-Belmonte, M.; Chiono, V.; Ferretti, C.; Baino, F.; Tonda-Turo, C.; Vitale-Brovarone, C.; Pashkuleva, I.; Reis, R.L.; Ciardelli, G. Bioactive Glass/Polymer Composite Scaffolds Mimicking Bone Tissue. *J. Biomed Mater. Res. A* **2012**, *100A*, 2654–2667. [CrossRef] [PubMed]
50. Meydani, B.; Vahedifar, A.; Askari, G.; Madadlou, A. Influence of the Maillard Reaction on the Properties of Cold-Set Whey Protein and Maltodextrin Binary Gels. *Int. Dairy J.* **2019**, *90*, 79–87. [CrossRef]
51. Fatimi, A.; Okoro, O.V.; Podstawczyk, D.; Siminska-Stanny, J.; Shavandi, A. Natural Hydrogel-Based Bio-Inks for 3D Bioprinting in Tissue Engineering: A Review. *Gels* **2022**, *8*, 179. [CrossRef]
52. Shavandi, A.; Hosseini, S.; Okoro, O.V.; Nie, L.; Eghbali Babadi, F.; Melchels, F. 3D Bioprinting of Lignocellulosic Biomaterials. *Adv. Healthc. Mater.* **2020**, *9*, 2001472. [CrossRef]
53. Shah, R.; Saha, N.; Saha, P. Influence of Temperature, PH and Simulated Biological Solutions on Swelling and Structural Properties of Biomineralized ($CaCO_3$) PVP–CMC Hydrogel. *Prog. Biomater.* **2015**, *4*, 123–136. [CrossRef]
54. Will, M.A.; Clark, N.A.; Swain, J.E. Biological PH Buffers in IVF: Help or Hindrance to Success. *J. Assist. Reprod. Genet.* **2011**, *28*, 711–724. [CrossRef] [PubMed]
55. Khoder, M.; Tsapis, N.; Domergue-Dupont, V.; Gueutin, C.; Fattal, E. Removal of Residual Colonic Ciprofloxacin in the Rat by Activated Charcoal Entrapped within Zinc-Pectinate Beads. *Eur. J. Pharm. Sci.* **2010**, *41*, 281–288. [CrossRef] [PubMed]
56. Hirsch, J.; Mossine, V.V.; Feather, M.S. The Detection of Some Dicarbonyl Intermediates Arising from the Degradation of Amadori Compounds (the Maillard Reaction). *Carbohydr. Res.* **1995**, *273*, 171–177. [CrossRef]
57. Zhang, M.; Li, H.; Lang, B.; O'Donnell, K.; Zhang, H.; Wang, Z.; Dong, Y.; Wu, C.; Williams, R.O. Formulation and Delivery of Improved Amorphous Fenofibrate Solid Dispersions Prepared by Thin Film Freezing. *Eur. J. Pharm. Biopharm.* **2012**, *82*, 534–544. [CrossRef] [PubMed]
58. Zhou, S.; Bismarck, A.; Steinke, J.H.G. Ion-Responsive Alginate Based Macroporous Injectable Hydrogel Scaffolds Prepared by Emulsion Templating. *J. Mater. Chem. B* **2013**, *1*, 4736. [CrossRef] [PubMed]
59. Afewerki, S.; Sheikhi, A.; Kannan, S.; Ahadian, S.; Khademhosseini, A. Gelatin-Polysaccharide Composite Scaffolds for 3D Cell Culture and Tissue Engineering: Towards Natural Therapeutics. *Bioeng. Transl. Med.* **2019**, *4*, 96–115. [CrossRef]
60. Shoichet, M.S.; Li, R.H.; White, M.L.; Winn, S.R. Stability of Hydrogels Used in Cell Encapsulation: An in Vitro Comparison of Alginate and Agarose. *Biotechnol. Bioeng.* **1996**, *50*, 374–381. [CrossRef]
61. Ye, Y.; Zhang, X.; Deng, X.; Hao, L.; Wang, W. Modification of Alginate Hydrogel Films for Delivering Hydrophobic Kaempferol. *J. Nanomater.* **2019**, *2019*, 9170732. [CrossRef]
62. Eral, H.B.; López-Mejías, V.; O'Mahony, M.; Trout, B.L.; Myerson, A.S.; Doyle, P.S. Biocompatible Alginate Microgel Particles as Heteronucleants and Encapsulating Vehicles for Hydrophilic and Hydrophobic Drugs. *Cryst. Growth Des.* **2014**, *14*, 2073–2082. [CrossRef]
63. Al-Husseini, J.K.; Stanton, N.J.; Selassie, C.R.D.; Johal, M.S. The Binding of Drug Molecules to Serum Albumin: The Effect of Drug Hydrophobicity on Binding Strength and Protein Desolvation. *Langmuir* **2019**, *35*, 17054–17060. [CrossRef] [PubMed]
64. Hazim, R.A.; Volland, S.; Yen, A.; Burgess, B.L.; Williams, D.S. Rapid Differentiation of the Human RPE Cell Line, ARPE-19, Induced by Nicotinamide. *Exp. Eye Res.* **2019**, *179*, 18–24. [CrossRef]
65. Hsu, Y.-J.; Lin, C.-W.; Cho, S.-L.; Yang, W.-S.; Yang, C.-M.; Yang, C.-H. Protective Effect of Fenofibrate on Oxidative Stress-Induced Apoptosis in Retinal–Choroidal Vascular Endothelial Cells: Implication for Diabetic Retinopathy Treatment. *Antioxidants* **2020**, *9*, 712. [CrossRef]
66. Deng, G.; Moran, E.P.; Cheng, R.; Matlock, G.; Zhou, K.; Moran, D.; Chen, D.; Yu, Q.; Ma, J.-X. Therapeutic Effects of a Novel Agonist of Peroxisome Proliferator-Activated Receptor Alpha for the Treatment of Diabetic Retinopathy. *Investig. Ophthalmol. Vis. Sci.* **2017**, *58*, 5030. [CrossRef]

67. Popescu, L.M.; Gherghiceanu, M.; Suciu, L.C.; Manole, C.G.; Hinescu, M.E. Telocytes and Putative Stem Cells in the Lungs: Electron Microscopy, Electron Tomography and Laser Scanning Microscopy. *Cell Tissue Res.* **2011**, *345*, 391–403. [CrossRef] [PubMed]
68. Uggeri, J.; Gatti, R.; Belletti, S.; Scandroglio, R.; Corradini, R.; Rotoli, B.M.; Orlandini, G. Calcein-AM Is a Detector of Intracellular Oxidative Activity. *Histochem. Cell Biol.* **2000**, *122*, 499–505. [CrossRef]
69. Stiefel, P.; Schmidt-Emrich, S.; Maniura-Weber, K.; Ren, Q. Critical Aspects of Using Bacterial Cell Viability Assays with the Fluorophores SYTO9 and Propidium Iodide. *BMC Microbiol.* **2015**, *15*, 36. [CrossRef]
70. Murphy, C.M.; O'Brien, F.J. Understanding the Effect of Mean Pore Size on Cell Activity in Collagen-Glycosaminoglycan Scaffolds. *Cell Adhes. Migr.* **2010**, *4*, 377–381. [CrossRef]
71. Choi, S.-W.; Xie, J.; Xia, Y. Chitosan-Based Inverse Opals: Three-Dimensional Scaffolds with Uniform Pore Structures for Cell Culture. *Adv. Mater.* **2009**, *21*, 2997–3001. [CrossRef] [PubMed]

Disclaimer/Publisher's Note: The statements, opinions and data contained in all publications are solely those of the individual author(s) and contributor(s) and not of MDPI and/or the editor(s). MDPI and/or the editor(s) disclaim responsibility for any injury to people or property resulting from any ideas, methods, instructions or products referred to in the content.

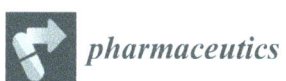 *pharmaceutics*

Article

Chitosan Hydrogels Cross-Linked with Trimesic Acid for the Delivery of 5-Fluorouracil in Cancer Therapy

Sravani Emani, Anil Vangala, Federico Buonocore, Niousha Yarandi and Gianpiero Calabrese *

School of Life Sciences, Pharmacy and Chemistry, Kingston University London, Kingston-upon-Thames KT1 2EE, UK
* Correspondence: g.calabrese@kingston.ac.uk; Tel.: +44-(0)-20-8417-7065

Abstract: Chitosan exhibits unique properties making it a suitable material for drug delivery. Considering the rising popularity of hydrogels in this field, this work offers a comprehensive study of hydrogels constituted by chitosan and cross-linked with 1,3,5-benzene tricarboxylic acid (BTC; also known as trimesic acid). Hydrogels were prepared by cross-linking chitosan with BTC in different concentrations. The nature of the gels was studied through oscillatory amplitude strain and frequency sweep tests within the linear viscoelastic region (LVE) limit. The flow curves of the gels revealed shear thinning behavior. High G′ values imply strong cross-linking with improved stability. The rheological tests revealed that the strength of the hydrogel network increased with the cross-linking degree. Hardness, cohesiveness, adhesiveness, compressibility, and elasticity of the gels were determined using a texture analyzer. The scanning electron microscopy (SEM) data of the cross-linked hydrogels showed distinctive pores with a pore size increasing according to increasing concentrations (pore size range between 3–18 µm). Computational analysis was performed by docking simulations between chitosan and BTC. Drug release studies employing 5-fluorouracil (5-FU) yielded a more sustained release profile with 35 to 50% release among the formulations studied in a 3 h period. Overall, this work demonstrated that the presence of BTC as cross-linker leads to satisfactory mechanical properties of the chitosan hydrogel, suggesting potential applications in the sustained release of cancer therapeutics.

Keywords: chitosan; 1,3,5-benzene tricarboxylic acid; hydrogels; rheology

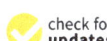

Citation: Emani, S.; Vangala, A.; Buonocore, F.; Yarandi, N.; Calabrese, G. Chitosan Hydrogels Cross-Linked with Trimesic Acid for the Delivery of 5-Fluorouracil in Cancer Therapy. *Pharmaceutics* 2023, 15, 1084. https://doi.org/10.3390/pharmaceutics15041084

Academic Editor: Giulia Bonacucina

Received: 15 January 2023
Revised: 21 March 2023
Accepted: 22 March 2023
Published: 28 March 2023

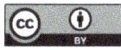

Copyright: © 2023 by the authors. Licensee MDPI, Basel, Switzerland. This article is an open access article distributed under the terms and conditions of the Creative Commons Attribution (CC BY) license (https://creativecommons.org/licenses/by/4.0/).

1. Introduction

Polymeric hydrogels are used in the field of drug delivery for the controlled release of therapeutic ingredients. Hydrogels are cross-linked networks and hold hydrophilic functional groups in their structure. Hydrophilic functional groups, such as amine (-NH$_2$), hydroxyl (-OH), sulfonates (-SO$_3$H), and amides (CONH$_2$), can absorb large amounts of water and are attached to polymeric networks [1]. They form a mesh-like structure that has a potential ability to hold and deliver drug molecules at the site of action [2,3]. The hydrogels can be formed from either natural (chitosan [4], collagen [5], fibrin [6], cellulose [7], hyaluronic acid [8]), synthetic (polyethylene glycol [9], polyvinyl alcohol [10], polyacrylamide [11], and poly-N-isopropylacrylamide [12]) or semisynthetic materials (PEG with other proteins) [13]. The polymeric chains establish a superficial 3D network with interstitial spaces that can port the physiological or aqueous fluids [14]. These fluids can facilitate the diffusion of oxygen as well as nutrients that play an important role in cell growth and proliferation [15].

Among several polymers, chitosan is extensively studied in drug delivery. A great number of applications have been proposed for chitosan, from HIV [16] and cancer therapy [17–22], to tissue engineering [23], biotechnology, agriculture [24], and wound dressings [25–28]. Chitosan is a cationic polymer made of repeated units of β-(1 → 4)-2-acetamido-D-glucose and β-(1 → 4)-2-amino-D-glucose units and formed via the process of deacetylation of chitin. The chemical structure of chitosan is composed of two main sugars, namely glucosamine and N-acetyl glucosamine (Figure 1). The chemical reactivity of the polymer is due to the presence of primary amino and hydroxy groups.

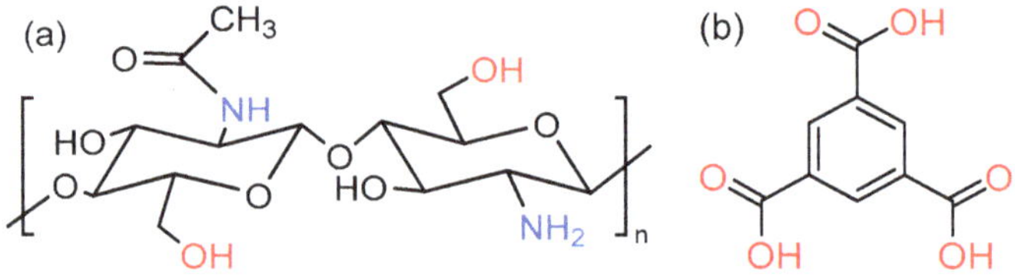

Figure 1. Structures of (**a**) chitosan and (**b**) 1,3,5-benzene tricarboxylic acid (BTC).

At physiological pH, chitosan acts as a mucoadhesive polymer. Here, the amino groups become protonated and act as a determining factor in chitosan's mucoadhesive properties [29]. When dissolved in protic solvents, such as water, chitosan possesses positively charged amine groups (NH_3^+), which account for its solubility [25] and its mucoadhesive properties (as it can favorably interact with the negatively charged mucus). The degree of deacetylation (DD) and the molecular weight of chitosan are also crucial in determining biological properties. The solubility of the polymer increases with an increase in DD of chitosan, but on the other hand, a low DD results in a slower diffusion of the drug through the polymeric network. Hence, chitosan with an approximate DD value of 75–85% is preferred [30].

Chitosan is in the form of either physical or chemically cross-linked hydrogels. Cross-linkers interact with the amine groups in the chitosan, forming molecular bridges in the chitosan chains. As novel chitosan and carrageenan nanoparticles-based gels showed a good potential for the sustained release of drugs in topical administration [31], more recently, research focused on the hydrogels produced by cross-linking chitosan with different materials, such as glutaraldehyde [32–34], genipin [35,36], and collagen [37,38]. One such material used for this purpose is 1,3,5-benzene tricarboxylic acid (BTC, Figure 1). Controlled drug release of the chitosan–BTC hydrogels have previously been reported by Yang et al. [39]. In addition, the positively charged chitosan in acidic medium can allow the attachment of nucleic acids, such as DNA and siRNA [40]. The reason for using BTC is to design a more stable system that can encapsulate both hydrophilic and lipophilic drugs in the polymeric networks [41]. Hydrogels with definite porous structures can be used as carriers for drug delivery [42]. The carboxylic acid (-COOH) groups of BTC undergo deprotonation and form ionic cross-links with the amine groups (NH_2) of chitosan. In addition, possible interactions, such as ionic, hydrogen, and π-π bonding, were reported in the literature [43].

When combining chitosan and BTC, gelation occurs at room temperature, and these gels can be used for encapsulating hydrophilic and lipophilic drugs for controlled or sustained drug release. In previously reported procedures, porous chitosan was prepared using BTC as a cross-linker [39] and supramolecular hydrogels from hydroxy pyridines [44]. In biomedical applications, there is a need for a stable hydrogel system that meets essential criteria of toughness and stability. However, most hydrogels formulated do not display these properties. Hence, there is a need to improve the gel characteristics either by physical or chemical alteration. The rheological studies of the viscoelastic materials provide the information about the mechanical strength of the hydrogels [45]. The dynamic changes in the microscopic structure and gelation can be monitored using a rheometer [46]. This aids in understanding the cross-linking degree, elasticity, flow, and viscosity of the gel material in response to applied stress and strain [47]. The rheological tests can be performed monitoring parameters, such as stress relaxation (when subjected to strain, there is decrease in stress), oscillatory amplitude strain sweep (amplitude of the deformation or shear stress is varied at constant frequency), frequency strain sweep within the linear viscoelastic region (LVE), rotational viscometry, and creep recovery [48].

Viscoelastic materials exhibit a reversible response that depends on the rate of applied load. This mechanism usually occurs in polymeric materials. These materials are time-dependent, which makes them strain-rate sensitive. Viscoelasticity is the property of a material that exhibits both viscous and elastic properties when deformed. When a viscoelastic material is subjected to stress, the response is composed of elastic deformation (which stores energy) and viscous flow (which releases energy). The profile of the frequency sweep data gives the degree of dispersion, whereas interparticle association frequency sweep curves can provide information about the product (gel) behavior during storage and application. At certain frequency, either the elastic or viscous seems dominant which indicates the elastic or viscous nature of the structured material (Figure 2). From Graph a (Figure 2), the particles were dispersed irregularly, and the viscous component dominated the elastic component [49]. In Graph b of the same figure, the loss modulus is greater than the viscous modulus, and complex viscosity (η^*) is dependent on frequency. In both cases, sedimentation is likely to occur, causing the instability of the gel structure. In Graph c (Figure 2), the particles are evenly spread and well-dispersed. The elastic modulus dominated the viscous modulus and independence of frequency.

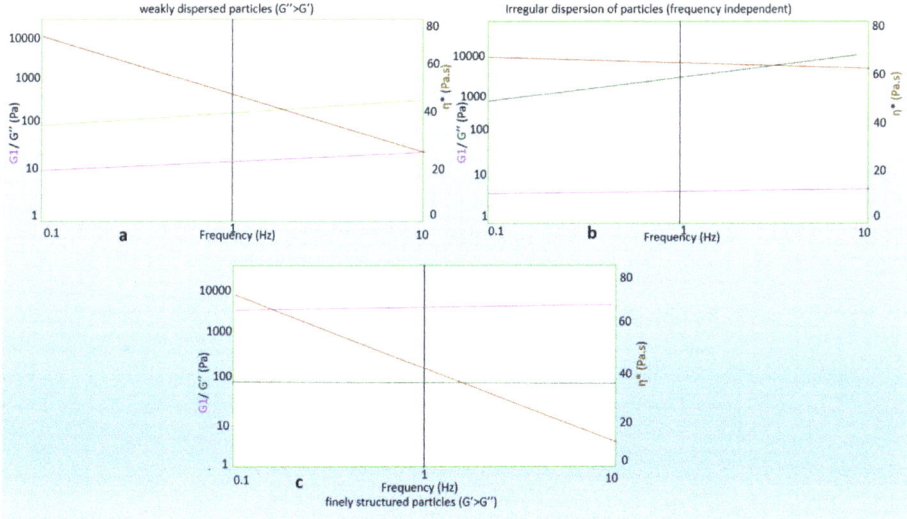

Figure 2. Graphs representing viscoelastic parameters: (**a**) weakly dispersed particles (G″ > G′); (**b**) irregular dispersion of particles; (**c**) fine structured particles (G′ > G″) [49]. Lines legend: purple for G′, elastic modulus; green for G″, viscous modulus; and orange for η^*, complex viscosity...

The phase angle reveals the material deformation to either solid or liquid. Low phase angle results can be seen in a solid, and a high phase angle corresponds to liquid. The gel point is another critical parameter that determines the dynamic viscoelastic properties of the polymer systems. The sudden change in viscosity of the fluid can be determined using the gelling point. At the gelling point, a solution becomes more resistant to flow due to a loss in fluidity. Winter and Chambon [50,51] explained that the gelling point can be identified from the dynamic viscoelastic parameters. They emphasized the rheological parameters of a new cross-linking system using end-linked poly dimethyl siloxane. The viscoelasticity of the material can be determined from the loss tangent (tan δ) which is a ratio of the energy lost to the total energy stored during the analysis [52]. These measurements are important to determine the mechanical strength of the material. Creep recovery can provide information about the recoverable viscoelastic deformation and viscous deformation (non-recoverable) [53].

Drugs are released from the polymeric network through four different mechanisms: stimulated release, degradation-controlled, solvent-controlled, and diffusion-controlled release [54]. Thus, the rate of drug release depends on the characteristics of the polymer, solvent used, and the physico–chemical properties of the drug. Researchers have found that 5-FU has a promising anticancer effect and can be used as a model drug [55]. The efficacy and safety of 5-FU can theoretically be improved by using drug delivery vehicles such as hydrogels. Indeed, the high water content of the porous three-dimensional structure of chitosan hydrogels (up to 99% w/w of water in some cases) facilitates the incorporation of hydrophilic drugs. The non-specific distribution of the drug in vivo, which affects non-target cells leading to side effects, can be overcome by the introduction of hydrogels to release drugs in a controlled manner [56,57]. In this study, hydrogels were prepared by mixing physical solutions of chitosan and BTC. The prepared hydrogels were characterized using NMR, Fourier-transformed infrared spectroscopy (FTIR), texture analysis, and rheological data to determine the mechanical and flow properties of the hydrogels. The release of 5-FU from the prepared hydrogels and the impact of variations in cross-linker amounts were also investigated.

2. Materials and Methods

2.1. Materials

Low molecular weight chitosan (>75% deacetylated, 20–300 cps (1% in 1% acetic acid)), 1,3,5-benzene tricarboxylic acid (BTC, trimesic acid, $C_9H_6O_6$, Mwt 210.14 g/mol), 5-fluorouracil (5-FU, ≥99% HPLC, powder, $C_4H_3FN_2O_2$, Mwt 130.08), dialysis tubing with an average flat width of 25 mm (1.0 inch) and molecular weight cut-off (MWCO) 3500 Da, glacial acetic acid, deuterium chloride, deuterium oxide, and ethanol were all purchased from Sigma-Aldrich, Gillingham (UK). Aluminium specimen stubs (0.5″) and carbon tabs (12 mm diameter) were purchased from Agar Scientific Ltd., Stanstead (UK). Deionised water was used for all preparations.

2.2. Preparation of Chitosan–BTC Hydrogels

Chitosan hydrogels with different concentrations were prepared according to a modification of the method previously reported by Yang et al. [39]. Briefly, chitosan solution (1 wt%, 2.50 g) was prepared by dissolving chitosan in acetic acid (250 mL of 0.6% v/v). This mixture was heated at 40 °C overnight. BTC solutions were prepared by dissolving BTC powder in ethanol in varying concentrations. Three different concentrations (M1, M2, M3) were, respectively, prepared by mixing:

- A combination of 1 wt% chitosan solution and 10 mM BTC-ethanol solution (M1);
- A combination of 1 wt% chitosan solution and 50 mM BTC-ethanol solution (M2);
- A combination of 0.5 wt% chitosan solution and 50 mM BTC-ethanol solution (M3).

The solutions of chitosan and BTC formed a gel at room temperature upon mixing.

A consistent amount of drug (15 mg) was loaded in all formulations to have a final concentration of 0.3 mg/mL of 5-FU.

2.3. Computational Study

The docking procedure for subsequent ligands was performed using AutoDock Vina (docking software) [58] and UCSF Chimera (software to display the docking) [59]. The SMILES strings for the molecules were obtained using SwissADME [60].

2.4. Nuclear Magnetic Resonance (NMR) Spectroscopy

The typical proton NMR spectra of chitosan and chitosan–BTC were performed on a Bruker Avance III 400 MHz two-channel FT-NMR spectrometer. An aliquot of lyophilized sample (c.a. 15 mg) was dissolved in DCl/D_2O (20%). After dissolution, the chitosan solution was transferred to an NMR tube (5 mm). The experiments were carried out at 70 °C, a temperature at which solvent peaks does not interfere with the chitosan's peaks. The chemical shifts of the chitosan and BTC protons were recorded using the spectra.

2.5. Fourier Transform INFRARED Spectroscopy (FTIR)

Hydrogel formulations were analyzed using a thermo-scientific Nicolet™ iS5 FTIR spectrophotometer in the range of 4000–400 cm^{-1} with an accumulation of 16 scans. The sample spectrum was collected and processed using OMNIC thermo scientific software.

2.6. Viscosity

The viscosity of the hydrogels was determined at room temperature using a Brookfield dial (DV-II + Pro) viscometer. The formulations were placed in beakers (25 mL), and measurements were taken using an LV spindle 64. The viscosity readings (in cP) were recorded at different shear rates (10, 20, 50, 60, 100 rpm) with the torque range between 10 and 100%. The viscometry parameters were measured at 25 ± 0.05 °C in triplicates.

2.7. Texture Profile Analysis

The texture profile analysis (TPA) of the hydrogels was carried out using a TA.XT.Plus texture analyser (Stable Micro System). This instrument can be used to determine the physical characteristics, cohesiveness, adhesiveness, consistency, and firmness of gels or other semisolid dosage forms [61,62]. The test results can be correlated to the therapeutic outcome of the drug formulation [63]. In addition, this is a simple and reproducible method that provides an easy method to perform the testing of the gels. The probe used for the analysis of the formulations was P/10. The probe was programmed at the selected speed of 2 mm/s, pre-test speed (1.0 mm/s), and post-test speed (10 mm/s) at 5 mm. The instrument was calibrated (including the probe height) before the sample was tested. Approximately, the gel formulation (25 mL) was placed in a standard beaker (50 mL), and care was taken to avoid air bubbles that can interfere with the results. The readings were taken in triplicates.

2.8. Rheological Characterization

Rheological measurements of the chitosan–BTC hydrogels were carried out using a rotational Malvern Kinexus Pro rheometer using rSpace software. The hydrogels were tested after 7 days of preparation using the probe CP4/40 SR4147SS. Measurements were taken at 37 °C for all samples. The samples were dispensed on the surface of the preheated lower plate, and the upper cone was allowed a gap of 0.1424 mm. The excess hydrogel was removed using a spatula. Then, the temperature was allowed to equilibrate to 37 °C. Once stabilized, the flow curves were recorded with varied shear rates at the same temperature. The tests were performed in triplicates.

Oscillation amplitude sweep and frequency sweep tests within the linear viscoelastic region (LVE) were carried out at 37 °C. Strain sweep tests were performed using a strain from 0.1 to 100% to the hydrogel once the gel was allowed to reach equilibrium. These tests measure the storage and loss modulus with respect to shear strain at constant temperature (37 °C) and frequency (1 Hz). In the frequency sweep, the frequency was varied (0.1 to 10%), while the amplitude of the deformation was kept constant. The storage and loss modulus of the hydrogels were plotted against frequency to determine the viscoelastic properties of the gels.

2.9. Scanning Electron Microscopy

The morphology of the hydrogels was analysed using a Zeiss EVO 50 scanning electron microscope (SEM). The hydrogels were freeze-dried and positioned on aluminum specimen stubs on which 12 mm diameter carbon tabs were placed. The gels were coated with gold using a sputter coater (SC7640) and scanned at an extra high-tension voltage of 10–20 kV. The specimen was adjusted to a height of 2 mm with a diameter of 35 mm. The samples were viewed using different magnifications, and the software used for SEM operation was Zeiss Smart SEM.

2.10. Drug Release Study

The release of 5-FU was studied at 37 °C. Briefly, samples (5 mL of hydrogel, concentration of 5-FU = 0.3 mg/mL) were placed in a dialysis bag and kept in phosphate buffered saline (PBS solution) (50 mL) at pH 7.4 [64]. At regular intervals, 2 mL of the release medium was removed from the solution and replaced with fresh medium (2 mL). The drug release study was monitored up to 180 min. The same method was employed for studying the release of 5-FU at pH = 6.5. UV-Vis spectrophotometry at 266 nm was used to determine the amount of 5-FU released. The total amount of 5-FU loaded and the cumulative release were calculated from different concentrations of drug solutions using a standard calibration curve at 266 nm (R^2 = 0.9912).

2.11. Statistical Analysis

Statistical differences in the drug release profile were assessed using an ANOVA test [65], and a value of $p < 0.05$ was considered statistically significant. The results from the experimental data were presented as mean ± standard deviation. The error bars in the graph represent the standard deviation (n = 3). The results attained were analyzed using SPSS® statistical software.

3. Results and Discussion

3.1. Interaction between Chitosan and BTC

Chitosan hydrogels were prepared by mixing different ratios of chitosan and BTC. Following a visual assessment, no differences in the appearance of the samples (M1–M3) were observed; a picture of M1 is reported in Figure 3 for illustrative purposes. The reactive amino groups on the chitosan can be oriented in the acetic acid solution and form hydrophilic active sites [66]. Then, BTC was dissolved in ethanol and used as cross-linking reagent to form the hydrogel. The interactions between carboxylic acids and chitosan were previously reported in the literature [67]. ^{1}H NMR analysis of chitosan–BTC was carried out using DCl/D$_2$O [68]. The neutralization reaction between chitosan and BTC can be seen in Figure 4.

The DDA was calculated using integrals of the proton peaks of the deacetylated monomer (H-D, 3.10 ppm) and protons of the acetyl group (H-A$_c$, 1.98 ppm) as proposed by Shigemasa et al. [69]. The DDA of chitosan was calculated as 68.84%. The solvent peak resonated at 4.80 ppm. The small peaks at 1.9 ppm, in both spectra of structures i and iv of Figure 4, originated from the acetyl protons of chitosan. The area between 3 and 4 ppm represents the proton peaks of the deacetylated monomers [70,71]. Furthermore, the singlet at 8.52 ppm confirms the aromatic signals from BTC that do not belong to the structure of chitosan.

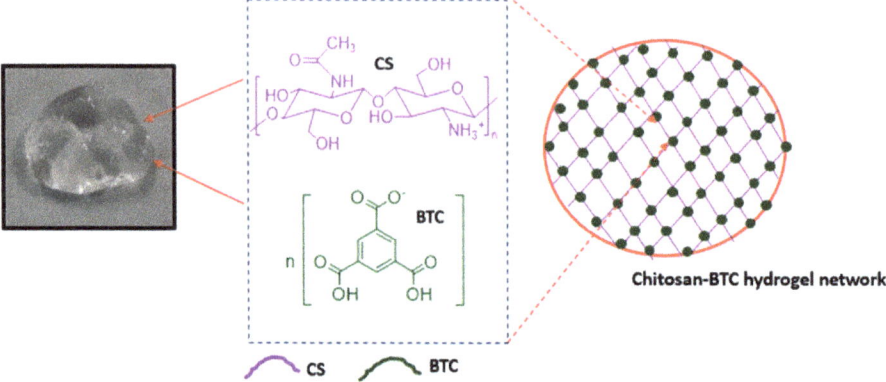

Figure 3. Chitosan–BTC hydrogel (M1).

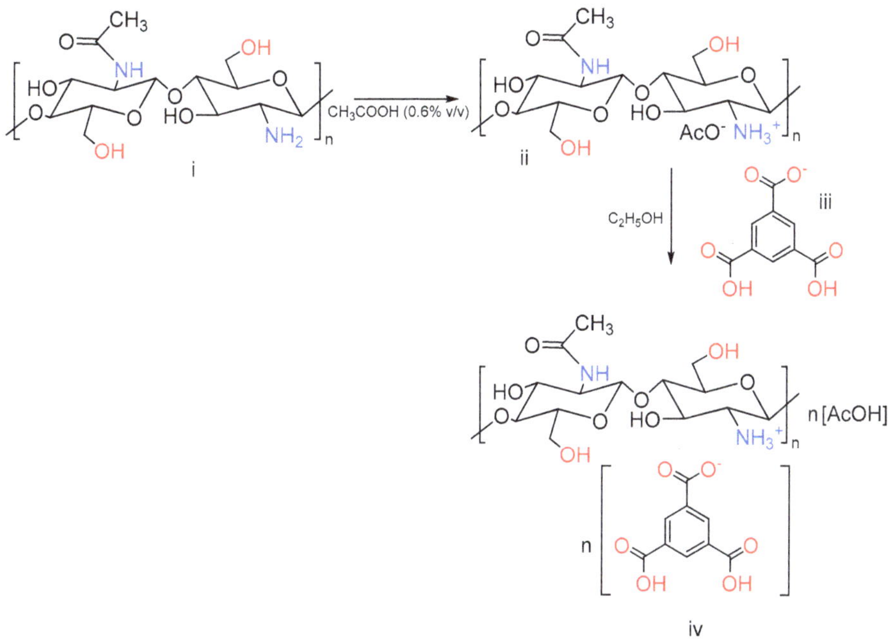

Figure 4. Schematic representation of the cross-linking effect of BTC in the formation of chitosan hydrogels: (**i**) chitosan; (**ii**) protonated chitosan; (**iii**) BTC; and (**iv**) chitosan glucosamine carboxylate salt.

3.2. Nuclear Magnetic Resonance (NMR) Spectroscopy

In relation to the chemical structures presented in Figure 4, NMR characterization was conducted, and results are as follows:

Chitosan (i): ^{1}H NMR (400 MHz, D$_2$O) δ 4.71 ppm (s, 24H), 3.75 ppm (d, *J* = 66.9 Hz, 5H), 3.10 ppm (s, 1H), 1.98 ppm (s, 1H).

BTC (iii): ^{1}H NMR (400 MHz, DMSO) δ 13.52 ppm (3H, s), 8.63 ppm (3H, s).

Chitosan glucosamine carboxylate salt (iv): ^{1}H NMR (400 MHz, D$_2$O) δ 8.52 ppm (s, 5H), 3.65 ppm (d, *J* = 80.0 Hz, 28H), 3.02 ppm (s, 6H), 1.90 ppm (s, 4H).

3.3. Computational Study

To further elucidate the interaction between the polymer (chitosan) and the cross-linked (BTC), a computational study was conducted. Docking is a computational procedure that helps in predicting the binding of one molecule to the pocket of another molecule [72]. This virtual-aided drug design can verify the library of compounds and elucidate the results using a scoring function. This technique is used in the identification of molecular properties using 3D structures [73]. The SMILES string for the chitosan and BTC were obtained using SwissADME software. Below is the SMILES string for the chitosan COC(=O)NC7C(O)C(OC6OC(CO)C(OC5OC(CO)C(OC4OC(CO)C(OC3OC(CO)C(OC2OC(CO)C(OC1OC(CO)C(O)C(O)C1N)C(O)C2N)C(O)C3N)C(O)C4N)C(O)C5N)C(O)C6N)C(CO)OC7OC8C(O)C(N)C(OC8CO)OC9C(O)C(N)C(O)OC9CO. The SMILES string for the BTC is OHC(=O) C1=CC(=CC(=C1) C(OH)=O) C(OH)=O. A table of docking scores appears in a small window, with the tightest binding docking pose for the ligand at the top. The docking poses between chitosan (brown) and BTC (green) can be seen in Figure 5.

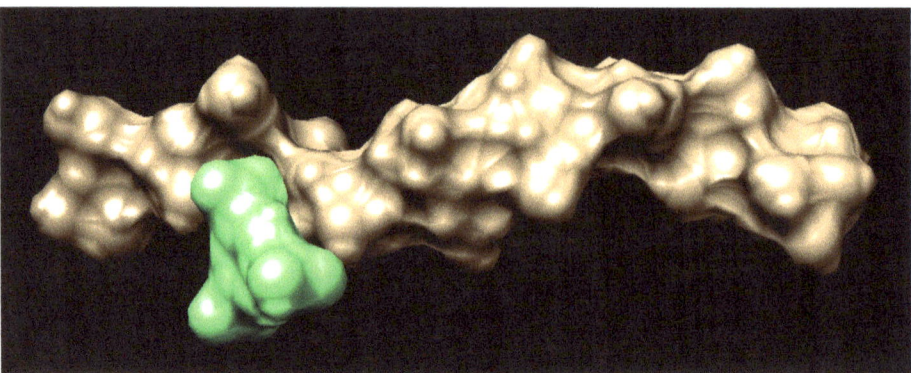

Figure 5. Docking pose (brown, chitosan; green, BTC docked).

REMARK VINA RESULT: −3.3 0.267 4.922

In the above-represented docking studies (Figure 6), the amine groups of the chitosan interacted with BTC by forming hydrogen bonds. The top ten binding poses from the docking video are remarkably similar in binding energy, i.e., several molecules of carboxylic acid groups were binding to the chitosan at the same time. Hence, all the interactions seem possible from the docking. Many of these interactions can separate the solvent (water) post-gelling. The docking suggests the intermolecular hydrogen bonding between the chitosan and carboxylic acid groups. In addition, there is a possibility of hydrogen bond formation between the carboxylic groups of BTC. The predicted binding energy for each conformation will be given as a docking score in kcal/mole. The two variables in the table are root mean square deviation (RMSD) l.b. (lower bound) and u.b. (upper bound). The docking scores predict the binding affinities of the two molecules once they are docked. The lower the RMSD score, the higher the precision of docking. A negative docking score corresponds to strong binding, and a less negative corresponds to weak binding of the polymer with the docking molecule. From the VINA result, 3.3 kcal/mole is the best binding score with lower bound limit of 0.267 Å and upper bound limit of 4.922 Å. The results also indicate that hydrogen bonding contributes significantly to the interactions between the polymer and the cross-linker.

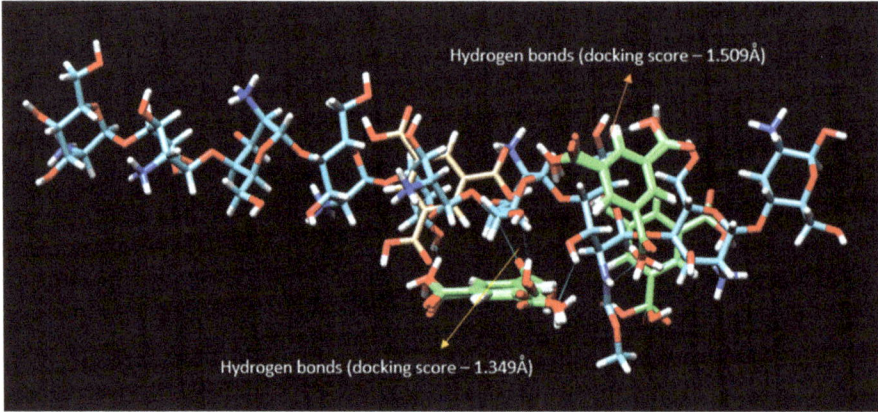

Figure 6. Chimera model. The binding energy of two different torsions (one having a score of −3.4 and another −3.3) are presented in this picture. The two green portions show possible binding of the polymer with BTC.

3.4. Fourier nTransform Infrared Spectroscopy (FTIR)

The FTIR spectrum of not cross-linked and of cross-linked hydrogels can be seen in Figure 7. The spectrum shows a band of 2884 cm^{-1} due to O-H and N-H bending (both overlapping in the same region). The band at 2556 cm^{-1} corresponds to the bending of the OH group of the carboxylic acid group (BTC), which cannot be seen in the uncross-linked chitosan hydrogel. In addition, weak C-H bending of the aromatic ring of BTC can be seen in the cross-linked gels. The bands at 1357 cm^{-1} and 1272 cm^{-1} are due to O-H and C-N bending vibrations. The band at 1429 cm^{-1} can be seen in both cross-linked and uncross-linked gels. The strong absorption band at 1549 cm^{-1} corresponds to amide bonds of chitosan. Another band at 1626 cm^{-1} can be due to amine N-H symmetrical vibration [74]. The hydrogels of concentrations 1–10 mM show greater absorption when compared to other concentrations. The carbonyl stretches (C=O) in less concentrated hydrogels showed more prominent peaks when compared to those having higher concentrations at 1706 cm^{-1} and further confirms the presence of BTC in the structure. The strong bending at 682, 741, and 899 cm^{-1} is attributed to aromatic C-H bending, which became less intense at increased concentrations. The C-O-C glycosidic linkage from the chitosan can be seen at 1065 cm^{-1}. The interaction between chitosan and BTC can also be proven from the presence of C-O-C bend in the cross-linked signals. These interpretations prove effective cross-linking of chitosan with BTC that takes place at the amino group of chitosan.

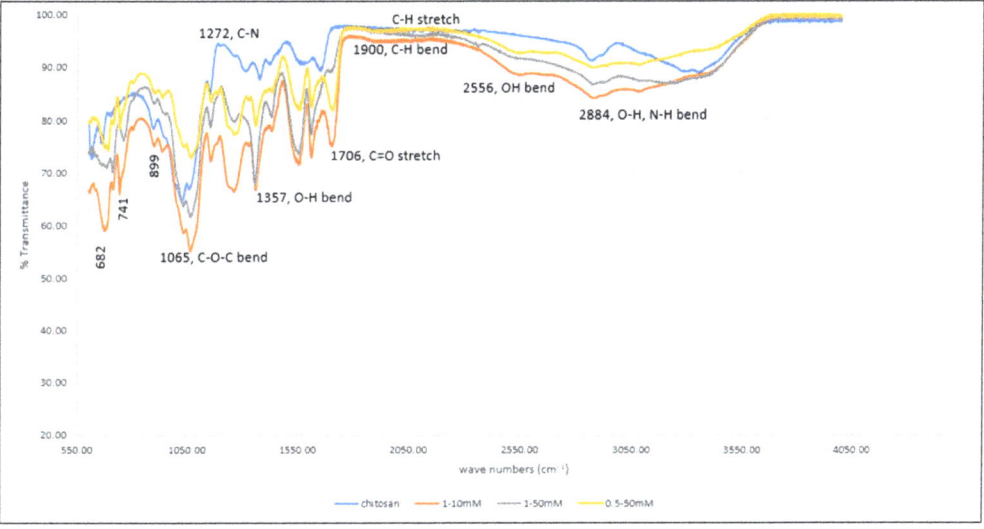

Figure 7. FTIR spectrum of uncross-linked and cross-linked chitosan hydrogel (in different concentrations).

3.5. Viscosity

The effect of the cross-linker on the polymer concentrations are listed in Table 1.

The values for the torque were recorded between 10 and 100%, and those for the viscosity of the hydrogels were recorded at different shear rates (rpm). An increase in shear rate makes the fluid layers slide over one another at high speed and influences the viscosity of the material. The viscosity of all the formulations decreased with an increase in shear rate which confirms the pseudoplastic behavior of the fluids. Pseudoplasticity is a characteristic feature of shear-thinning fluids and is time-independent. Shear thinning behavior of hydrogel systems are great for biomedical applications. The non-Newtonian behavior is related to the structural reformation of molecules due to flow. High shear rates can cause the breakdown of fluid structures leading to reduced viscosity. This property influences the performance of the hydrogel during drug delivery via injection [75]. In addition, the viscosity of sample M1 is higher than other concentrations. The high viscosity of formulations often affects the injectability and syringeability performance while injecting the hydrogel [76]. Presumably, the viscosity data shows greater and more efficient cross-linking at lower BTC concentrations as opposed to high concentrations.

Table 1. Viscosities of hydrogels with different concentrations (M1, M2, and M3).

Samples	Viscosity 10 rpm		Viscosity 20 rpm		Viscosity 50 rpm		Viscosity 60 rpm		Viscosity 100 rpm	
	Torque (%)	cP	Torque (%)	cP	Torque (%)	cP	Torque (%)	cP	Torque (%)	cP
M1	11.4	135.6	13.5	81	14.7	43.5	17.5	21	21.3	12.7
M2	11.1	66.6	12.8	38	14	16.6	15.6	15.6	17	10.2
M3	10.2	57	10.5	32.4	13.3	16	14	14	17.4	10.4

3.6. Texture Analysis

Table 2 reports the results of texture analysis of the hydrogels at three different concentrations (M1, M2, and M3). The instrument can measure the forward and backward extrusions and present the recorded forces (A and B) in response to the contraction and retraction of the probe. Initially, the instrument was calibrated for force and height measurement. The probe was programmed as per the optimized test conditions, and measurements were taken.

Table 2. Texture properties of the hydrogel formulations under the optimized test conditions.

Sample	Force A1 (g) (Max. Compressing Force, Hardness)	Area A1 (g*sec) Cohesiveness	Force B1 (g) Min. Retracting Force	Area B1 (g*sec) Adhesiveness
M1	7.201	6.717	1.200	1.466
M2	8.120	16.348	1.820	3.321
M3	6.810	6.073	1.000	2.142

During the test, the probe traveled at a speed of 2 mm/s downwards into the gel and was then withdrawn. Gel parameters, including hardness, cohesiveness, and adhesiveness, were evaluated using a standard force-time plot (as seen in Figure S7). The readings were taken in triplicates. The variables from the table show retracting, compressing, cohesiveness, and adhesiveness, which cumulatively determine the texture of the material. Area A1 shows the cohesiveness of the gel, while area B1 shows the adhesiveness of the hydrogel to the probe [61]. Cohesiveness is a feature where particles stick to each other and influence the flow properties. An increase in cohesiveness causes a decrease in the flow due to agglomeration of the gel molecules [77]. In Table 2, M2 shows high cohesiveness, hence retarding the flow of the hydrogels. The adhesiveness of the gels was represented by the retracting force B1. This is the work required to overcome the forces between the surface of the gel and the probe [78]. The cohesiveness and adhesiveness of different concentrations of gels were plotted against the area as shown in Figure 8. Though the difference in adhesiveness is not significant, a slight increase is observed for M2, which might be attributed to the higher ability of the gel to chemically interact with the probe. The hardness of the gels was measured from the maximum compressing force of the gel formulations. It gives the force required to deform the gels. The hydrogel's hardness values can be verified based on the area of the application. The hydrogel concentrations with low compressing force showed less cohesiveness.

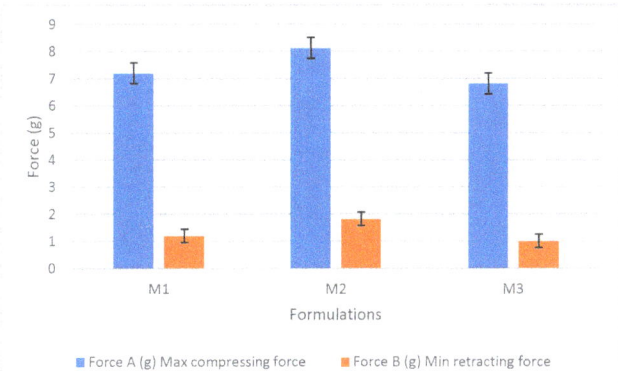

Figure 8. The compressing and retracting forces of the three hydrogel formulations (M1, M2, and M3). Results represent mean values ± SD. n = 3.

3.7. Oscillation Amplitude Strain Sweep Experiments

The oscillation amplitude strain tests provide information regarding the effect of BTC and polymer concentration on the sample structures. The influence of stress amplitude on the hydrogels can be seen in Figure 9. The tests were conducted under constant stress and strain and help to determine the hydrogels' viscoelastic properties. Strain sweep tests confirmed the gel-like behavior since the data of all the samples showed the elastic (storage) modulus G′ higher than the loss (viscous) modulus G″ (as shown in the figures). In addition, the flow properties of the gels can be determined from the complex modulus (G*) and the phase angle (δ). The complex modulus determines the stiffness of the material.

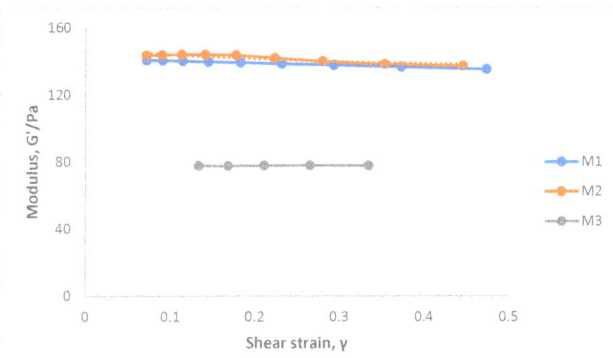

Figure 9. Amplitude strain sweep for hydrogels prepared with different concentrations of chitosan–BTC. (See Supplementary Tables S2–S4).

The LVE region of the hydrogels can be seen in Figures S8–S10. This region implies a stress range over which G′ is independent of applied shear stress. For evaluating the mechanical strength of the hydrogels, the elastic modulus from the LVE region was compared with the strain values. Hydrogels with less amount of chitosan (M3) have the elastic modulus value of 77.15 Pa when compared to high G′ 135.7 Pa (M2) and medium G′ of 134.7 Pa (M1). The high level of polymer in the cross-linked network has given a stronger hydrogel when compared to low levels of chitosan and BTC. From the above high and medium G′ values, we can see little difference due to the comparable concentrations of the polymer in both samples (M1 and M2). In case of M2, the G′ values decreased abruptly at a shear strain of 0.5%. This evidence suggests cross-linking of these hydrogels resulted in the following observations: (1) an increase of elastic modulus of G′ that refers to the material deformation, i.e., of the intermolecular networks in the gel structure; and (2) an increase in shear stress is observed in M2 in the linear viscoelastic region.

The rheological data from the oscillation tests provided the calculated shear stress and strain as seen in Table 3. In theory, the shear modulus is defined as the ratio of shear stress to the shear strain. When the shear modulus of the material is higher than the other, then the material is known to have high rigidity. The shear modulus of the hydrogels with M2 was found to be higher than other samples. Therefore, the material is found to have high rigidity.

Table 3. The calculated shear stress and strain results from within the LVE range.

Sample	Shear Stress (Pa)	Shear Strain	Shear Modulus
M1	6.4297×10^{-2}	4.7421×10^{-2}	1.35587609
M2	2.033×10^{-1}	1.4887×10^{-1}	1.36562101
M3	2.5966×10^{-2}	3.344×10^{-2}	$7.76495215 \times 10^{-1}$

3.8. Frequency Strain Sweep Experiments

Frequency strain sweep experiments for the hydrogels were performed within the LVE region to determine the frequency dependence. The distribution of frequencies in Tables S5–S7 clearly shows the dispersion and association of particles in the hydrogel structure. The stability of the cross-linked networks can be studied using these tests. Figure 10 represents the graph plotted between the elastic modulus and the frequency. The angular frequency of the test material was set as ranging between 0.1 and 10 rad/s. Both G′ and G″ were frequency-dependent, which can be attributed to the viscoelastic properties of the hydrogel network. At a high frequency of 10 Hz, the shear viscosity of M1 was 2.9 Pa s, which increased with increasing concentrations of both polymer and cross-linker.

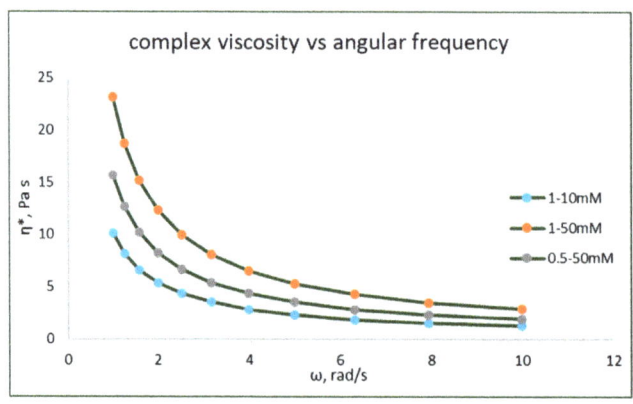

Figure 10. Frequency sweep (ω) and complex viscosity (η) of hydrogels at different concentrations. (See Supplementary Tables S5–S7).

Interestingly, with an increase in complex viscosity, the angular frequency of the hydrogels decreased. This confirms that the hydrogels show a shear-thinning behavior, thus proving that the hydrogels prepared were pseudoplastic fluids. In addition, the elastic modulus G′ of the hydrogels was higher than the loss modulus G″ and thus confirms the behavior.

3.9. Scanning Electron Microscopy

The scanning electron microscopy (SEM) images of chitosan–BTC gels demonstrated the presence of interconnected pores between the gel networks as seen in Figure 11. The lyophilized gels have highly connected pores, which can allow the passage of nutrients and drugs to the site of action. The gels with concentrations M1, M2, and M3 have pore size ranging from 2.8–3.3 µm, 14–16 µm, and 5–18 µm, respectively. Here, it can be noted that hydrogels with low concentrations of BTC present smaller pore sizes when compared to higher concentrations. The higher the porosity, the higher the rate of drug release [79]. M1 with low BTC depicts long streaks of branched out polymer network, while M2 and M3 with relatively high BTC appear to have formed more tortuous pores. So, from the previous observations, the hydrogels with higher BTC concentrations were found suitable for drug delivery applications.

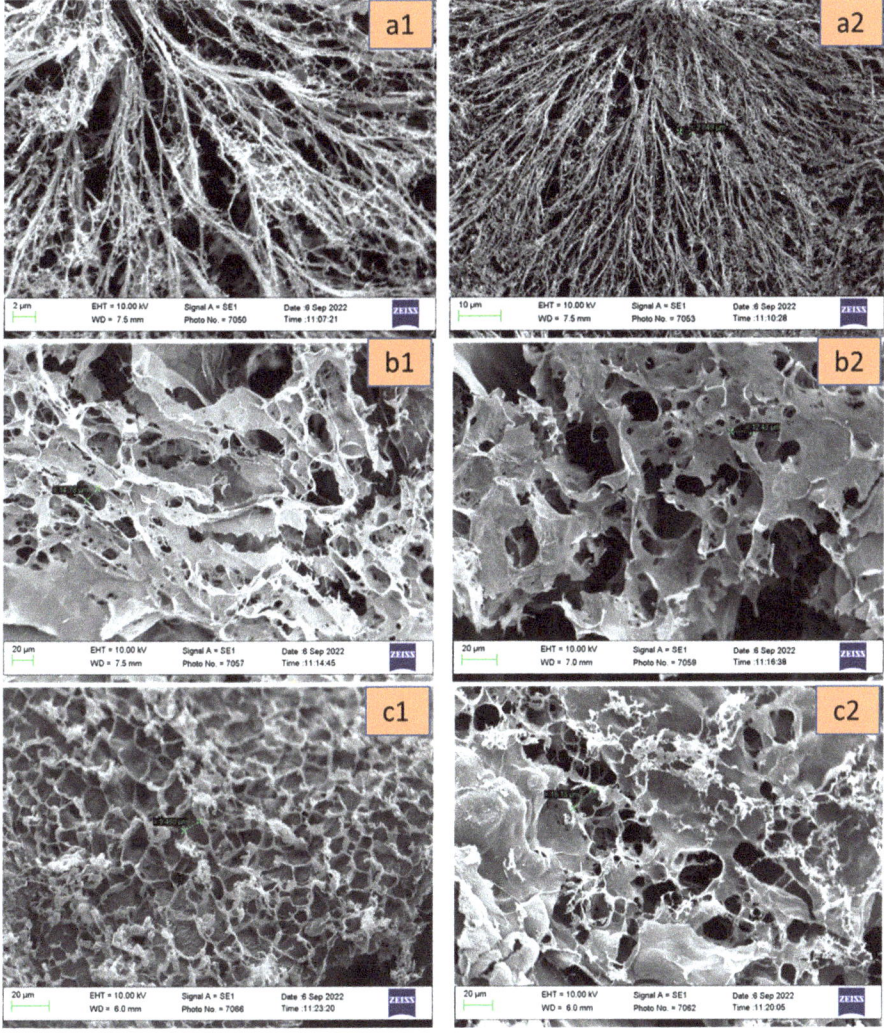

Figure 11. SEM structures of freeze-dried chitosan hydrogels M1 (**a1,a2**), M2 (**b1,b2**), and M3 (**c1,c2**) at different magnifications.

3.10. Drug Release Studies

Figure 12 shows the in vitro release behavior of the three samples (namely: M1, M2, and M3) of BTC-cross-linked chitosan hydrogels loaded with 5-FU. The rate of drug release from the hydrogels was noted to be more pronounced in the first 20 min, followed by a more gradual release, amounting to an overall release between 35% and 50% within the study period of 180 min [39,54]. The amino groups of chitosan are not protonated at pH 7.4, resulting in the formation of physical networks in the hydrogels. These networks are responsible for the controlled release of the drug in PBS medium as reported in the literature [80]. In addition, the degree of cross-linking of the polymer influenced the release capacity of the hydrogel matrix. In general, high levels of cross-linker improve drug loading effectiveness, while slowing the rate at which entrapped drugs are released. Interestingly, the concentrations of chitosan and BTC influenced the pattern of 5-FU release from the hydrogel matrix. The drug release profiles of chitosan–BTC at 37 °C can be seen in Figure 12. A higher concentration of BTC, which in turn results in a greater extent of cross-linking in M2, caused a retarded drug release in the first 60 min. On the other hand, when chitosan concentration was reduced from 1% to 0.5% (i.e., comparing M2 with M3), a 'burst-effect' in drug release was noted within the first 20 min. A lower amount of chitosan in the M3 hydrogel, yielding less cross-linking with BTC, may have enabled more pronounced drug release. According to ANOVA, statistically significant differences in drug release were observed between hydrogels with different chitosan/BTC ratios. In the case of M1 and M2, the t-test ($p = 0.21$) indicates no significant difference in time required for drug release. However, there is a significant difference in time for drug release between M2 and M3 ($p = 0.007$). Based on these studies, the prepared hydrogel can be used for drug delivery systems and other biomedical applications.

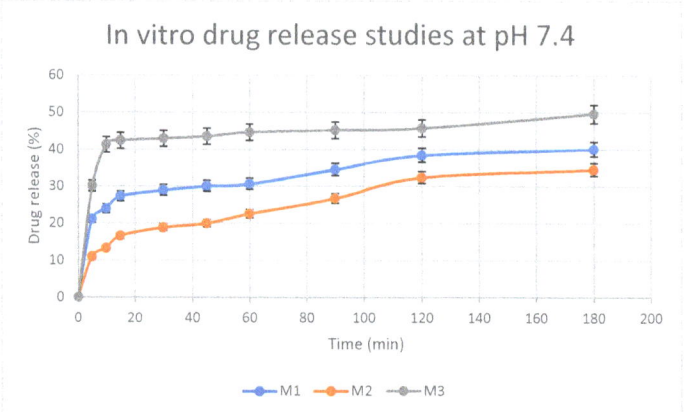

Figure 12. Release profile of 5-FU incorporated in chitosan–BTC hydrogels (M1, M2, and M3) investigated in phosphate-buffered saline (PBS) medium, pH 7.4. Results represent mean values ± SD; n = 3 (For M1 and M2: $p > 0.05$; M1 and M3: $p < 0.05$).

At pH 6.5, rapid release of the drug occurs from 0 to 5 min, and then the drug is released gradually from 5 to 180 min (as seen in Figure 13). In addition, there is not a significant difference in time for drug release between the gel concentrations (M1, M2, and M3) at this pH.

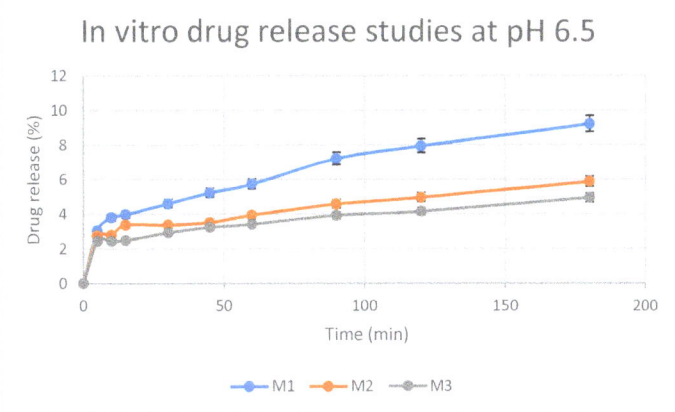

Figure 13. Release profile of 5-FU incorporated in chitosan–BTC hydrogels (M1, M2, and M3) investigated in phosphate-buffered saline (PBS) medium, pH 6.5 Results represent mean values ± SD; n = 3 (For M1 and M2: $p < 0.05$; M1 and M3: $p < 0.05$).

When comparing the 2 release profiles at different pH values, it is evident that at pH = 7.4 there is a higher extent of drug (cumulative) release than at pH 6.5. This might suggest that 5-FU is not released via erosion of the hydrogel, (i.e., the polymer is solubilized, and the hydrogel is disassembled); 5-FU is rather released via diffusion which is favoured in non-acidic environments.

4. Conclusions

The current research aimed to develop BTC-cross-linked chitosan hydrogels containing 5-FU for cancer therapy. Using different ratios of BTC/chitosan, flow curves of the hydrogels revealed shear thinning behavior of the resulting hydrogels. With an increase in the shear rate, there is a decline in the apparent viscosity, which is a characteristic feature of shear-thinning fluids. Viscoelastic investigations of the hydrogels revealed the elastic (G') modulus values were higher than the viscous (G'') values, hence confirming the elastic behavior of all prepared hydrogels. Further oscillatory tests (strain and frequency sweep) confirmed the stable hydrogels' behavior since all exhibited a plateau in the range of 0.1–10 Hz. Under physiological conditions, the gel behaviour can be tuned by changing the cross-linker concentrations. The low G' (77.15 Pa) and G'' (8.711 Pa) values of M2 indicate poor mechanical strength when compared to other samples. Spectroscopic and structural investigations of the formulated hydrogels (NMR, FTIR, and SEM) confirmed the presence of glycosidic bonds signals in all the spectra. The cross-sectional freeze-dried images exhibited porous, compact, and homogenous distribution of hydrogel networks. This provides a scope for encapsulating drugs in the hydrogel matrix. The hydrogels exhibited slow drug release in PBS (<50%) that provides a scope for sustained drug release. Additionally, the release at slightly acidic pH showed a slower and more prolonged release of the drug, which might be explained in light of the porous structure of the hydrogel matrix, coupled with the ionization of chitosan in acidic pH environments. The drug release also appeared to have a direct correlation with the extent of polymer cross-linking, thus facilitating a sustained drug delivery. This is a desired characteristic of hydrogels which tends to enhance the safety and efficacy of drug therapy.

Overall, the data from this study on the properties of hydrogels and their behavior in vitro demonstrates a great potential for enhanced biological performance and thus warrant further investigations.

Supplementary Materials: The following supporting information can be downloaded at: https://www.mdpi.com/article/10.3390/pharmaceutics15041084/s1, Figure S1: ^{1}H NMR spectra of chitosan (i). Figure S2. 1H NMR spectra of BTC (iii). Figure S3. 1H NMR spectra of chitosan glucosamine carboxylate salt (iv). Figure S4. IR spectra of M1 hydrogel. Figure S5. IR of M2 hydrogel. Figure S6. IR spectra of M3 hydrogel. Figure S7. Force vs. time plot of chitosan–BTC hydrogels in three different concentrations: M1, M2, and M3. Figure S8. Oscillation dynamics of elastic and viscous moduli of chitosan cross-linked with BTC (M1 hydrogel). Figure S9. Oscillation dynamics of elastic and viscous moduli of chitosan cross-linked with BTC (M2 hydrogel). Figure S10. Oscillation dynamics of elastic and viscous moduli of chitosan cross-linked with BTC (M3 hydrogel). Table S1. Hydrogels compositions. Table S2. Amplitude strain sweep for hydrogels with chitosan–BTC concentration 1–10 Mm (sup-plementary material). Table S3. Amplitude strain sweep for hydrogels with chitosan–BTC concentration 1–50 mM (sup-plementary material). Table S4. Amplitude strain sweep for hydrogels with chitosan–BTC concentration 0.5–50 Mm (supplementary material). Table S5. Frequency sweep for hydrogels with chitosan–BTC concentration 1–10 mM (supple-mentary material). Table S6. Frequency strain sweep for hydrogels with chitosan–BTC concentration 1–50 mM (supplementary material). Table S7. Frequency strain sweep for hydrogels with chitosan–BTC concentration 0.5–50 mM (supple-mentary material). Table S8. Frequency strain sweep for hydrogels with chitosan–BTC concentration 0.5–50 mM (supplementary material).

Author Contributions: Conceptualization, G.C. and F.B.; methodology, N.Y. and S.E..; software, S.E.; validation, F.B., N.Y. and S.E.; formal analysis, S.E.; investigation, S.E.; resources, G.C.; data curation, A.V.; writing—original draft preparation, S.E.; writing, S.E.; review and editing, G.C. and A.V.; visualization, G.C.; supervision, G.C.; project administration, S.E. All authors have read and agreed to the published version of the manuscript.

Funding: This research received no external funding.

Institutional Review Board Statement: Not applicable.

Informed Consent Statement: Data supporting reported results can be found in the manuscript.

Data Availability Statement: Data are available upon request.

Conflicts of Interest: The authors declare no conflict of interest.

References

1. Ahmed, E.M. Hydrogel: Preparation, characterization, and applications: A review. *J. Adv. Res.* **2015**, *6*, 105–121. [CrossRef] [PubMed]
2. Sharpe, A.L.; Daily, A.M.; Horava, S.D.; A Peppas, N. Therapeutic applications of hydrogels in oral drug delivery. *Expert Opin. Drug Deliv.* **2014**, *11*, 901–915. [CrossRef] [PubMed]
3. Narayanaswamy, R.; Torchilin, V.P. Hydrogels and their applications in targeted drug delivery. *Molecules* **2019**, *24*, 603. [CrossRef] [PubMed]
4. Ishihara, M.; Obara, K.; Nakamura, S.; Fujita, M.; Masuoka, K.; Kanatani, Y.; Takase, B.; Hattori, H.; Morimoto, Y.; Ishihara, M.; et al. Chitosan hydrogel as a drug delivery carrier to control angiogenesis. *J. Artif. Organs* **2006**, *9*, 8–16. [CrossRef] [PubMed]
5. Moeinzadeh, S.; Park, Y.; Lin, S.; Yang, Y.P. In-situ stable injectable collagen-based hydrogels for cell and growth factor delivery. *Materialia* **2020**, *15*, 100954. [CrossRef]
6. Yu, Z.; Li, H.; Xia, P.; Kong, W.; Chang, Y.; Fu, C.; Wang, K.; Yang, X.; Qi, Z. Application of fibrin-based hydrogels for nerve protection and regeneration after spinal cord injury. *J. Biol. Eng.* **2020**, *14*, 22. [CrossRef]
7. Zainal, S.H.; Mohd, N.H.; Suhaili, N.; Anuar, F.H.; Lazim, A.M.; Othaman, R. Preparation of cellulose-based hydrogel: A review. *J. Mater. Res. Technol.* **2021**, *10*, 935–952. [CrossRef]
8. Xu, X.; Jha, A.K.; Harrington, D.A.; Farach-Carson, M.C.; Jia, X. Hyaluronic acid-based hydrogels: From a natural polysaccharide to complex networks. *Soft Matter* **2012**, *8*, 3280–3294. [CrossRef]
9. Oh, Y.; Cha, J.; Kang, S.-G.; Kim, P. A polyethylene glycol-based hydrogel as macroporous scaffold for tumorsphere formation of glioblastoma multiforme. *J. Ind. Eng. Chem.* **2016**, *39*, 10–15. [CrossRef]
10. Jensen, B.E.B.; Dávila, I.; Zelikin, A.N. Poly(vinyl alcohol) physical hydrogels: Matrix-mediated drug delivery using spontaneously eroding substrate. *J. Phys. Chem. B* **2016**, *120*, 5916–5926. [CrossRef]
11. Sharifzadeh, G.; Hezaveh, H.; Muhamad, I.I.; Hashim, S.; Khairuddin, N. Montmorillonite-based polyacrylamide hydrogel rings for controlled vaginal drug delivery. *Mater. Sci. Eng. C* **2019**, *110*, 110609. [CrossRef] [PubMed]
12. Qiu, Y.; Park, K. Environment-Sensitive Hydrogels for Drug Delivery. 2001. Available online: www.elsevier.com/locate/drugdeliv (accessed on 1 February 2020).

13. Berkovitch, Y.; Seliktar, D. Semi-synthetic hydrogel composition and stiffness regulate neuronal morphogenesis. *Int. J. Pharm.* **2017**, *523*, 545–555. [CrossRef] [PubMed]
14. Rossi, B.; Venuti, V.; D'Amico, F.; Gessini, A.; Mele, A.; Punta, C.; Melone, L.; Crupi, V.; Majolino, D.; Masciovecchio, C. Guest-matrix interactions affect the solvation of cyclodextrin-based polymeric hydrogels: A UV Raman scattering study. *Soft Matter* **2016**, *12*, 8861–8868. [CrossRef]
15. Concheiro, A.; Alvarez-Lorenzo, C. Chemically cross-linked and grafted cyclodextrin hydrogels: From nanostructures to drug-eluting medical devices. *Adv. Drug Deliv. Rev.* **2013**, *65*, 1188–1203. [CrossRef] [PubMed]
16. Naveed, M.; Phil, L.; Sohail, M.; Hasnat, M.; Baig, M.M.F.A.; Ihsan, A.U.; Shumzaid, M.; Kakar, M.U.; Khan, T.M.; Akabar, M.D.; et al. Chitosan oligosaccharide (COS): An overview. *Int. J. Biol. Macromol.* **2019**, *129*, 827–843. [CrossRef]
17. Kim, J.H.; Lee, J.-H.; Kim, K.-S.; Na, K.; Song, S.-C.; Lee, J.; Kuh, H.-J. Intratumoral delivery of paclitaxel using a thermosensitive hydrogel in human tumor xenografts. *Arch. Pharmacal Res.* **2013**, *36*, 94–101. [CrossRef]
18. Pesoa, J.I.; Rico, M.J.; Rozados, V.R.; Scharovsky, O.G.; Luna, J.A.; Mengatto, L.N. Paclitaxel delivery system based on poly(lactide-co-glycolide) microparticles and chitosan thermosensitive gel for mammary adenicarcinoma treatment. *J. Pharm. Pharmacol.* **2018**, *70*, 1494–1502. [CrossRef] [PubMed]
19. Zhang, N.; Xu, X.; Zhang, X.; Qu, D.; Xue, L.; Mo, R.; Zhang, C. Nanocomposite hydrogel incorporating gold nanorods and paclitaxel-loaded chitosan micelles for combination photothermal chemotherpay. *Int. J. Pharm.* **2016**, *497*, 210–221. [CrossRef]
20. Jiang, Y.; Meng, X.; Wu, Z.; Qi, X. Modified chitosan thermosensitive hydrogel enables sustained and efficient anti-tumor therapy via intratumoral injection. *Carbohydr. Polym.* **2016**, *144*, 245–253. [CrossRef]
21. Ishihara, M.; Fujita, M.; Obara, K.; Hattori, H.; Nakamura, S.; Nambu, M.; Kiyosawa, T.; Kanatani, Y.; Takase, B.; Kikuchi, M.; et al. Controlled releases of FGF-2 and Paclitaxel from Chitosan Hydrogels and their Subsequent Effects on Wound Repair, Angiogenesis and Tumor Growth. *Curr. Drug Deliv.* **2006**, *3*, 351–358. [CrossRef]
22. Liu, J.; Zhang, L.; Yang, Z.; Zhao, X. Controlled release of paclitaxel from a self-assembling peptide hydrogel formed insitu and antitumor study in vitro. *Int. J. Nanomed.* **2011**, *6*, 2143–2153. [CrossRef]
23. Croisier, F.; Jérôme, C. Chitosan-based biomaterials for tissue engineering. *Eur. Polym. J.* **2013**, *49*, 780–792. [CrossRef]
24. Bandara, S.; Du, H.; Carson, L.; Bradford, D.; Kommalapati, R. Agricultural and biomedical applications of chitosan-based nanomaterials. *Nanomaterials* **2020**, *10*, 1903. [CrossRef] [PubMed]
25. Elieh-Ali-Komi, D.; Hamblin, M.R.; Daniel, E.-A.-K. Chitin and Chitosan: Production and Application of Versatile Biomedical Nanomaterials. *Int. J. Adv. Res.* **2016**, *4*, 411–427.
26. Hamedi, H.; Moradi, S.; Hudson, S.M.; Tonelli, A.E. Chitosan based hydrogels and their applications for drug delivery in wound dressings: A review. *Carbohydr. Polym.* **2018**, *199*, 445–460. [CrossRef] [PubMed]
27. Safer, A.-M.; Leporatti, S. Chitosan Nanoparticles for Antiviral Drug Delivery: A Novel Route for COVID-19 Treatment. *Int. J. Nanomed.* **2021**, *16*, 8141–8158. [CrossRef] [PubMed]
28. Cao, Y.; Tan, Y.F.; Wong, Y.S.; Liew, M.W.J.; Venkatraman, S. Recent advances in chitosan-based carriers for gene delivery. *Mar. Drugs* **2019**, *17*, 381. [CrossRef] [PubMed]
29. Sandri, S.R.G.; Bonferoni, M.; Ferrari, F.; Mori, M.; Caramella, C. The role of chitosan as a mucoadhesive agent in mucosal drug delivery. *J. Drug Deliv. Sci. Technol.* **2012**, *22*, 275–284. [CrossRef]
30. Aranaz, I.; Alcántara, A.R.; Civera, M.C.; Arias, C.; Elorza, B.; Caballero, A.H.; Acosta, N. Chitosan: An overview of its properties and applications. *Polymers* **2021**, *13*, 3256. [CrossRef]
31. Snoreen, S.; Pervaiz, F.; Ashames, A.; Buabeid, M.; Fahelelbom, K.; Shoukat, H.; Maqbool, I.; Murtaza, G. Optimization of novel naproxen-loaded chitosan/carrageenan nanocarrier-based gel for topical delivery: Ex vivo, histopathological, and in vivo evaluation. *Pharmaceuticals* **2021**, *14*, 557. [CrossRef]
32. Beppu, M.; Vieira, R.; Aimoli, C.; Santana, C. Crosslinking of chitosan membranes using glutaraldehyde: Effect on ion permeability and water absorption. *J. Membr. Sci.* **2007**, *301*, 126–130. [CrossRef]
33. Monteiro, O.A., Jr.; Airoldi, C. Some studies of crosslinking chitosan-glutaraldehyde interaction in a homogeneous system. *Int. J. Biol. Macromol.* **1999**, *26*, 119–128. [CrossRef] [PubMed]
34. Kildeeva, N.R.; Perminov, P.A.; Vladimirov, L.V.; Novikov, V.V.; Mikhailov, S.N. About mechanism of chitosan cross-linking with glutaraldehyde. *Russ. J. Bioorganic Chem.* **2009**, *35*, 360–369. [CrossRef]
35. Vo, N.T.N.; Huang, L.; Lemos, H.; Mellor, A.L.; Novakovic, K. Genipin-crosslinked chitosan hydrogels: Preliminary evaluation of the in vitro biocompatibility and biodegradation. *J. Appl. Polym. Sci.* **2021**, *138*, 50848. [CrossRef]
36. Muzzarelli, R.A. Genipin-crosslinked chitosan hydrogels as biomedical and pharmaceutical aids. *Carbohydr. Polym.* **2009**, *77*, 1–9. [CrossRef]
37. Jayakumar, R.; Reis, R.L.; Mano, J.F. Phosphorous containing chitosan beads for controlled oral drug delivery. *J. Bioact. Compat. Polym.* **2006**, *21*, 327–340. [CrossRef]
38. Kaur, K.; Paiva, S.S.; Caffrey, D.; Cavanagh, B.L.; Murphy, C.M. Injectable chitosan/collagen hydrogels nano-engineered with functionalized single wall carbon nanotubes for minimally invasive applications in bone. *Mater. Sci. Eng. C* **2021**, *128*, 112340. [CrossRef]
39. Yang, Y.; Chen, G.; Murray, P.; Zhang, H. Porous chitosan by crosslinking with tricarboxylic acid and tuneable release. *SN Appl. Sci.* **2020**, *2*, 1–10. [CrossRef]

40. Buschmann, M.D.; Merzouki, A.; Lavertu, M.; Thibault, M.; Jean, M.; Darras, V. Chitosans for delivery of nucleic acids. *Adv. Drug Deliv. Rev* **2013**, *65*, 1234–1270. [CrossRef]
41. Larrañeta, E.; Stewart, S.; Ervine, M.; Al-Kasasbeh, R.; Donnelly, R.F. Hydrogels for Hydrophobic Drug Delivery. Classification, Synthesis and Applications. *J. Funct. Biomater.* **2018**, *9*, 13. [CrossRef]
42. Vashist, A.; Ahmad, S. Hydrogels: Smart Materials for Drug Delivery. *Orient. J. Chem.* **2013**, *29*, 861–870. [CrossRef]
43. Bhatt, R.; Sreedhar, B.; Padmaja, P. Chitosan supramolecularly cross linked with trimesic acid—Facile synthesis, characterization and evaluation of adsorption potential for chromium(VI). *Int. J. Biol. Macromol.* **2017**, *104*, 1254–1266. [CrossRef]
44. Tang, L.M.; Wang, Y.J. Highly stable supramolecular hydrogels formed from 1,3,5-benzenetricarboxylic acid and hydroxyl pyridines. *Chin. Chem. Lett.* **2009**, *20*, 1259–1262. [CrossRef]
45. Goudoulas, T.B.; Germann, N. Phase transition kinetics and rheology of gelatin-alginate mixtures. *Food Hydrocoll.* **2017**, *66*, 49–60. [CrossRef]
46. Pai, V.; Srinivasarao, M.; Khan, S.A. Evolution of microstructure and rheology in mixed polysaccharide systems. *Macromolecules* **2002**, *35*, 1699–1707. [CrossRef]
47. Richa; Choudhury, A.R. Synthesis and rheological characterization of a novel thermostable quick setting composite hydrogel of gellan and pullulan. *Int. J. Biol. Macromol.* **2018**, *125*, 979–988. [CrossRef] [PubMed]
48. Zuidema, J.M.; Rivet, C.J.; Gilbert, R.J.; Morrison, F.A. A protocol for rheological characterization of hydrogels for tissue engineering strategies. *J. Biomed. Mater. Res. Part B Appl. Biomater.* **2013**, *102*, 1063–1073. [CrossRef]
49. Malvern Panalytical. *Rheological Analysis of Dispersions by Frequency Sweep Testing*; AZoM, 2023. Available online: https://www.azom.com/article.aspx?ArticleID=2884 (accessed on 23 January 2023).
50. Ferry, J.D. *Viscoelastic Properties of Polymers*; John Wiley & Sons: New York, NA, USA, 1980.
51. Matricardi, P.; Dentini, M.; Crescenzi, V. Porphyrin Amphiphiles as Templates for the Nucleation of Calcium Carbonate. 1987. Available online: https://pubs.acs.org/sharingguidelines (accessed on 5 February 2023).
52. Montembault, A.; Viton, C.; Domard, A. Rheometric Study of the Gelation of Chitosan in Aqueous Solution without Cross-Linking Agent. *Biomacromolecules* **2005**, *6*, 653–662. [CrossRef]
53. Laukkanen, O.-V.; Winter, H.H. Strain accumulation in bituminous binders under repeated creep-recovery loading predicted from small-amplitude oscillatory shear (SAOS) experiments. *Mech. Time-Depend. Mater.* **2017**, *22*, 499–518. [CrossRef]
54. Gull, N.; Khan, S.M.; Butt, M.T.Z.; Khalid, S.; Shafiq, M.; Islam, A.; Asim, S.; Hafeez, S.; Khan, R.U. In vitro study of chitosan-based multi-responsive hydrogels as drug release vehicles: A preclinical study. *RSC Adv.* **2019**, *9*, 31078–31091. [CrossRef]
55. Zhang, D.-Y.; Shen, X.-Z.; Wang, J.-Y.; Dong, L.; Zheng, Y.-L.; Wu, L.-L. Preparation of chitosan-polyaspartic acid-5-fluorouracil nanoparticles and its anti-carcinoma effect on tumor growth in nude mice. *World J. Gastroenterol.* **2008**, *14*, 3554–3562. [CrossRef] [PubMed]
56. Hou, Q.; De Bank, P.A.; Shakesheff, K.M. Injectable scaffolds for tissue regeneration. *J. Mater. Chem.* **2004**, *14*, 1915–1923. [CrossRef]
57. Lee, S.-Y.; Tae, G. Formulation and in vitro characterization of an in situ gelable, photo-polymerizable Pluronic hydrogel suitable for injection. *J. Control. Release* **2007**, *119*, 313–319. [CrossRef] [PubMed]
58. Trott, O.; Olson, A.J. AutoDock Vina: Improving the speed and accuracy of docking with a new scoring function, efficient optimization, and multithreading. *J. Comput. Chem.* **2010**, *31*, 455–461. [CrossRef] [PubMed]
59. Pettersen, E.F.; Goddard, T.D.; Huang, C.C.; Couch, G.S.; Greenblatt, D.M.; Meng, E.C.; Ferrin, T.E. UCSF Chimera? A visualization system for exploratory research and analysis. *J. Comput. Chem.* **2004**, *25*, 1605–1612. [CrossRef] [PubMed]
60. Daina, A.; Michielin, O.; Zoete, V. SwissADME: A free web tool to evaluate pharmacokinetics, drug-likeness and medicinal chemistry friendliness of small molecules. *Sci. Rep.* **2017**, *7*, 42717. [CrossRef] [PubMed]
61. Jones, D.S.; Woolfson, A.; Brown, A.F. Textural, viscoelastic and mucoadhesive properties of pharmaceutical gels composed of cellulose polymers. *Int. J. Pharm.* **1997**, *151*, 223–233. [CrossRef]
62. Jones, D.S.; Andrews, G.P.; Gorman, S.P. Characterization of crosslinking effects on the physicochemical and drug diffusional properties of cationic hydrogels designed as bioactive urological biomaterials. *J. Pharm. Pharmacol.* **2005**, *57*, 1251–1259. [CrossRef]
63. Hurler, J.; Engesland, A.; Kermany, B.P.; Škalko-Basnet, N. Improved texture analysis for hydrogel characterization: Gel cohesiveness, adhesiveness, and hardness. *J. Appl. Polym. Sci.* **2011**, *125*, 180–188. [CrossRef]
64. Noreen, S.; Pervaiz, F.; Ijaz, M.; Shoukat, H. Synthesis and characterization of pH-sensitive chemically crosslinked block copolymer [Hyaluronic acid/Poloxamer 407-co-poly (Methacrylic acid)] hydrogels for colon targeting. *Polym. Technol. Mater.* **2022**, *61*, 1071–1087. [CrossRef]
65. Obata, Y.; Nishino, T.; Kushibiki, T.; Tomoshige, R.; Xia, Z.; Miyazaki, M.; Abe, K.; Koji, T.; Tabata, Y.; Kohno, S. HSP47 siRNA conjugated with cationized gelatin microspheres suppresses peritoneal fibrosis in mice. *Acta Biomater.* **2012**, *8*, 2688–2696. [CrossRef]
66. Shamov, M.; Bratskaya, S.; Avramenko, V. Interaction of Carboxylic Acids with Chitosan: Effect of pK and Hydrocarbon Chain Length. *J. Colloid Interface Sci.* **2002**, *249*, 316–321. [CrossRef]
67. Mitani, T.; Yamashita, T.; Okumura, C.; Ishii, H. Adsorption of Benzoic Acid and Its Derivatives to Swollen Chitosan Beads. *Biosci. Biotechnol. Biochem.* **1995**, *59*, 927–928. [CrossRef]
68. Shapiro, Y.E. Structure and dynamics of hydrogels and organogels: An NMR spectroscopy approach. *Prog. Polym. Sci.* **2011**, *36*, 1184–1253. [CrossRef]

69. Lavertu, M.; Xia, Z.; Serreqi, A.; Berrada, M.; Rodrigues, A.; Wang, D.; Buschmann, M.; Gupta, A. A validated 1H NMR method for the determination of the degree of deacetylation of chitosan. *J. Pharm. Biomed. Anal.* **2003**, *32*, 1149–1158. [CrossRef]
70. Vårum, K.M.; Anthonsen, M.W.; Grasdalen, H.; Smidsrød, O. Determination of the degree of N-acetylation and the distribution of N-acetyl groups in partially N-deacetylated chitins (chitosans) by high-field n.m.r. spectroscopy. *Carbohydr. Res.* **1991**, *211*, 17–23. [CrossRef] [PubMed]
71. Shigemasa, Y.; Matsuura, H.; Sashiwa, H.; Saimoto, H. Biological Macromolecules Evaluation of different absorbance ratios from infrared spectroscopy for analyzing the degree of deacetylation in chitin. *Int. J. Biol. Macromol.* **1996**, *18*, 237–242. [CrossRef] [PubMed]
72. Azam, S.S.; Abbasi, S.W. Molecular docking studies for the identification of novel melatoninergic inhibitors for acetylserotonin-O-methyltransferase using different docking routines. *Theor. Biol. Med. Model.* **2013**, *10*, 63. [CrossRef]
73. Mani, S.; Supriya, T.; Shankar, M.; Lalitha, S.K.; Dastgiri, J.; Babu, M.N. A Over View on Molecular Docking American Journal of Biological and Pharmaceutical Research a over View on Molecular Docking. *Am. J. Biol. Pharm. Res.* **2016**, *3*, 83–89.
74. Altinisik, A.; Yurdakoç, K. Chitosan/poly(vinyl alcohol) hydrogels for amoxicillin release. *Polym. Bull.* **2013**, *71*, 759–774. [CrossRef]
75. Muthu, M.S.; Rawat, M.K.; Mishra, A.; Singh, S. PLGA nanoparticle formulations of risperidone: Preparation and neuropharmacological evaluation. *Nanomedicine* **2009**, *5*, 323–333. [CrossRef] [PubMed]
76. Zhang, Q.; Fassihi, M.A.; Fassihi, R. Delivery Considerations of Highly Viscous Polymeric Fluids Mimicking Concentrated Biopharmaceuticals: Assessment of Injectability via Measurement of Total Work Done "WT". *AAPS PharmSciTech* **2018**, *19*, 1520–1528. [CrossRef] [PubMed]
77. Tobin, A.B.; Heunemann, P.; Wemmer, J.; Stokes, J.R.; Nicholson, T.; Windhab, E.J.; Fischer, P. Cohesiveness and flowability of particulated solid and semi-solid food systems. *Food Funct.* **2017**, *8*, 3647–3653. [CrossRef] [PubMed]
78. Cevher, E.; Taha, M.A.; Orlu, M.; Araman, A. Evaluation of Mechanical and Mucoadhesive Properties of Clomiphene Citrate Gel Formulations Containing Carbomers and Their Thiolated Derivatives. *Drug Deliv.* **2008**, *15*, 57–67. [CrossRef] [PubMed]
79. Varghese, J.S.; Chellappa, N.; Fathima, N.N. Gelatin–carrageenan hydrogels: Role of pore size distribution on drug delivery process. *Colloids Surf. B Biointerfaces* **2014**, *113*, 346–351. [CrossRef] [PubMed]
80. Butt, A.; Jabeen, S.; Nisar, N.; Islam, A.; Gull, N.; Iqbal, S.S.; Khan, S.M.; Yameen, B. Controlled release of cephradine by biopolymers based target specific crosslinked hydrogels. *Int. J. Biol. Macromol.* **2018**, *121*, 104–112. [CrossRef]

Disclaimer/Publisher's Note: The statements, opinions and data contained in all publications are solely those of the individual author(s) and contributor(s) and not of MDPI and/or the editor(s). MDPI and/or the editor(s) disclaim responsibility for any injury to people or property resulting from any ideas, methods, instructions or products referred to in the content.

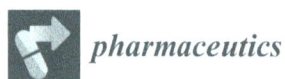 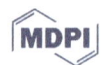

Article

Corneal Permeability and Uptake of Twenty-Five Drugs: Species Comparison and Quantitative Structure–Permeability Relationships

Cleildo P. Santana [1,2], Brock A. Matter [1], Madhoosudan A. Patil [1], Armando Silva-Cunha [2] and Uday B. Kompella [1,3,4,5,*]

[1] Department of Pharmaceutical Sciences, University of Colorado Anschutz Medical Campus, Aurora, CO 80045, USA; cleildopsantana@gmail.com (C.P.S.); brock.matter@cuanschutz.edu (B.A.M.); madhoosudan.patil@cuanschutz.edu (M.A.P.)
[2] Faculty of Pharmacy, Federal University of Minas Gerais, Belo Horizonte 31270-901, MG, Brazil; armando@ufmg.br
[3] Department of Ophthalmology, University of Colorado Anschutz Medical Campus, Aurora, CO 80045, USA
[4] Department of Bioengineering, University of Colorado Anschutz Medical Campus, Aurora, CO 80045, USA
[5] Colorado Center for Nanomedicine and Nanosafety, University of Colorado Anschutz Medical Campus, Aurora, CO 80045, USA
* Correspondence: uday.kompella@cuanschutz.edu

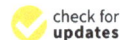

Citation: Santana, C.P.; Matter, B.A.; Patil, M.A.; Silva-Cunha, A.; Kompella, U.B. Corneal Permeability and Uptake of Twenty-Five Drugs: Species Comparison and Quantitative Structure–Permeability Relationships. *Pharmaceutics* 2023, 15, 1646. https://doi.org/10.3390/pharmaceutics15061646

Academic Editor: Francisco Javier Otero-Espinar

Received: 22 April 2023
Revised: 28 May 2023
Accepted: 29 May 2023
Published: 2 June 2023

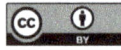

Copyright: © 2023 by the authors. Licensee MDPI, Basel, Switzerland. This article is an open access article distributed under the terms and conditions of the Creative Commons Attribution (CC BY) license (https:// creativecommons.org/licenses/by/ 4.0/).

Abstract: The purpose of this study was to determine corneal permeability and uptake in rabbit, porcine, and bovine corneas for twenty-five drugs using an N-in-1 (cassette) approach and relate these parameters to drug physicochemical properties and tissue thickness through quantitative structure permeability relationships (QSPRs). A twenty-five-drug cassette containing β-blockers, NSAIDs, and corticosteroids in solution at a micro-dose was exposed to the epithelial side of rabbit, porcine, or bovine corneas mounted in a diffusion chamber, and the corneal drug permeability and tissue uptake were monitored using an LC-MS/MS method. Data obtained were used to construct and evaluate over 46,000 quantitative structure–permeability (QSPR) models using multiple linear regression, and the best-fit models were cross-validated by Y-randomization. Drug permeability was generally higher in rabbit cornea and comparable between bovine and porcine corneas. Permeability differences between species could be explained in part by differences in corneal thickness. Corneal uptake between species correlated with a slope close to 1, indicating generally similar drug uptake per unit weight of tissue. A high correlation was observed between bovine, porcine, and rabbit corneas for permeability and between bovine and porcine corneas for uptake ($R^2 \geq 0.94$). MLR models indicated that drug characteristics such as lipophilicity (LogD), heteroatom ratio (HR), nitrogen ratio (NR), hydrogen bond acceptors (HBA), rotatable bonds (RB), index of refraction (IR), and tissue thickness (TT) are of great influence on drug permeability and uptake. When data for all species along with thickness as a parameter was used in MLR, the best fit equation for permeability was Log (% transport/cm$^2 \cdot$ s) = 0.441 LogD − 8.29 IR + 8.357 NR − 0.279 HBA − 3.833 TT + 10.432 ($R^2 = 0.826$), and the best-fit equation for uptake was Log (%/g) = 0.387 LogD + 4.442 HR + 0.105 RB − 0.303 HBA − 2.235 TT + 1.422 ($R^2 = 0.750$). Thus, it is feasible to explain corneal drug delivery in three species using a single equation.

Keywords: β-blockers; NSAIDs; corticosteroids; drug delivery; ocular delivery; drug permeability; QSPR; MLR

1. Introduction

Ophthalmic drug products can be administered by systemic, periocular, intraocular, or topical routes [1,2]. The oral route, a noninvasive, systemic route, although convenient for dosing, is not a viable option for most ophthalmic drugs due to hepatic first-pass metabolism, extensive drug dilution in the blood, and the presence of blood–tissue barriers that limit ocular drug bioavailability. The blood–aqueous barrier, which limits drug transport from the systemic circulation to the anterior chamber [3], is constituted by the tight junctions of the ciliary non-pigmented epithelium and the endothelial layers of the iris and the inner wall of Schlemm's canal. The blood–retina barrier, which limits drug transport from the systemic circulation to the retina [4], is constituted by the tight junctions of retinal endothelial cells (inner blood–retinal barrier) and retinal pigment epithelial cells (outer blood–retinal barrier). Both blood–tissue barriers are mainly imposed by tight junctions, with the blood–retinal barrier being more formidable, similar to the blood–brain barrier [4]. While the periocular and intraocular routes are invasive, the topical route allows noninvasive dosing to the eye.

The topical ophthalmic route, wherein the drug product is dosed noninvasively to the ocular surface, is widely used in treating eye diseases afflicting the anterior segment of the eye. Eye drops are the most commonly used topical ophthalmic drug products [5]. Although the eye is a readily accessible organ and eye drops are widely used, topical ocular drug delivery remains limited and challenging. This is due to a series of anatomical and physiological barriers of the eye, which can be broadly categorized as static or permeability barriers and dynamic or fluid flow barriers that limit drug delivery [6]. Static barriers for topical drug delivery to the anterior segment include the cornea and conjunctiva, especially tight junctions containing epithelial layers in these tissues. Dynamic barriers include blinking, nasolacrimal drainage, and blood and lymphatic flows. Additionally, metabolic barriers of eye tissues, including cytochrome P450 systems, proteases, and nucleases, may degrade topically applied drugs. The above barriers, in particular nasolacrimal drainage and epithelial permeability barriers, contribute the most towards low bioavailability of drugs to the anterior segment of the eye. In general, much less than 10% of the topically applied drug reaches intraocular tissues from an eye drop [7–10], and the bioavailability is predicted to be 1 to 5% for lipophilic drugs and less than 0.5% for hydrophilic drugs [11]. Currently, there are no FDA-approved eye drops to treat back-of-the-eye diseases due to inadequate delivery [5].

After topical administration of an eye drop in the precorneal area, it tends to accumulate in the conjunctival cul-de-sac and mix with the lacrimal fluid [3,4,12]. In the time interval between the administration and its complete drainage into the nasal cavity, the drop is expected to spread on the eye surface by the blinking movement [13]. The lacrimal fluid is composed of an external lipidic layer, a middle aqueous layer, and an internal mucin layer, and the components include electrolytes, lipids, proteins, and glycoproteins that may interact with drugs. The tear turnover time is about 1 to 2 min [14], and after this time, the majority of the drug administered can be lost through the nasal cavity or the conjunctiva into the systemic circulation [15].

The cornea is the main static barrier for drug absorption into the aqueous humor following topical administration. It is highly specialized, with three key regions: epithelium, stroma, and endothelium, which are lipophilic, hydrophilic, and lipophilic, respectively. The epithelium is composed of five layers of epithelial cells with tight junctions that form an important barrier to avoid fluid loss and pathogen penetration into the eye. Due to their highly lipophilic character, hydrophilic drugs show limited permeability across the corneal epithelium. Through this layer, drugs can permeate passively either between the cells via the paracellular pathway or through the cell or transcellular pathway. While the paracellular pathway prefers small hydrophilic drugs, the transcellular pathway prefers small lipophilic drugs. The corneal stroma is a highly hydrophilic layer that behaves like a liquid with a viscosity of about 1.5 times that of water for the diffusion of dextrans, allowing a permeability of dextrans as large as 34 nm [2]. Stroma is rate limiting for the transport of lipophilic drugs [11,16,17]. The endothelium, constituted by a leaky monolayer of cells, is less of a barrier than the epithelium. The corneal penetration of drugs is limited to compounds with a molecular weight typically lower than 500 Da; the average molecular weight of approved topical ophthalmic drugs is 392 Da, with a range of 111 to 1811 Da [18].

Aqueous solutions usually have the simplest manufacturing process and may result in high tissue concentrations since the soluble drug is at a molecular level and typically near the solubility limit of the drug. Corneal permeability is known to depend on drug properties such as lipophilicity, molecular size, charge, and shape [6,16,19–21] as well as formulation composition [9,22]. Understanding the factors affecting corneal permeability is expected to benefit the development of eye drops with enhanced bioavailability.

For the evaluation of corneal permeability of drugs, rabbit, porcine, and bovine corneas have been investigated [23,24], with rabbit being [23,25] the most commonly used animal model due to extensive ocular pharmacokinetic data availability [25]. The work herein employed the simultaneous analysis of 25 drug compounds of three different pharmacological classes using an innovative LC-MS/MS method to determine their tissue permeability and develop a predictive QSPR relationship of drug permeability in bovine, porcine, and rabbit corneas.

2. Materials and Methods

2.1. Chemicals

Alprenolol hydrochloride, atenolol, betaxolol hydrochloride, bromfenac sodium, calcium chloride, difluprednate, formic acid, flupirtine maleate, D-glucose, dimethyl sulfoxide (DMSO), HEPES (4-(2-hydroxyethyl)-1-piperazinethanesulfonic acid), indoprofen, ketoprofen, magnesium chloride, magnesium sulfate, mefenamic acid, methanol, metoprolol tartrate, nadolol, naproxen, nepafenac, pindolol, prednisolone, propranolol hydrochloride, sotalol hydrochloride, timolol maleate, tolmetin sodium salt dihydrate, and triamcinolone were purchased from Sigma-Aldrich, St. Louis, MO, USA. Acetonitrile, hydrochloric acid, potassium chloride, potassium phosphate dibasic, sodium chloride, and sodium phosphate dibasic were purchased from Fisher Scientific, Pittsburgh, PA, USA. Amfenac sodium monohydrate was purchased from VWR International LLC, Radnor, PA, USA. Sodium bicarbonate was purchased from Mallinckrodt Inc., Dublin, Leinster, Ireland. Budesonide, fluocinolone acetonide, and triamcinolone hexacetonide were purchased from Spectrum Chemical, New Brunswick, NJ, USA. Dexamethasone was purchased from Sigma-Aldrich, St. Louis, MO, USA, and Shanxi Jinjin Chemical Co., Ltd., Hejin, Shanxi, China. Oxprenolol hydrochloride was purchased from MP Biomedicals, Santa Ana, CA, USA. Dexamethasone-4,6,21,21-d4 was purchased from CDN Isotopes, QC, Canada. Flupirtine-d4 hydrochloride and timolol-d5 maleate were purchased from Santa Cruz Biotechnology, Santa Cruz, CA, USA.

2.2. Dosing Solution Preparation

The dosing solution was prepared from a drug cassette stock solution containing 25 drugs dissolved in DMSO at a final concentration of 200 ng μL^{-1}. To prepare the dosing solution, 10 µL of the drug cassette stock solution was diluted to 10 mL in assay buffer (NaCl 122.0 mM, NaHCO3 25.0 mM, MgSO4 1.2 mM, K2HPO4 0.4 mM, CaCl2 1.4 mM, HEPES 10.0 mM and glucose 10.0 mM in water) (pH = 7.4) to achieve a final concentration of 200 ng mL^{-1}.

2.3. Tissue Preparation

Bovine and porcine corneas were collected from freshly excised eyes purchased from local abattoirs (Elizabeth Locker Plant, Elizabeth, CO, USA). Freshly isolated rabbit corneas were shipped overnight from Pel-Freez (Rogers, AR, USA). The eyes were immersed in refrigerated HBSS solution during transport to the laboratory. The corneas were isolated from the eyes and mounted in NaviCyte Vertical Ussing chambers (San Diego, CA, USA), with their epithelial side facing the donor compartment.

2.4. Test Conditions

The dosing solution (1.5 mL) was placed in the donor side of the chambers, while plain assay buffer (1.5 mL) was placed in the acceptor side of the chambers. Both solutions and chambers were kept at 37 °C during the duration of the experiment (6 h). The aeration of the medium was performed using 5% CO_2 and 95% air with slow bubbling. At 15, 30, 60,

120, 180, 240, 300, and 360 min, 50 µL samples were withdrawn from the acceptor side of the chambers, with immediate replacement of the volume with fresh assay buffer. Aliquots of the donor solution were also withdrawn at the end of the study from the donor side of the chambers. All samples were spiked with the internal standard solution immediately after collection.

2.5. Permeability Evaluation

The drug amount in the samples was quantified using LC-MS/MS, with sample data corrected for acceptor solution replenishment. Drug amounts in all samples were normalized as percent values of the initial amount of drug quantified in the dosing solution. The permeability of the drugs was compared using the apparent permeability coefficient [26] (P_{app}), given by Equation (1):

$$P_{app} = \frac{(dm/dt) \cdot V_0}{A \cdot m_0} \quad (1)$$

where dm/dt is the derivative of the cumulative drug amount transported through the tissue as a function of time, V_0 is the volume on the acceptor side, A is the contact area of the tissue with the solutions, and m_0 is the initial drug amount in the donor solution.

Permeability can be related to diffusivity [26] (Equation (2)) as follows:

$$D = \frac{P_{app} \cdot h}{k} \quad (2)$$

where P_{app} is the apparent permeability coefficient, h is the tissue thickness, and k is the partition coefficient of the drug between the tissue and dosing solution. Tissue thickness was calculated from results reported in the literature by different groups for bovine, porcine, and rabbit corneas (Table 1).

Table 1. Corneal thickness reported in the literature for each tissue tested.

Corneal Thickness (µm)		
Bovine	Porcine	Rabbit
800 [27]	950 [28]	480 [28]
1530 [28]	1188 [29]	370 [27]
1015 [30]	955 [31]	381 [32]
1024 [33]	850 [34]	500 [35]
1160 [36]	851 [37]	422 [38]
1105.8 *	958.8 *	430.6 *

* Average value.

Drug flux [39] across the tissues was also used to compare tissue permeability (Equation (3)):

$$J = \frac{dm/dt}{A} \quad (3)$$

where dm/dt is the derivative of the cumulative drug amount transported through the tissue as a function of time, and A is the contact area of the tissue with the solutions.

2.6. Drug Extraction

To extract the drugs from the cornea, the method developed by Matter, Bourne, and Kompella [40] was used. At the end of the experiment, the portion of the cornea exposed to the donor and acceptor solutions was taken from the chambers and submitted to a liquid–liquid extraction protocol before LC-MS/MS analysis. First, 50 ± 5 mg of each tissue was placed into fresh tubes. Briefly, 100 µL of fresh PBS and 10 µL of the internal standard were added to the tubes, and the content was homogenized using a glass-glass homogenizer. The samples were subjected to three freeze–thaw cycles, using liquid nitrogen (−196 °C) to freeze followed by room temperature thawing. Then, 300 µL of a solution of methanol and acetonitrile (2:1) was added to each tube, and after 30 min at room temperature, the samples were vortexed for 10 min and sonicated for 5 min. Afterwards, the tubes were centrifuged for 10 min, and the supernatant was collected into fresh tubes. The samples were evaporated (Savant SpeedVac SC100, Holbrook, NY, USA) until the sample volumes were less than 100 µL.

2.7. LC-MS/MS Analysis

For drug quantification, the method developed by Matter, Bourne, and Kompella [40] was used. An AB Sciex Qtrap 4500/Shimadzu HPLC was used, and the mobile phase consisted of a mixture of 0.1% formic acid in water (A) and 0.1% formic acid in 9:1 acetonitrile:water (B). The gradient elution was performed at 40 °C as follows: 99.4% of A (0–2 min), 94% of A (2.5 min), 47% of A (10.5 min), 6% of A (14 min), and 99.4% of A (14.5–18 min) using a Phenomenex Kinetex column. In the MS detector, the following transitions were monitored: 272.9/255 (sotalol), 267/190 (atenolol), 249/116 (pindolol), 309.9/254 (nadolol), 316.9/261 (timolol), 267.9/116 (metoprolol), 265.9/116 (oxprenolol), 304.9/196 (flupirtine), 395/375.1 (triamcinolone), 259.9/116 (propranolol), 249.9/116 (alprenolol), 308/116 (betaxolol), 361/343.1 (prednisolone), 254.8/238 (nepafenac), 393/373.2 (dexamethasone), 281.9/236 (indoprofen), 256/210 (amfenac), 453/433.2 (fluocinolone acetonide), 257.8/119 (tolmetin), 254.9/209 (ketoprofen), 231/185.1 (naproxen), 431/413.1 (budesonide), 333.8/316 (bromfenac), 509.1/303.1 (difluprednate), 241.9/224 (mefenamic acid) and 533.2/415.1 (triamcinolone hexacetonide). The equipment was operated at 500 °C with a spray voltage of 5 k and curtain and ion source gas pressures of 45 and 50 psi, respectively, along with an entrance and collision cell exit potential of 10 and 14 V, respectively.

2.8. Multiple Linear Regression (MLR) Modelling

LC-MS/MS quantification data were used to obtain predictive linear models of cumulative transport, permeability, and drug uptake for each tissue. Multiple linear regressions were performed using the least squares method with Microsoft Excel® Professional 2016. The following molecular descriptors were calculated for each drug with ACDLabs® (version 2019) and used as independent variables (Supplementary Materials Table S1): molecular weight, number of hydrogen bond donors, number of hydrogen bond acceptors, number of hydrogen bond donors and acceptors, total polar surface area, number of rotatable bonds, carbon ratio, nitrogen ratio, nitric oxide ratio, heteroatom ratio, halogen ratio, number of rings, number of aromatic rings, number of 5 atom rings, number of non-aromatic 6 atom rings, log(BCF), parachor, index of refraction, surface tension, density, polarizability, molar volume, molecular volume, molar refractivity, LogS, LogP, and LogD at pH of 7.2, 7.3, 7.4, 7.5, and 7.6.

To select the best-fit models, all possible collinearity-free models with four, three, and two independent variables were obtained, as described in Figure 1.

Only models presenting significant ($p < 0.05$) coefficients for all independent variables were selected and evaluated by R^2, adjusted R^2, and F values.

Best-fit models for each of the three parameters evaluated were submitted to internal cross-validation using the Q^2 coefficient. Once the applicability domain of the models was defined [41], the Q^2 coefficient was obtained with Microsoft Excel® by sample splitting, where ≈20% of the samples constituted the test set. The splitting was repeated 1000 times for each model. The coefficient calculation followed the relationship [42] described by Equation (4):

$$Q^2 = 1 - \frac{\left[\sum_{i=1}^{test}(\hat{y}_i - y_i)^2\right]/n_{test}}{\left[\sum_{i=1}^{tr}(\hat{y}_i - \overline{y}_{tr})^2\right]/n_{tr}} \quad (4)$$

where n_{test} and n_{tr} refer to the number of samples in the test and training sets, respectively, y represents the experimental value, $\hat{y}$ represents the predicted value, and $\overline{y}$ represents the average value.

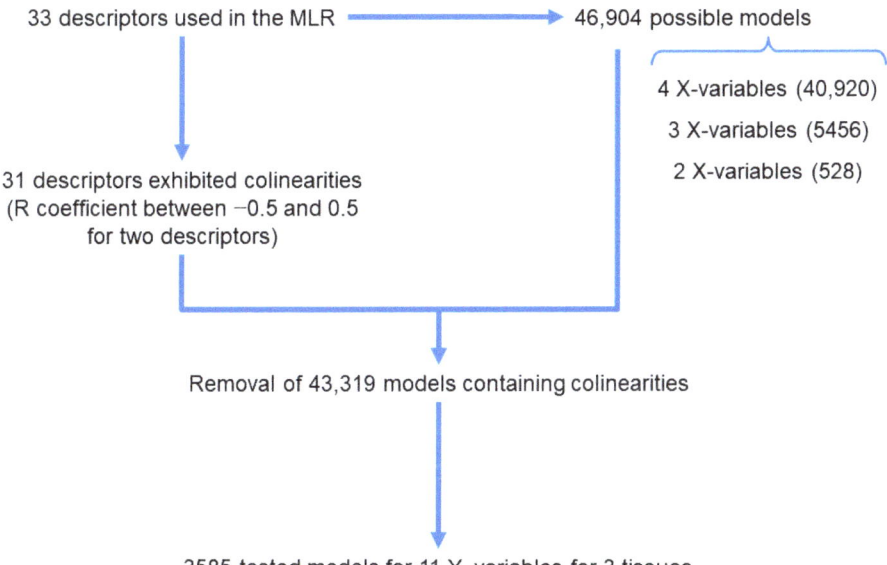

Figure 1. Rationale for the obtaining of MLR models.

2.9. Bioavailability Estimation

Systemic and aqueous humor bioavailability values were calculated based on apparent permeability coefficients measured in the porcine cornea in the present study and those estimated for porcine conjunctiva. The conjunctival permeability was estimated using regression models and equations developed for each drug class based on a correlation of corneal and conjunctival permeability values reported in the literature [24,43]. In this step, only experimental articles simultaneously reporting data from porcine cornea and conjunctiva were considered.

P_{app} values through porcine cornea or conjunctiva were each used to calculate the clearance through human tissues by multiplying the values with the human corneal (1.04 cm^2) or conjunctival (17.64 cm^2) total surface areas, unlike a prior study reporting the following equations, which used half of the conjunctival surface area [43]. From cornea and conjunctiva, the clearance (µL min^{-1}) into human aqueous humor and into human systemic circulation were calculated, respectively. These values were then used to calculate bioavailability using the following relationships [43]:

$$CL_{Topical} = CL_{Cornea} + CL_{Conjunctiva} + Q_{Tear} \tag{5}$$

$$BA_{Aqueous} = \frac{CL_{Cornea}}{CL_{Topical}} \cdot 100 \tag{6}$$

$$BA_{Systemic} = \frac{CL_{Conjunctiva}}{CL_{Topical}} \cdot 100 \tag{7}$$

where $CL_{Topical}$ represents the total clearance through the ocular surface, CL_{Cornea} represents the clearance through cornea, $CL_{Conjunctiva}$ represents the clearance through conjunctiva, Q_{Tear} represents the human tear flow rate (1.2 µL min^{-1}) and the associated clearance [44], $BA_{Aqueous}$ represents the dose bioavailability in aqueous humor, and $BA_{Systemic}$ represents the dose bioavailability in systemic circulation.

2.10. Statistical Analysis

All the values are described as the mean ± standard deviation. Comparisons between groups were performed using a one-way ANOVA with GraphPad Prism 5.04, considering $\alpha = 0.05$.

3. Results

3.1. Cumulative Transport and Permeability Coefficient

The values of cumulative transport found for the drugs evaluated are presented in Figure 2.

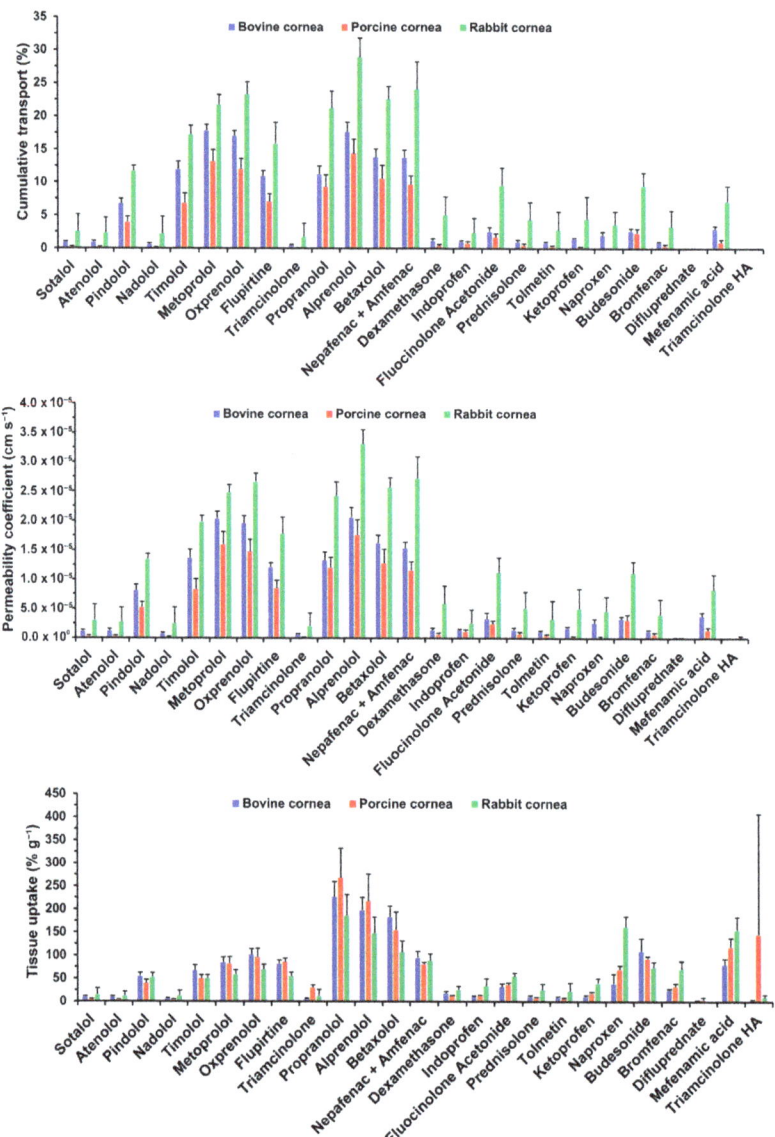

Figure 2. Cumulative transport, apparent permeability coefficient, and tissue uptake values. Mean ± STD is reported for 5 corneas.

The β-blockers were the drug class that showed the largest extent of transport across all corneas. For bovine cornea, the extent of transport was given as metoprolol, oxprenolol, and alprenolol > betaxolol > timolol and propranolol > pindolol > atenolol, nadolol, and sotalol. The drug extent of transport across porcine cornea was lower than that of bovine cornea, with alprenolol, metoprolol, and oxprenolol > betaxolol and propranolol > timolol and pindolol > sotalol, atenolol, and nadolol. Rabbit cornea showed a higher extent of β-blocker transport, with alprenolol > metoprolol, oxprenolol, propranolol, and betaxolol > timolol > pindolol > sotalol, atenolol, and nadolol. No significant differences were detected for sotalol, atenolol, or nadolol between the tissues, nor for pindolol between bovine and porcine corneas.

For the steroids, the extent of transport through the bovine cornea was budesonide and fluocinolone acetonide > dexamethasone and prednisolone > triamcinolone and difluprednate. In porcine tissue, the rank order was budesonide and fluocinolone acetonide > triamcinolone, dexamethasone, prednisolone, and difluprednate. In rabbit cornea, the extent of transport was higher than that of bovine and porcine tissues, with the rank order being fluocinolone acetonide and budesonide > triamcinolone, dexamethasone, and prednisolone > triamcinolone hexacetonide. No transport was detected for triamcinolone hexacetonide through bovine or porcine corneas or for difluprednate through rabbit cornea. Bovine and porcine corneas showed comparable results for all steroids. On the other hand, both tissues showed significantly lower transport of dexamethasone, fluocinolone acetonide, prednisolone, and budesonide than that observed in rabbit cornea.

In bovine cornea, the NSAIDs showed the extent of transport as nepafenac > flupirtine > mefenamic acid > indoprofen, tolmetin, ketoprofen, naproxen, and bromfenac. Porcine cornea showed the extent of transport as nepafenac > flupirtine > indoprofen, tolmetin, ketoprofen, naproxen, bromfenac, and mefenamic acid, with the overall extent lower than half of that for bovine. Rabbit cornea showed a higher extent of transport than that of bovine tissue, observed as nepafenac > flupirtine > indoprofen, tolmetin, ketoprofen, naproxen, bromfenac, and mefenamic acid. Flupirtine and nepafenac transport through porcine cornea was significantly lower than through bovine cornea, and both were lower than those observed for rabbit cornea. Mefenamic acid transport was comparable between bovine and porcine corneas but significantly lower than that observed for rabbit cornea.

Permeability coefficients for all drugs followed the same trends observed for cumulative transport, including significant differences. Data are presented in Figure 2. Therefore, differences between P_{app} of drugs will not be described here to avoid redundancy.

3.2. Tissue Uptake

The tissue uptake data is presented in Figure 2.

Besides cumulative transport, β-blockers showed high uptake by the tissues. In bovine cornea, the amounts detected were higher for propranolol, alprenolol, and betaxolol > pindolol, timolol, metoprolol, and oxprenolol > sotalol, atenolol, and nadolol. In porcine and rabbit corneas, the extent of β-blocker uptake was propranolol > alprenolol and betaxolol > pindolol, timolol, metoprolol, and oxprenolol > sotalol, atenolol, and nadolol. The extent of β-blocker uptake was comparable between bovine and porcine corneas but significantly lower for propranolol, alprenolol, and betaxolol in rabbit cornea.

The extent of steroid uptake by bovine cornea was observed as budesonide > all the other steroids. In porcine cornea, steroid uptake was observed as budesonide > fluocinolone acetonide > triamcinolone, dexamethasone, prednisolone, difluprednate, and triamcinolone hexacetonide. Rabbit cornea showed an overall higher extent of steroid uptake, with budesonide > fluocinolone acetonide > triamcinolone, dexamethasone, and prednisolone > triamcinolone hexacetonide. No tissue uptake was quantifiable for difluprednate in rabbit cornea. Bovine and porcine corneas showed comparable extents of steroid uptake. Rabbit cornea showed higher fluocinolone acetonide uptake than bovine cornea and, on the other hand, lower budesonide uptake than bovine and porcine corneas.

Regarding bovine cornea, the extent of uptake of NSAIDs was nepafenac and mefenamic acid > flupirtine and naproxen > indoprofen, tolmetin, ketoprofen, and bromfenac. In porcine cornea, the extent of uptake of NSAIDs was in the order: mefenamic acid > flupirtine, nepafenac, and naproxen > indoprofen, tolmetin, ketoprofen, and bromfenac. Rabbit cornea showed a higher extent of uptake for the NSAIDs, with naproxen and mefenamic acid > nepafenac and bromfenac > flupirtine, indoprofen, tolmetin, and ketoprofen. Rabbit cornea showed higher uptake of naproxen and bromfenac than porcine cornea, which in turn showed higher uptake of naproxen and mefenamic acid than bovine cornea. Rabbit cornea showed higher uptake compared to bovine cornea regarding indoprofen, ketoprofen, naproxen, bromfenac, and mefenamic acid.

3.3. Correlation Plots

Various correlations were verified by R^2 determination, with the graphs and results presented in Figure 3a,b.

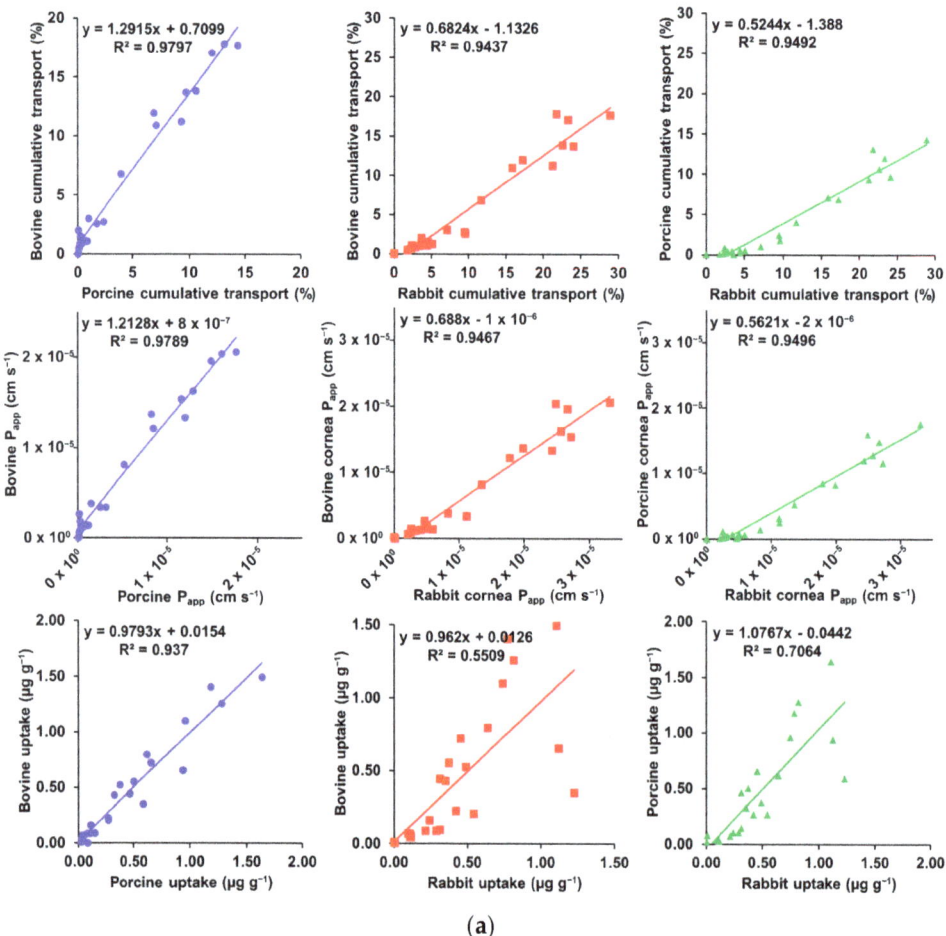

(a)

Figure 3. Cont.

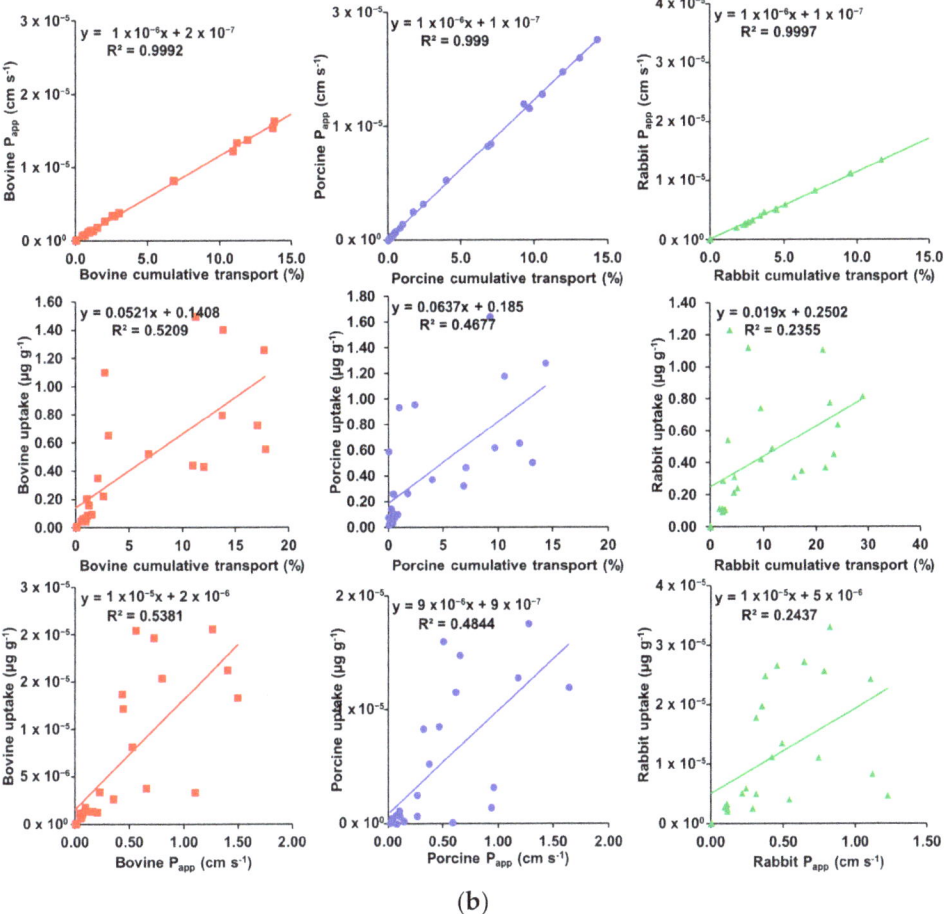

Figure 3. (a) Inter-species correlation plots for cumulative transport, P_{app}, and tissue uptake. (b) Within species correlations for P_{app} vs. cumulative transport, tissue uptake vs. cumulative transport, and tissue uptake vs. P_{app}.

Bovine vs. porcine cornea showed a high correlation for cumulative transport ($R^2 = 0.9797$), P_{app} ($R^2 = 0.9789$), and tissue uptake ($R^2 = 0.9370$), where the first two bovine corneas showed higher values and the last, lower values. When correlated to rabbit cornea, bovine and porcine corneas showed a high correlation for cumulative transport ($R^2 = 0.9437$ and 0.9492, respectively) and for P_{app} ($R^2 = 0.9467$ and 0.9496, respectively), with both measurements showing higher values in rabbit cornea. However, bovine and porcine corneas showed weak or good correlation, respectively, with rabbit cornea for tissue uptake ($R^2 = 0.5509$ and 0.7064, respectively).

Tissue uptake did not show a high correlation with P_{app} or cumulative transport in bovine ($R^2 = 0.5381$ and 0.5209, respectively), porcine ($R^2 = 0.4844$ and 0.4677, respectively), or rabbit ($R^2 = 0.2437$ and 0.2355, respectively) corneas. On the other hand, a high correlation ($R^2 \geq 0.9990$) was observed between P_{app} and cumulative transport for all tissues.

The permeability and tissue uptake also showed good correlation with LogD at pH 7.4, following sigmoidal relationships, which are presented in Figure 4.

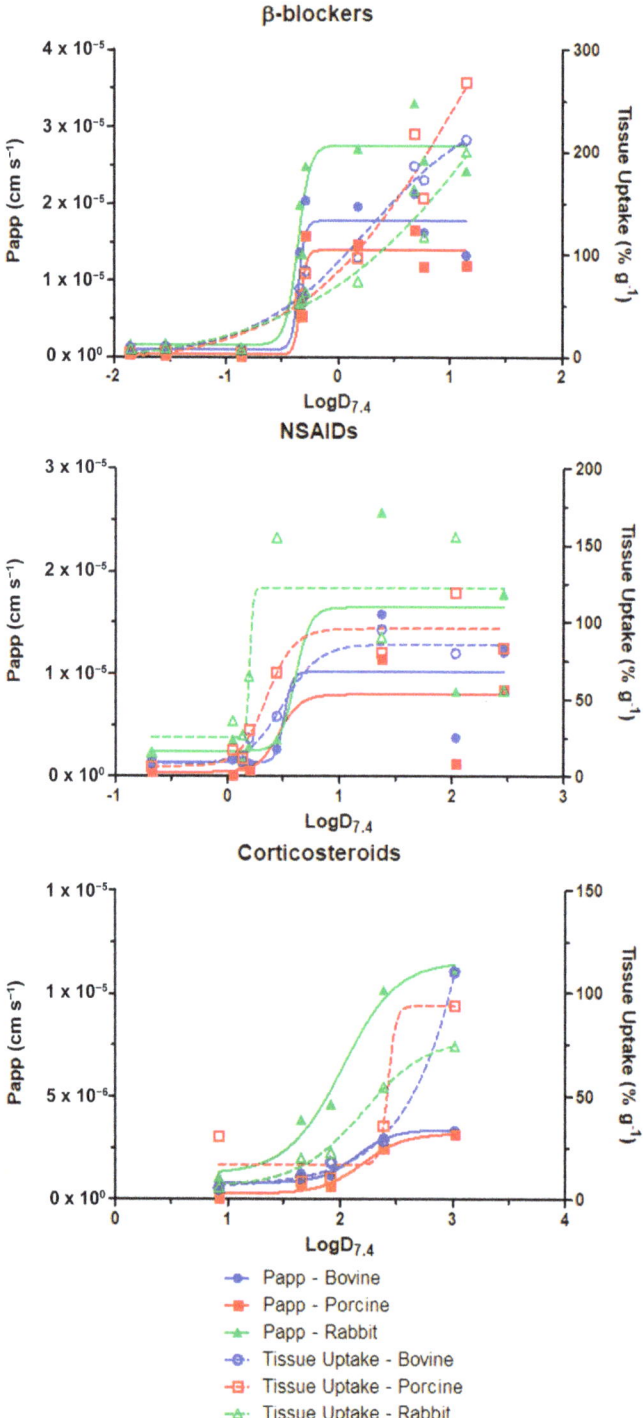

Figure 4. Correlation plots of permeability and tissue uptake with LogD at pH 7.4.

To compare the behavior of the sigmoidal curves, Table 2 presents $LogD_{7.4}$ values at half-maximum for each parameter:

Table 2. $LogD_{7.4}$ at half-maximum of the sigmoidal curves obtained for permeability and tissue uptake.

Tissue	Parameter	LogD7.4 at Half-Maximum		
		β-Blockers	NSAIDs	Corticosteroids
Bovine	Papp (cm s^{-1})	−0.3521	0.5118	2.145
	Tissue uptake (% g^{-1})	0.2783	0.5068	5.61
Porcine	Papp (cm s^{-1})	−0.3327	0.4692	2.202
	Tissue uptake (% g^{-1})	1.093	0.3586	2.43
Rabbit	Papp (cm s^{-1})	−0.3578	0.6092	2.023
	Tissue uptake (% g^{-1})	1.758	0.2055	2.204

3.4. MLR Modeling

The best-fit models obtained were ranked considering R^2 and Q^2 coefficients, and the models with the best performance for each tissue are described in Table 3:

Table 3. Best-fit predictive models obtained for each tissue and each parameter evaluated.

Parameter	Tissue	Unit	Coefficients	R^2	Q^2
Permeability	Bovine	Flux (log % s^{-1}/cm^2)	(8.312) + (−0.236·HBA) + (7.254·NR) + (−7.192·IR) + (0.348·LogD7.4)	0.87	0.735
		Papp (log cm s^{-1})	(−5.84) + (−0.101·HBDA) + (0.141·RB) + (3.994·NR) + (0.274·LogD7.4)	0.812	0.632
	Porcine	Flux (log % s^{-1}/cm^2)	(11.882) + (−0.319·HBA) + (10.175·NR) + (−9.504·IR) + (0.503·LogD7.4)	0.857	0.704
		Papp (log cm s^{-1})	(−24.374) + (−0.329·HBDA) + (8.346·Log MV) + (14.591·NR) + (0.227·LogD7.4)	0.722	0.462
	Rabbit	Flux (log % s^{-1}/cm^2)	(10.143) + (−0.279·HBA) + (7.64·NR) + (−8.174·IR) + (0.47·LogD7.4)	0.884	0.748
		Papp (log cm s^{-1})	(−5.496) + (−0.061·HBDA) + (0.11·RB) + (2.308·NR) + (0.245·LogD7.4)	0.781	0.537
Cumulative transport	Bovine	Amount (%)	(179.182) + (−2.468·HBA) + (81.565·NR) + (−106.291·IR) + (3.247·LogD7.4)	0.764	0.529
		Amount (%)	(−6.868) + (2.251·RB) + (2.282·LogD7.4)	0.676	0.492
	Porcine	Amount (%)	(142.4) + (−1.956·HBA) + (57.287·NR) + (−84.66·IR) + (2.559·LogD7.4)	0.75	0.522
		Amount (%)	(−6.025) + (1.754·RB) + (1.857·LogD7.4)	0.691	0.5
	Rabbit	Amount (%)	(253.788) + (−3.628·HBA) + (110.828·NR) + (−149.001·IR) + (5.481·LogD7.4)	0.801	0.617
		Amount (%)	(−7.379) + (3.048·RB) + (4.057·LogD7.4)	0.675	0.493
Tissue uptake	Bovine	Amount (% g^{-1})	(0.763) + (−0.293·HBA) + (0.145·RB) + (5.139·HR) + (0.426·LogD7.4)	0.863	0.69
	Porcine	Amount (% g^{-1})	(7.694) + (−2.834·Log MW) + (0.118·RB) + (0.419·LogD7.4)	0.728	0.562
	Rabbit	Amount (% g^{-1})	(2.23) + (−0.146·HBDA) + (0.041·RB) + (2.376·NR) + (0.216·LogD7.4)	0.807	0.657

HBA: hydrogen bond acceptors; HBDA: hyd. bond donors + acceptors; NR: N ratio; RB: rotatable bonds; HR: heteroatom ratio; IR: index of refraction; LogD: LogD at pH = 7.4; Log MV: log molar volume; Log MW: log molecular weight.

Corneal thickness was considered a parameter to include the structure of the tissue as an x-variable in modeling. Results showed that considering the nature of the tissue in regression caused the resulting models to present higher robustness, as presented in Table 4.

3.5. Bioavailability Estimation

The regression equations (Table 5) used to estimate P_{app} values through the conjunctiva had high coefficients of determination for all drug classes, and the values for clearance obtained are presented in Figure 5.

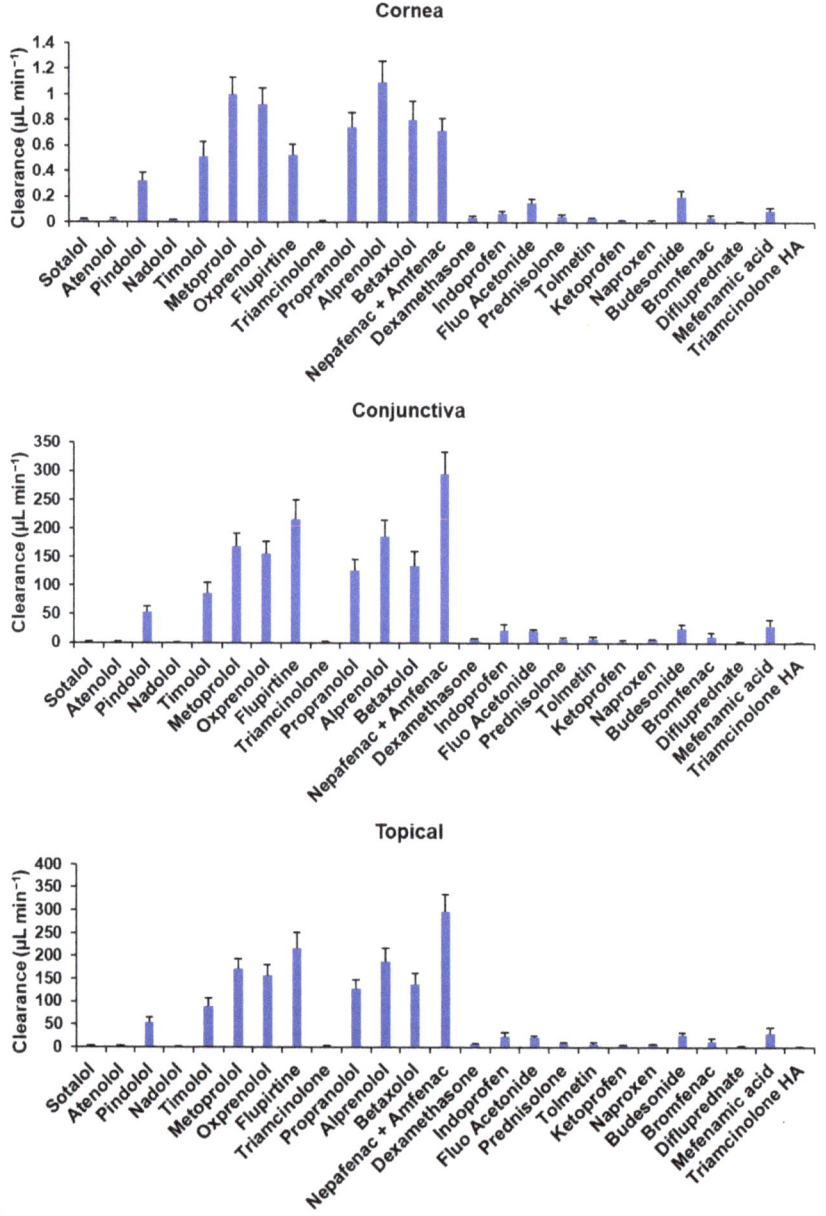

Figure 5. Calculated values of clearance through human cornea, human conjunctiva, and total topical clearance. Mean ± STD is reported for 5 estimates.

The bioavailability values in aqueous humor and in systemic circulation are presented in Figure 6. The magnitude is close to what is expected for ocular bioavailability, but generally higher for conjunctiva based systemic bioavailability. The trends for different drugs did not follow what is anticipated based on drug lipophilicity and literature reports, consistent with the limitation of the bioavailability estimation methods in this study.

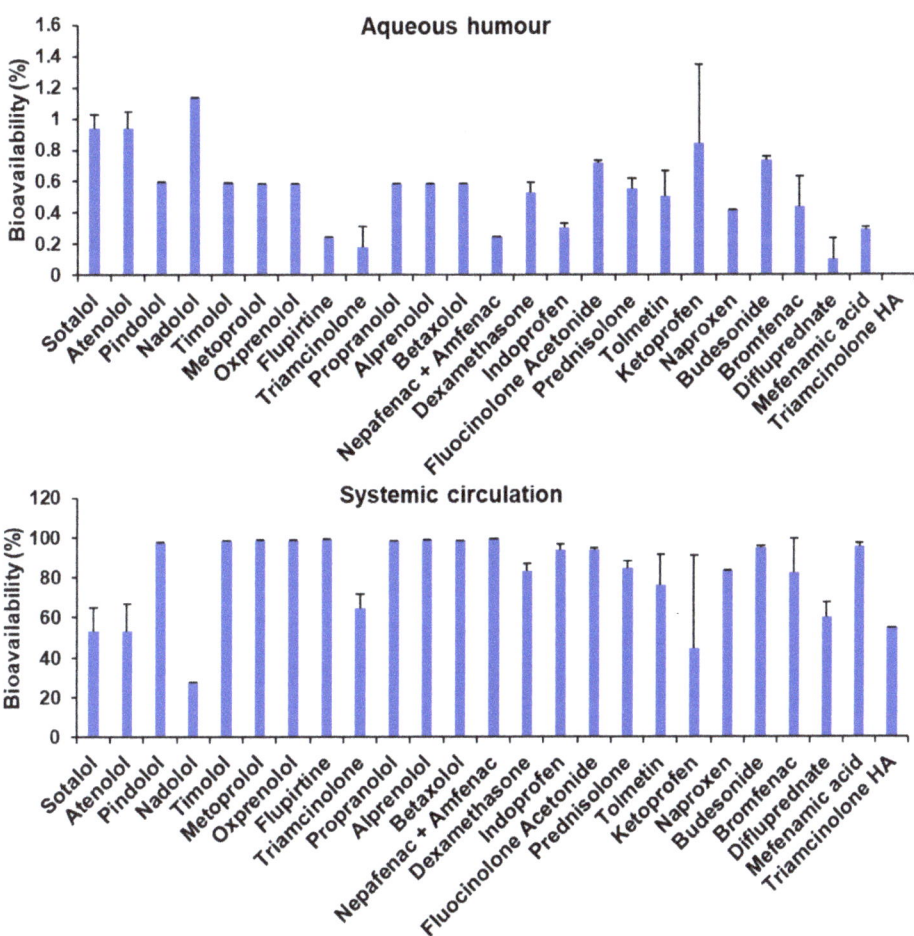

Figure 6. The estimated bioavailability values in aqueous humor and in systemic circulation for the human eye using porcine tissue permeability values. Mean ± STD is reported for 5 estimates.

Table 4. Best-fit predictive models obtained for each parameter evaluated, considering tissue thickness.

Parameter	Unit	Model	R^2	Q^2
Flux	$-\log \% \cdot s^{-1}/cm^2$	$(3.474) + (3.833 \cdot TT) + (0.138 \cdot HBDA) + (-0.135 \cdot RB) + (-5.07 \cdot NR) + (-0.375 \cdot LogD)$	0.781	0.719
Flux	$-\log \% \cdot s^{-1}/cm^2$	$(-10.432) + (3.833 \cdot TT) + (0.279 \cdot HBA) + (-8.357 \cdot NR) + (8.29 \cdot IR) + (-0.441 \cdot LogD)$	0.826	0.780
P_{app}	$-\log cm\ s^{-1}$	$(5.41) + (7.257 \cdot TT) + (0.086 \cdot HBDA) + (-0.151 \cdot RB) + (-3.872 \cdot NR) + (-0.315 \cdot LogD)$	0.691	0.608
P_{app}	$-\log cm\ s^{-1}$	$(-9.001) + (7.256 \cdot TT) + (0.207 \cdot HBA) + (-7.687 \cdot NR) + (8.548 \cdot IR) + (-0.374 \cdot LogD)$	0.716	0.650

Table 4. Cont.

Parameter	Unit	Model	R^2	Q^2
Cumulative transport	%	$(6.118) + (-84.079 \cdot TT) + (-1.383 \cdot HBA) + (2.093 \cdot RB) + (25.45 \cdot NR) + (3.029 \cdot LogD)$	0.700	0.610
Cumulative transport	%	$(198.783) + (-84.079 \cdot TT) + (-2.685 \cdot HBA) + (83.227 \cdot NR) + (-113.318 \cdot IR) + (3.763 \cdot LogD)$	0.734	0.662
Tissue uptake	$\log \% \ g^{-1}$	$(1.422) + (-2.235 \cdot TT) + (-0.303 \cdot HBA) + (0.105 \cdot RB) + (4.442 \cdot HR) + (0.387 \cdot LogD)$	0.750	0.684
Tissue uptake	$\log \% \ g^{-1}$	$(1.853) + (-2.235 \cdot TT) + (-0.13 \cdot HBDA) + (0.097 \cdot RB) + (2.615 \cdot NR) + (0.308 \cdot LogD)$	0.748	0.678

TT: tissue thickness; HBA: hydrogen bond acceptors; HBDA: hyd. bond donors + acceptors; NR: N ratio; RB: rotatable bonds; HR: heteroatom ratio; IR: index of refraction; LogD: LogD at pH = 7.4.

Table 5. Models used to estimate conjunctival Papp values for porcine cornea.

Drug Class	R^2	Model
β-blockers	0.934	$P_{app}\text{Conjunctiva} = (10.141 \cdot P_{app}\text{Cornea}) + (-0.00000267)$
NSAIDs	0.979	$P_{app}\text{Conjunctiva} = (24.645 \cdot P_{app}\text{Cornea}) + (-0.00000633)$
Corticosteroids	0.999	$P_{app}\text{Conjunctiva} = (7.150 \cdot P^{app}\text{Cornea}) + (0.00000136)$

4. Discussion

Rabbit cornea has been widely used in ocular research, with the permeation behavior of many drugs well characterized, as summarized by Prausnitz and Noonan [45]. However, the porcine cornea holds important similarities with the human cornea, suggesting that it might be a more appropriate model to assess drug permeation. Van den Berghe, Guillet, and Compan [28] compared the central corneal thickness and number of layers of the epithelium of porcine, human, bovine, and rabbit corneas and indicated that porcine and human corneas are similar in this regard, while the bovine cornea is much thicker with more epithelial cell layers, and rabbit cornea is thinner with a similar number of cell layers in the corneal epithelium. Greiner et al. [46] suggested that human and porcine corneas had more comparable phosphate metabolism, relative to rabbit [47]. Porcine and rabbit corneas have significantly higher collagen fibrillar diameter, interfibrillar distance, and interlamellar distance compared to human cornea, but the magnitudes are of a similar order [48]. The presence of a Bowman's layer in porcine cornea, previously an object of controversy among specialists [49], has also been demonstrated in more recent studies [48,50], marking another similarity with human, rabbit, and bovine corneas [51].

In this study, rabbit cornea showed higher transport and P_{app} values than bovine and porcine corneas, which had values closer to each other. This finding might be related to the lower thickness of the rabbit cornea, which can deliver drugs to the anterior chamber faster than thicker tissues. For all tissues, permeability was higher for drugs with intermediate lipophilicity, mostly β-blockers, flupirtine, and nepafenac. Permeability might also be affected by drug ionization in the medium since charged molecules remain in the aqueous medium to a greater degree. By observing data through this prism, we can notice that the highest transported amounts were observed for drugs with a higher pKa, behaving as weak bases that tend to be ionized at pH 7.4. For most drugs, the bovine and porcine permeabilities were comparable. However, β-blockers, flupirtine, and nepafenac showed higher permeability through the bovine cornea. Differences have been reported in the conformation of collagen packaging between these two tissues, with porcine displaying more regular, approximately orthogonal layers and bovine displaying more randomly interwoven layers [52]. These differences might also have a role in the behavior of the cornea as a barrier since regular packaging may provide higher fiber density to the tissue, thereby increasing barrier capacity.

Tissue uptake behaved like cumulative transport, with the influence of the epithelium layer more noticeable. The lipophilic character of this layer increases the retention of lipophilic drugs, which was the case for all species. It is possible to notice that bovine and porcine corneas showed higher uptake of drugs with intermediate lipophilicity, while rabbit cornea showed higher uptake of drugs with higher lipophilicity. Rabbit cornea has a lower thickness than the other tissues, with this difference observed mainly for the hydrophilic stroma. Therefore, it is possible that in rabbit cornea, the lipophilic character of the epithelium is more prominent, thus favoring the uptake of lipophilic drugs per unit of tissue weight. On the other hand, for bovine and porcine corneas, the stroma might have a higher influence, allowing for the uptake of less lipophilic drugs.

A high correlation was found between P_{app} and cumulative transport for all species. This correlation is expected since P_{app} is obtained from the slope of the cumulative transport curve, and all cumulative transport data were normalized to the percent of the initial amount. The same degree of correlation was not observed between cumulative transport or P_{app} and tissue uptake, with weak to no correlation observed for all species, which indicates the influence of different factors on these two phenomena.

When comparing species, a high correlation was also found for cumulative transport and P_{app} between the species. A good to weak correlation was found between porcine or bovine and rabbit for tissue uptake, although the uptake across species was similar based on a slope close to 1. A high correlation was observed between bovine and porcine cornea for this parameter. It is important to note that bovine and porcine corneas showed not only a high correlation for the parameters measured but also that the correlation slopes were close to 1, indicating that the values observed were of the same order. Generally, the permeability differed between the species more than the tissue uptake, consistent with differences in tissue thickness.

P_{app} and tissue uptake showed a good correlation with $LogD_{7.4}$ (Figure 4), which was the most relevant molecular descriptor indicated by modeling. The correlation followed a sigmoidal relationship, also reported by some authors [17,53,54]. In this relationship, the $LogD_{7.4}$ value at half-maximum was taken as a comparison parameter (Table 2) and showed that, for β-blockers and steroids, optimal $LogD_{7.4}$ values for tissue permeation were lower than those for uptake. NSAIDs, on the other hand, showed the opposite behavior of β-blockers and steroids, with higher half-maximum $LogD_{7.4}$ values for P_{app} than for tissue uptake and higher maximum uptake for rabbit cornea. While permeability for the three drug classes and uptake for NSAIDs appeared to reach a more definite maximum in all species, tissue uptake of β-blockers in all species and corticosteroids in bovine cornea appeared to have more room for accumulation with a further increase in LogD beyond what was tested. The lack of saturation of corticosteroid uptake in the bovine eye might be due to the greater number of epithelial cell layers in this species. In general, the highest uptake and permeability were observed for β-blockers.

Data modeling using MLR provided models with a high degree ($0.822 \leq R \leq 0.940$) of correlation for all parameters tested. For the permeability and cumulative transport parameters, the best-fit models contained as x-variables the number of hydrogen bond sites, the nitrogen atom ratio in the molecule, the number of rotatable bonds, the molar volume, the index of refraction, and the LogD at a pH of 7.4. It is important to note that for the permeability parameter, although the apparent permeability coefficient (P_{app}) was calculated, better models were obtained with flux as the y-variable.

For permeability and cumulative transport models, the number of hydrogen bond acceptor or donor sites is a variable frequently reported [55–57]. This parameter is directly related to the degree of polarity of the molecule, and, therefore, these sites can limit to a certain degree the permeation of a molecule through the barrier of the corneal epithelium, which is strongly lipophilic.

The nitrogen atom ratio in the molecule can also be a factor of strong influence on its permeability since these atoms can form polar groups in the molecule, participating in the formation of hydrogen bonds. Furthermore, nitrogen atoms are often present in these molecules as amine groups, which have a direct influence on the ionization state of the molecules at the pH of the medium. The ionization of molecules is a determining factor for their permeability not only through the cornea but also through any biological membrane [48].

The variable LogD at a pH of 7.4 was present in the most relevant models not only for cumulative transport and permeability but also for tissue uptake, being identified as the most relevant variable among those tested. Since LogD describes the octanol/water partition coefficient at experimental pH, this variable combines the influence of molecular structure and ionizable groups in its hydrophobicity, showing better experimental applicability than LogP in this context.

The refractive index is defined as the ratio between the speed of light in each substance and in a vacuum. The modification of the light speed when passing through a substance is due to the interaction between the electric field of light and the electronic cloud of the molecules. If the oscillation frequency of the incident light is like that of a particular atom, group, or molecule, the greater the interaction between them, the greater the refraction of light. Rocquefelte et al. [58] pointed out that the refractive index of a substance is closely related to its mass density, electron density, and the presence of chromophore groups and excitable electrons in the molecules. Several electron-dense groups are present in the molecules studied and contribute to the refraction of light since, in addition to absorbing radiation, these groups also enable greater attraction between drug molecules, such as nitrogen and oxygen heteroatoms, amine, carboxyl, carbonyl, and hydroxyl groups, as well as halogens.

Another factor that was shown to be relevant for the three tissues tested was the count of rotatable bonds in the molecules. Rotatable bonds comprise any single bond, not in a ring, bound to a nonterminal heavy (non-hydrogen and non-nitrogen) atom [59]. The influence of this variable has been described by some authors as either limiting or contributing to drug absorption, e.g., Veber et al. [59], Zakeri-Milani et al. [60], Iyer et al. [61], and Davis, Gerry, and Tan [62]. Either way, the presence of rotatable bonds can lead to conformational changes in the molecules, and these shape changes can determine the molecule's ability to pass through or be retained in densely packed barriers such as corneal epithelium [63].

Modeling results have indicated the influence of molar volume on permeability through the cornea. This size-related descriptor has also been used [64,65] as a correction factor for permeability through other biological and artificial membranes, since size may be a determinant property for permeability limited by porous structures.

Data modeling for the tissue uptake parameter showed the relevance of different variables for the different tissues evaluated, although it is possible to highlight some similarities between them. First, it is possible to verify the influence of the presence of polar regions in the molecules, represented by the variables of hydrogen bond acceptor sites for bovine and the sum of hydrogen bond donor and acceptor sites in the rabbit cornea, as well as by the ratios of nitrogen and of heteroatoms in the molecules. The influence of polarity is also represented by the variable LogD at pH 7.4 in all the models obtained. Structural properties also had an influence on the uptake, as evidenced by the relevance of rotatable bonds and molecular weight. It is important to notice that, regarding size-related properties such as molar volume and molecular weight, the latter might account better for the presence of oxygen and nitrogen atoms since these atoms might increase the molecular weight without significantly altering the molar volume [66].

Bioavailability assessment represents a crucial step in drug feasibility evaluation. When considering ocular drug delivery, bioavailability is restricted by barriers present in the eye. For topical drug delivery to the anterior chamber, three main barriers may be considered: blinking and tear fluid drainage, cornea, and conjunctiva, each presenting unique absorption-limiting characteristics.

The conjunctival epithelium is composed of 2 to 3 stratified cell layers bound by tight junctions, but different from corneal epithelium, conjunctiva presents a higher density of pores ranging from 4.9 to 3.0 nm in diameter, thus permitting the paracellular absorption of hydrophilic and large molecules, according to Lawrence and Miller [67]. These structural properties make the conjunctiva more permeable than the cornea for many drug classes.

However, the permeability properties of the conjunctiva depend on isolation and tissue mounting techniques, with poor isolation techniques resulting in the loss of integrity of the conjunctival barrier and the associated trans-tissue electrical resistance [68]. Thus, in vitro studies are inherently limited. Although a precise prediction of the in vivo pharmacokinetics of a drug will remain elusive, some useful information can be gathered from in vitro permeability data. Assuming that conjunctival permeability predominantly accounts for systemic availability while corneal permeability contributes predominantly to aqueous humor bioavailability, we estimated the bioavailability for various drugs in this study. Our estimates indicated that overall bioavailability in aqueous humor after corneal absorption would be limited, with values ranging from 0.00 to 1.13%. The range observed is related to corneal barrier properties and perm-selectivity, which allow restricted and differential permeability to different compounds. Low aqueous humor bioavailability is expected for most drugs administered topically due to corneal barrier properties discussed previously in this article. It is apparent that systemic availability did not follow the previously reported trend. A limitation of the present approach is that blink-induced rapid tear drainage was not considered. Additionally, nasal absorption contributes 50% or more to the systemic absorption of β-blockers [15]. Thus, nasal permeability and blink-induced drainage rates should be factored in to better estimate the systemic as well as topical bioavailability of ophthalmic drugs. Further, most literature-reported permeabilities for the conjunctiva may be overestimates due to improper tissue isolation, magnifying the conjunctival clearance of drugs estimated in this study.

For β-blockers, diffusion and partition coefficients in the conjunctiva are reportedly higher than in the cornea [69]. Results indicated that systemic bioavailability would be more than 96% for β-blockers, except for sotalol, atenolol, and nadolol, hydrophilic β-blockers, which would be more susceptible to tear drainage but less permeable. This result agrees with the ones by Lee, Kompella, and Lee [15], in which the authors describe lower systemic bioavailability for hydrophilic β-blockers such as atenolol (41%). The authors also determined that nasal drainage contributes more to systemic absorption than the conjunctival pathway for systemic absorption. Corticosteroids, however, being predominantly lipophilic, showed possibly more limited conjunctival absorption than β-blockers, reflected mainly in triamcinolone, difluprednate, and triamcinolone hexacetonide. It is important to note that in rabbit conjunctival epithelial cells, the presence of p-glycoprotein efflux pumps was reported, which might hinder the absorption of lipophilic drugs [70]. Such mechanisms are described also for human and rabbit corneas [71] and might also be present in porcine cornea, thus explaining the lower slope observed for this drug class in the model obtained (Table 5). NSAIDs, on the other hand, would benefit from the presence of a sodium-dependent monocarboxylate transport process in the mucosal side of the conjunctiva [72], which would facilitate absorption. The influence of this mechanism might be reflected in the high model slope and bioavailability values found for this drug class, with ketoprofen being the only NSAID with an estimated systemic bioavailability lower than 80%.

5. Conclusions

Ex vivo corneal models for drug permeability are relevant in the preclinical stages of drug evaluation to identify drug candidates or formulations with superior permeability and to predict drug bioavailability in vivo. Different species have been used to evaluate the permeation of drugs through the cornea, including rabbit, porcine, and bovine. The present study compared the permeability of twenty-five drugs across the corneas of these three species and developed predictive equations as well as interspecies correlations for drug permeability and tissue uptake. This study established a single equation to predict corneal drug delivery in multiple species based on tissue thickness and drug properties such as lipophilicity and polar intermolecular interactions. Such equations help explain species differences in drug permeability and delivery.

A high correlation was observed between bovine, porcine, and rabbit corneas for permeability, with the permeability being comparable for bovine and porcine eyes and higher for the rabbit cornea. Permeability differences between species could be explained in part by differences in corneal thickness. Although tissue uptakes in all three species were similar, a high correlation was observed for tissue uptake between bovine and porcine corneas. The correlations between the properties observed in bovine and porcine corneas indicate that bovine cornea is acceptable for drug or formulation screening since it can provide data like porcine tissues, which are reportedly similar to human corneal tissue.

Estimation of drug bioavailability using ex vivo data indicated that topical absorption into aqueous humor would be limited for all drugs considered, with most of the dose being absorbed into the systemic circulation. Although the order of magnitude of bioavailability in aqueous humor may be comparable to literature-reported values, the trends may not be as reported. There is room to improve bioavailability predictions.

Bovine cornea has significantly higher thickness [36] than porcine and rabbit corneas, with more cell layers in the epithelium [28]. Stroma is also responsible for the higher thickness of bovine cornea [33]. Bovine cornea was established as a model for ocular irritancy by Gautheron et al. in 1992 [73], and in 1994 [74], it was assessed as a model for permeability by the same group. However, since then, bovine cornea has been used mainly for the evaluation of ocular irritancy. Thus, this work presents an important contribution to the literature since it evaluated bovine corneal permeability and the uptake of several drugs.

Future studies will evaluate in vivo delivery of the cassette, the effect of the cassette on barrier integrity, and enhance mathematical models to predict in vivo delivery based on in vitro delivery.

Supplementary Materials: The following supporting information can be downloaded at: https://www.mdpi.com/article/10.3390/pharmaceutics15061646/s1, Table S1: Physicochemical properties of drugs used in building quantitative structure-permeability relationships for bovine, porcine, and rabbit corneas.

Author Contributions: Conceptualization, U.B.K.; Methodology, C.P.S., B.A.M., M.A.P. and U.B.K.; Software, C.P.S. and B.A.M.; Validation, C.P.S. and B.A.M.; Formal analysis, C.P.S., B.A.M., M.A.P., A.S.-C. and U.B.K.; Investigation, C.P.S., B.A.M., A.S.-C. and U.B.K.; Resources, A.S.-C. and U.B.K.; Data curation, B.A.M. and U.B.K.; Writing—original draft, C.P.S.; Writing—review & editing, U.B.K., C.P.S., B.A.M., A.S.-C. and M.A.P.; Visualization, C.P.S. and U.B.K.; Supervision, U.B.K.; Project administration, A.S.-C. and U.B.K.; Funding acquisition, A.S.-C. and U.B.K. All authors have read and agreed to the published version of the manuscript.

Funding: This study was financed in part by the Coordenação de Aperfeiçoamento de Pessoal de Nível Superior—Brasil (CAPES)—Finance Code 001.

Institutional Review Board Statement: Not applicable.

Data Availability Statement: The data presented in this study are available within the article or in the Supplementary Material.

Acknowledgments: The authors are thankful to Rachel R. Hartman for her data review and assistance in the preparation of this manuscript.

Conflicts of Interest: The authors declare no conflict of interest.

References

1. Gaballa, S.A.; Kompella, U.B.; Elgarhy, O.; Alqahtani, A.M.; Pierscionek, B.; Alany, R.G.; Abdelkader, H. Corticosteroids in ophthalmology: Drug delivery innovations, pharmacology, clinical applications, and future perspectives. *Drug Deliv. Transl. Res.* **2021**, *11*, 866–893. [CrossRef] [PubMed]
2. Rajapakshal, A.; Fink, M.; Todd, B.A. Size-Dependent Diffusion of Dextrans in Excised Porcine Corneal Stroma. *Mol. Cell. Biomech.* **2015**, *12*, 215–230.
3. Coca-Prados, M. The blood-aqueous barrier in health and disease. *J. Glaucoma* **2014**, *23*, S36–S38. [CrossRef] [PubMed]
4. Cunha-Vaz, J.; Bernardes, R.; Lobo, C. Blood-retinal barrier. *Eur. J. Ophthalmol.* **2011**, *21* (Suppl. S6), S3–S9. [CrossRef] [PubMed]
5. Maurice, D.M. Drug delivery to the posterior segment from drops. *Surv. Ophthalmol.* **2002**, *47* (Suppl. S1), S41–S52. [CrossRef]

6. Yavuz, B.; Kompella, U. Ocular Drug Delivery. In *Handbook of Experimental Pharmacology*; Springer: Berlin/Heidelberg, Germany, 2017; Volume 242, pp. 57–93. [CrossRef]
7. Tang-Liu, D.D.; Liu, S.; Neff, J.; Sandri, R. Disposition of levobunolol after an ophthalmic dose to rabbits. *J. Pharm. Sci.* **1987**, *76*, 780–783. [CrossRef]
8. Tang-Liu, D.D.; Liu, S.S.; Weinkam, R.J. Ocular and systemic bioavailability of ophthalmic flurbiprofen. *J. Pharm. Biopharm.* **1984**, *12*, 611–626. [CrossRef]
9. Naageshwaran, V.; Ranta, V.P.; Toropainen, E.; Tuomainen, M.; Gum, G.; Xie, E.; Bhoopathy, S.; Urtti, A.; Del Amo, E.M. Topical pharmacokinetics of dexamethasone suspensions in the rabbit eye: Bioavailability comparison. *Int. J. Pharm.* **2022**, *615*, 121515. [CrossRef]
10. Fayyaz, A.; Ranta, V.P.; Toropainen, E.; Vellonen, K.S.; Valtari, A.; Puranen, J.; Ruponen, M.; Gardner, I.; Urtti, A.; Jamei, M.; et al. Topical ocular pharmacokinetics and bioavailability for a cocktail of atenolol, timolol and betaxolol in rabbits. *Eur. J. Pharm. Sci.* **2020**, *155*, 105553. [CrossRef]
11. Zhang, W.; Prausnitz, M.R.; Edwards, A. Model of transient drug diffusion across cornea. *J. Control Release* **2004**, *99*, 241–258. [CrossRef]
12. Tsubota, K. Tear dynamics and dry eye. *Prog. Retin. Eye Res.* **1998**, *17*, 565–596. [CrossRef]
13. Pflugfelder, S.C.; Stern, M.E. Biological functions of tear film. *Exp. Eye Res.* **2020**, *197*, 108115. [CrossRef]
14. Garaszczuk, I.K.; Montes Mico, R.; Iskander, D.R.; Expósito, A.C. The tear turnover and tear clearance tests—A review. *Expert. Rev. Med. Devices* **2018**, *15*, 219–229. [CrossRef]
15. Lee, Y.H.; Kompella, U.B.; Lee, V.H. Systemic absorption pathways of topically applied beta adrenergic antagonists in the pigmented rabbit. *Exp. Eye Res.* **1993**, *57*, 341–349. [CrossRef]
16. Schoenwald, R.D.; Huang, H.S. Corneal penetration behavior of beta-blocking agents I: Physiochemical factors. *J. Pharm. Sci.* **1983**, *72*, 1266–1272. [CrossRef]
17. Huang, H.S.; Schoenwald, R.D.; Lach, J.L. Corneal penetration behavior of beta-blocking agents II: Assessment of barrier contributions. *J. Pharm. Sci.* **1983**, *72*, 1272–1279. [CrossRef]
18. Karami, T.K.; Hailu, S.; Feng, S.; Graham, R.; Gukasyan, H.J. Eyes on Lipinski's Rule of Five: A New "Rule of Thumb" for Physicochemical Design Space of Ophthalmic Drugs. *J. Ocul. Pharm.* **2022**, *38*, 43–55. [CrossRef]
19. Grass, G.M.; Robinson, J.R. Mechanisms of corneal drug penetration I: In vivo and in vitro kinetics. *J. Pharm. Sci.* **1988**, *77*, 3–14. [CrossRef]
20. Eller, M.G.; Schoenwald, R.D.; Dixson, J.A.; Segarra, T.; Barfknecht, C.F. Topical Carbonic Anhydrase Inhibitors III: Optimization Model for Corneal Penetration of Ethoxzolamide Analogues. *J. Pharm. Sci.* **1985**, *74*, 155–160. [CrossRef]
21. Kidron, H.; Vellonen, K.S.; del Amo, E.M.; Tissari, A.; Urtti, A. Prediction of the Corneal Permeability of Drug-Like Compounds. *Pharm. Res.* **2010**, *27*, 1398–1407. [CrossRef]
22. Ashton, P.; Podder, S.K.; Lee, V.H.L. Formulation influence on conjunctival penetration of 4-beta blockers in the pigmented rabbit—A comparison with corneal penetration. *Pharm. Res.* **1991**, *8*, 1166–1174. [CrossRef] [PubMed]
23. Brock, D.J.; Kondow-McConaghy, H.; Allen, J.; Brkljača, Z.; Kustigian, L.; Jiang, M.; Zhang, J.; Rye, H.; Vazdar, M.; Pellois, J.P. Mechanism of Cell Penetration by Permeabilization of Late Endosomes: Interplay between a Multivalent TAT Peptide and Bis(monoacylglycero)phosphate. *Cell. Chem. Biol.* **2020**, *27*, 1296–1307.e1295. [CrossRef] [PubMed]
24. Loch, C.; Zakelj, S.; Kristl, A.; Nagel, S.; Guthoff, R.; Weitschies, W.; Seidlitz, A. Determination of permeability coefficients of ophthalmic drugs through different layers of porcine, rabbit and bovine eyes. *Eur. J. Pharm. Sci.* **2012**, *47*, 131–138. [CrossRef] [PubMed]
25. Chan, T.; Payor, S.; Holden, B.A. Corneal thickness profiles in rabbits using an ultrasonic pachometer. *Investig. Ophthalmol. Vis. Sci.* **1983**, *24*, 1408–1410.
26. Missel, P.; Chastain, J.; Mitra, A.; Kompella, U.; Kansara, V.; Duvvuri, S.; Amrite, A.; Cheruvu, N. In vitro transport and partitioning of AL-4940, active metabolite of angiostatic agent anecortave acetate, in ocular tissues of the posterior segment. *J. Ocul. Pharm.* **2010**, *26*, 137–146. [CrossRef]
27. Oliveira, G.A.; Ducas Rdo, N.; Teixeira, G.C.; Batista, A.C.; Oliveira, D.P.; Valadares, M.C. Short Time Exposure (STE) test in conjunction with Bovine Corneal Opacity and Permeability (BCOP) assay including histopathology to evaluate correspondence with the Globally Harmonized System (GHS) eye irritation classification of textile dyes. *Toxicol. Vitr.* **2015**, *29*, 1283–1288. [CrossRef]
28. Van den Berghe, C.; Guillet, M.C.; Compan, D. Performance of porcine corneal opacity and permeability assay to predict eye irritation for water-soluble cosmetic ingredients. *Toxicol. Vitr.* **2005**, *19*, 823–830. [CrossRef]
29. Pescina, S.; Govoni, P.; Potenza, A.; Padula, C.; Santi, P.; Nicoli, S. Development of a convenient ex vivo model for the study of transcorneal permeation of drugs: Histological and permeability evaluation. *J. Pharm. Sci.* **2015**, *104*, 63–71. [CrossRef]
30. Doughty, M.J.; Petrou, S.; Macmillan, H. Anatomy and morphology of the cornea of bovine eyes from a slaughterhouse. *Can. J. Zool.* **1995**, *73*, 2159–2165. [CrossRef]
31. Elsheikh, A.; Alhasso, D. Mechanical anisotropy of porcine cornea and correlation with stromal microstructure. *Exp. Eye Res.* **2009**, *88*, 1084–1091. [CrossRef]
32. Li, H.F.; Petroll, W.M.; Møller-Pedersen, T.; Maurer, J.K.; Cavanagh, H.D.; Jester, J.V. Epithelial and corneal thickness measurements by in vivo confocal microscopy through focusing (CMTF). *Curr. Eye Res.* **1997**, *16*, 214–221. [CrossRef]

33. Kim, Y.L.; Walsh, J.T., Jr.; Goldstick, T.K.; Glucksberg, M.R. Variation of corneal refractive index with hydration. *Phys. Med. Biol.* **2004**, *49*, 859–868. [CrossRef]
34. Wollensak, G.; Spoerl, E.; Seiler, T. Stress-strain measurements of human and porcine corneas after riboflavin–ultraviolet-A-induced cross-linking. *J. Cataract. Refract. Surg.* **2003**, *29*, 1780–1785. [CrossRef]
35. Goskonda, V.R.; Hill, R.A.; Khan, M.A.; Reddy, I.K. Permeability of chemical delivery systems across rabbit corneal (SIRC) cell line and isolated corneas: A comparative study. *Pharm. Dev. Technol.* **2000**, *5*, 409–416. [CrossRef]
36. Boyce, B.L.; Grazier, J.M.; Jones, R.E.; Nguyen, T.D. Full-field deformation of bovine cornea under constrained inflation conditions. *Biomaterials* **2008**, *29*, 3896–3904. [CrossRef]
37. Wollensak, G.; Aurich, H.; Pham, D.T.; Wirbelauer, C. Hydration behavior of porcine cornea crosslinked with riboflavin and ultraviolet A. *J. Cataract. Refract. Surg.* **2007**, *33*, 516–521. [CrossRef]
38. Wollensak, G.; Iomdina, E. Long-term biomechanical properties of rabbit cornea after photodynamic collagen crosslinking. *Acta Ophthalmol.* **2009**, *87*, 48–51. [CrossRef]
39. Attama, A.A.; Reichl, S.; Müller-Goymann, C.C. Diclofenac sodium delivery to the eye: In vitro evaluation of novel solid lipid nanoparticle formulation using human cornea construct. *Int. J. Pharm.* **2008**, *355*, 307–313. [CrossRef]
40. Matter, B.; Bourne, D.W.A.; Kompella, U.B. A High-Throughput LC-MS/MS Method for the Simultaneous Quantification of Twenty-Seven Drug Molecules in Ocular Tissues. *Aaps PharmSciTech* **2022**, *23*, 14. [CrossRef]
41. Roy, K.; Kar, S.; Ambure, P. On a simple approach for determining applicability domain of QSAR models. *Chemom. Intell. Lab. Syst.* **2015**, *145*, 22–29. [CrossRef]
42. Consonni, V.; Ballabio, D.; Todeschini, R. Evaluation of model predictive ability by external validation techniques. *J. Chemometr.* **2010**, *24*, 194–201. [CrossRef]
43. Ramsay, E.; Del Amo, E.M.; Toropainen, E.; Tengvall-Unadike, U.; Ranta, V.P.; Urtti, A.; Ruponen, M. Corneal and conjunctival drug permeability: Systematic comparison and pharmacokinetic impact in the eye. *Eur. J. Pharm. Sci.* **2018**, *119*, 83–89. [CrossRef] [PubMed]
44. Lee, V.H.; Robinson, J.R. Topical ocular drug delivery: Recent developments and future challenges. *J. Ocul. Pharm.* **1986**, *2*, 67–108. [CrossRef] [PubMed]
45. Prausnitz, M.R.; Noonan, J.S. Permeability of cornea, sclera, and conjunctiva: A literature analysis for drug delivery to the eye. *J. Pharm. Sci.* **1998**, *87*, 1479–1488. [CrossRef] [PubMed]
46. Greiner, J.V.; Kopp, S.J.; Lass, J.H.; Gold, J.B.; Glonek, T. Metabolic compatibility of abattoir and human corneas: An ex vivo 31P nuclear magnetic resonance spectroscopic study of intact tissues. *Cornea* **1993**, *12*, 461–465. [CrossRef]
47. Greiner, J.V.; Lass, J.H.; Glonek, T. Interspecies analysis of corneal phosphate metabolites. *Exp. Eye Res.* **1989**, *49*, 523–529. [CrossRef]
48. Subasinghe, S.K.; Ogbuehi, K.C.; Mitchell, L.; Dias, G.J. Animal model with structural similarity to human corneal collagen fibrillar arrangement. *Anat. Sci. Int.* **2021**, *96*, 286–293. [CrossRef]
49. Sanchez, I.; Martin, R.; Ussa, F.; Fernandez-Bueno, I. The parameters of the porcine eyeball. *Graefes Arch. Clin. Exp. Ophthalmol.* **2011**, *249*, 475–482. [CrossRef]
50. Hammond, G.M.; Young, R.D.; Muir, D.D.; Quantock, A.J. The microanatomy of Bowman's layer in the cornea of the pig: Changes in collagen fibril architecture at the corneoscleral limbus. *Eur. J. Anat.* **2020**, *24*, 399–406.
51. Hayashi, S.; Osawa, T.; Tohyama, K. Comparative observations on corneas, with special reference to Bowman's layer and Descemet's membrane in mammals and amphibians. *J. Morphol.* **2002**, *254*, 247–258. [CrossRef]
52. Bueno, J.M.; Gualda, E.J.; Artal, P. Analysis of corneal stroma organization with wavefront optimized nonlinear microscopy. *Cornea* **2011**, *30*, 692–701. [CrossRef]
53. Wang, W.; Sasaki, H.; Chien, D.S.; Lee, V.H. Lipophilicity influence on conjunctival drug penetration in the pigmented rabbit: A comparison with corneal penetration. *Curr. Eye Res.* **1991**, *10*, 571–579. [CrossRef]
54. Toropainen, E.; Ranta, V.P.; Vellonen, K.S.; Palmgrén, J.; Talvitie, A.; Laavola, M.; Suhonen, P.; Hämäläinen, K.M.; Auriola, S.; Urtti, A. Paracellular and passive transcellular permeability in immortalized human corneal epithelial cell culture model. *Eur. J. Pharm. Sci.* **2003**, *20*, 99–106. [CrossRef]
55. Over, B.; Matsson, P.; Tyrchan, C.; Artursson, P.; Doak, B.C.; Foley, M.A.; Hilgendorf, C.; Johnston, S.E.; Lee, M.D.; Lewis, R.J.; et al. Structural and conformational determinants of macrocycle cell permeability. *Nat. Chem. Biol.* **2016**, *12*, 1065–1074. [CrossRef]
56. Diukendjieva, A.; Tsakovska, I.; Alov, P.; Pencheva, T.; Pajeva, I.; Worth, A.P.; Madden, J.C.; Cronin, M.T.D. Advances in the prediction of gastrointestinal absorption: Quantitative Structure-Activity Relationship (QSAR) modelling of PAMPA permeability. *Comput. Toxicol.* **2019**, *10*, 51–59. [CrossRef]
57. Janicka, M.; Sztanke, M.; Sztanke, K. Predicting the Blood-Brain Barrier Permeability of New Drug-Like Compounds via HPLC with Various Stationary Phases. *Molecules* **2020**, *25*, 487. [CrossRef]
58. Rocquefelte, X.; Goubin, F.; Koo, H.J.; Whangbo, M.H.; Jobic, S. Investigation of the origin of the empirical relationship between refractive index and density on the basis of first principles calculations for the refractive indices of various TiO_2 phases. *Inorg. Chem.* **2004**, *43*, 2246–2251. [CrossRef]
59. Veber, D.F.; Johnson, S.R.; Cheng, H.Y.; Smith, B.R.; Ward, K.W.; Kopple, K.D. Molecular properties that influence the oral bioavailability of drug candidates. *J. Med. Chem.* **2002**, *45*, 2615–2623. [CrossRef]

60. Zakeri, M.P.; Tajerzadeh, H.; Eslamboulchilar, Z.; Barzegar, S.; Valizadeh, H. The relation between molecular properties of drugs and their transport across intestinal membrane. *DARU J. Pharm. Sci.* **2006**, *14*, 164–171.
61. Iyer, M.; Tseng, Y.J.; Senese, C.L.; Liu, J.Z.; Hopfinger, A.J. Prediction and mechanistic interpretation of human oral drug absorption using MI-QSAR analysis. *Mol. Pharm.* **2007**, *4*, 218–231. [CrossRef]
62. Davis, T.D.; Gerry, C.J.; Tan, D.S. General platform for systematic quantitative evaluation of small-molecule permeability in bacteria. *ACS Chem. Biol.* **2014**, *9*, 2535–2544. [CrossRef] [PubMed]
63. Suenderhauf, C.; Hammann, F.; Huwyler, J. Computational prediction of blood-brain barrier permeability using decision tree induction. *Molecules* **2012**, *17*, 10429–10445. [CrossRef] [PubMed]
64. Genty, M.; Gonzalez, G.; Clere, C.; Desangle-Gouty, V.; Legendre, J.Y. Determination of the passive absorption through the rat intestine using chromatographic indices and molar volume. *Eur. J. Pharm. Sci.* **2001**, *12*, 223–229. [CrossRef] [PubMed]
65. Yoon, C.H.; Shin, B.S.; Chang, H.S.; Kwon, L.S.; Kim, H.Y.; Yoo, S.E.; Yoo, S.D. Rapid screening of drug absorption potential using the immobilized artificial membrane phosphatidylcholine column and molar volume. *Chromatographia* **2004**, *60*, 399–404. [CrossRef]
66. Ghafourian, T.; Fooladi, S. The effect of structural QSAR parameters on skin penetration. *Int. J. Pharm.* **2001**, *217*, 1–11. [CrossRef]
67. Lawrence, M.S.; Miller, J.W. Ocular tissue permeabilities. *Int. Ophthalmol. Clin.* **2004**, *44*, 53–61. [CrossRef]
68. Kompella, U.B.; Kim, K.J.; Lee, V.H. Active chloride transport in the pigmented rabbit conjunctiva. *Curr. Eye Res.* **1993**, *12*, 1041–1048. [CrossRef]
69. Sasaki, H.; Igarashi, Y.; Nagano, T.; Yamamura, K.; Nishida, K.; Nakamura, J. Penetration of β-blockers through ocular membranes in a1bino rabbits. *J. Pharm. Pharmacol.* **1995**, *47*, 17–21. [CrossRef]
70. Saha, P.; Yang, J.J.; Lee, V.H.L. Existence of a p-glycoprotein drug efflux pump in cultured rabbit conjunctival epithelial cells. *Investig. Ophthalmol. Vis. Sci.* **1998**, *39*, 1221–1226.
71. Dey, S.; Gunda, S.; Mitra, A.K. Pharmacokinetics of erythromycin in rabbit corneas after single-dose infusion: Role of P-glycoprotein as a barrier to in vivo ocular drug absorption. *J. Pharmacol. Exp. Ther.* **2004**, *311*, 246–255. [CrossRef]
72. Horibe, Y.; Hosoya, K.; Kim, K.J.; Lee, V.H.L. Carrier-mediated transport of monocarboxylate drugs in the pigmented rabbit conjunctiva. *Investig. Ophthalmol. Vis. Sci.* **1998**, *39*, 1436–1443.
73. Gautheron, P.; Dukic, M.; Alix, D.; Sina, J.F. Bovine corneal opacity and permeability test: An in vitro assay of ocular irritancy. *Fundam. Appl. Toxicol.* **1992**, *18*, 442–449. [CrossRef]
74. Gautheron, P.; Giroux, J.; Cottin, M.; Audegond, L.; Morilla, A.; Mayordomo-Blanco, L.; Tortajada, A.; Haynes, G.; Vericat, J.A.; Pirovano, R.; et al. Interlaboratory assessment of the bovine corneal opacity and permeability (BCOP) assay. *Toxicol. In Vitro* **1994**, *8*, 381–392. [CrossRef]

Disclaimer/Publisher's Note: The statements, opinions and data contained in all publications are solely those of the individual author(s) and contributor(s) and not of MDPI and/or the editor(s). MDPI and/or the editor(s) disclaim responsibility for any injury to people or property resulting from any ideas, methods, instructions or products referred to in the content.

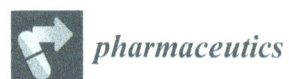

Article

Exploration of the Safety and Solubilization, Dissolution, Analgesic Effects of Common Basic Excipients on the NSAID Drug Ketoprofen

Heba A. Abou-Taleb [1], Mai E. Shoman [2], Tarek Saad Makram [3], Jelan A. Abdel-Aleem [4] and Hamdy Abdelkader [5,*]

[1] Department of Pharmaceutics and Industrial Pharmacy, Faculty of Pharmacy, Merit University (MUE), Sohag 82755, Egypt
[2] Department of Medicinal Chemistry, Faculty of Pharmacy, Minia University, Minia 61519, Egypt
[3] Department of Pharmaceutics and Industrial Pharmacy, Faculty of Pharmacy, October 6 University, October 6 12585, Egypt
[4] Department of Industrial Pharmacy, Faculty of Pharmacy, Assiut University, Assiut 71526, Egypt
[5] Department of Pharmaceutics, College of Pharmacy, King Khalid University, Abha 61441, Saudi Arabia
* Correspondence: habdelkader@kku.edu.sa

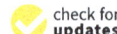

Citation: Abou-Taleb, H.A.; Shoman, M.E.; Makram, T.S.; Abdel-Aleem, J.A.; Abdelkader, H. Exploration of the Safety and Solubilization, Dissolution, Analgesic Effects of Common Basic Excipients on the NSAID Drug Ketoprofen. *Pharmaceutics* **2023**, *15*, 713. https://doi.org/10.3390/pharmaceutics15020713

Academic Editor: Peter Timmins

Received: 25 January 2023
Revised: 16 February 2023
Accepted: 17 February 2023
Published: 20 February 2023

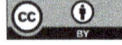

Copyright: © 2023 by the authors. Licensee MDPI, Basel, Switzerland. This article is an open access article distributed under the terms and conditions of the Creative Commons Attribution (CC BY) license (https://creativecommons.org/licenses/by/4.0/).

Abstract: Since its introduction to the market in the 1970s, ketoprofen has been widely used due to its high efficacy in moderate pain management. However, its poor solubility and ulcer side effects have diminished its popularity. This study prepared forms of ketoprofen modified with three basic excipients: tris, L-lysine, and L-arginine, and investigated their ability to improve water solubility and reduce ulcerogenic potential. The complexation/salt formation of ketoprofen and the basic excipients was prepared using physical mixing and coprecipitation methods. The prepared mixtures were studied for solubility, docking, dissolution, differential scanning calorimetry (DSC), Fourier transform infrared spectroscopy (FTIR), in vivo evaluation for efficacy (the writhing test), and safety (ulcerogenic liability). Phase solubility diagrams were constructed, and a linear solubility (AL type) curve was obtained with tris. Docking studies suggested a possible salt formation with L-arginine using Hirshfeld surface analysis. The order of enhancement of solubility and dissolution rates was as follows: L-arginine > L-lysine > tris. In vivo analgesic evaluation indicated a significant enhancement of the onset of action of analgesic activities for the three basic excipients. However, safety and gastric protection indicated that both ketoprofen arginine and ketoprofen lysine salts were more favorable than ketoprofen tris.

Keywords: ketoprofen; L-arginine; L-lysine; tris; basic amino acids; writhing; gastric ulcer

1. Introduction

An estimated 40% of commercially available drugs and up to 90% of newly discovered drug candidates have poor water solubility [1,2]. As a result, the development of solubilization techniques, as well as the search for new hydrotropes and potential water-soluble excipients to enhance the solubility and dissolution rates of poorly soluble drugs, has been an ongoing endeavor for formulation scientists [3,4]. Ketoprofen (Figure 1) is a non-steroidal anti-inflammatory drug (NSAID) that was discovered in 1968 [5]. It is the most commonly prescribed NSAID for various acute and chronic pain conditions, such as moderate to severe dental pain and osteoarthritis [5]. Ketoprofen is sold worldwide under different brand names, including as Orudis® capsules in the USA and as the over-the-counter (OTC) medication Ketofan® (25 mg immediate-release tablets and 50 mg capsules) on the Egyptian market. However, poor water solubility and dissolution rates of ketoprofen have resulted in erratic drug absorption and inconsistent bioavailability, especially in the first part of the gastrointestinal tract. As a weak acid, the solubility of ketoprofen in acidic gastric fluid is minimal [6,7].

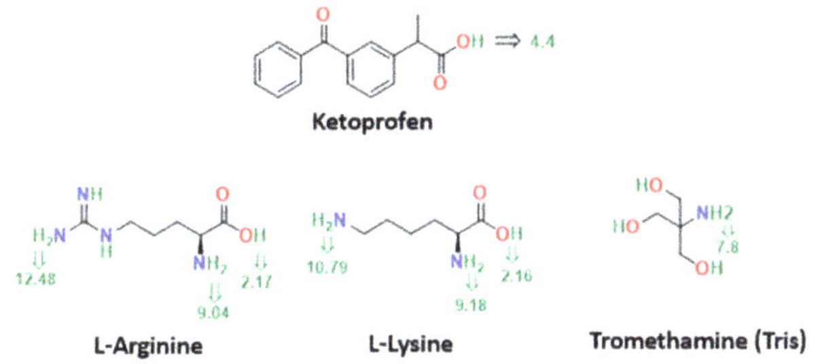

Figure 1. Structures and pKa values of ketoprofen, tris, L-lysine, and L-arginine.

Numerous solubilization techniques have been employed to improve solubility and dissolution rates of different water-insoluble drugs. These techniques include particle size reduction, solid dispersion, complexation, salt formation, cocrystallization, and nanoparticle encapsulation [8–10]. In addition, many water-soluble excipients have been used to improve the solubility and bioavailability of poorly soluble drugs. These include water-soluble macromolecules and hydrophilic polymers, such as polysaccharides, polyvinylpyrrolidone, polyethylene glycol, and cyclodextrins [10]. While these excipients have successfully enhanced the solubility of many drugs, their solubilizing capacity can be limited and require that they be used in large amounts, which can raise toxicological and regulatory concerns [3,10]. Low-molecular-weight excipients, such as urea and sugars, have also been extensively investigated. However, their solubilizing capacity is limited due to both their chemical neutrality and their lack of sufficient binding sites and ionizable groups [11].

In recent years, there has been a growing interest in investigating and utilizing amino acids due to their safety and tolerability. Amino acids are classified as GRAS (Generally Recognized as Safe) and are used as dietary supplements [4]. In addition, amino acids have been successfully used to solubilize both ionizable and non-ionizable drugs. They are small molecules with diverse chemical structures, and can be broadly classified into mainly amphoteric (e.g., glycine and alanine), acidic (e.g., aspartic acid and glutamic acid), or basic (e.g., arginine and lysine) amino acids (Figure 1). Additional side chains, such as hydroxyl and sulfhydryl groups, can boost their solubilizing capacity [4,12].

Ketoprofen-L-lysine can exist in salt or cocrystal forms, depending on the preparation method. Both forms have enhanced dissolution characteristics, but the bitterness scores for these two forms of ketoprofen-L-lysine were higher than that of the parent drug [13]. In another study, ketoprofen–tromethamine was prepared by a coprecipitation method, resulting in a new crystalline state with significantly enhanced solubility and dissolution rates [14].

Tromethamine (also known as tris aminomethane) is a basic excipient and a widely used buffering agent in biochemistry and protein assays. Tris has been used to form water-soluble salts from weak acids such as ketorolac and nimesulide [15].

This study explored the impact of three basic excipients (lysine, arginine, and tromethamine, or tris) with different basicity and pKa values (Figure 1) on the solubility, dissolution rates, and analgesic efficacy of ketoprofen, as well as ulcer side effects. The aim was to rank and showcase any particular advantages of these basic excipients in improving the biopharmaceutical properties and safety profile of the NSAID drug ketoprofen.

The specific objectives of the study included the formation of solid dispersions and physical mixtures, the construction of phase solubility diagrams, thermal and dissolution studies, spectral and docking analysis, analgesic evaluation using the writhing test in mice, gastric ulcer liability, and histopathological examination.

2. Materials and Methods
2.1. Materials

Ketoprofen was provided by Pharco Pharmaceuticals (Alexandria, Egypt). L-arginine was purchased from Fluka AG (Buchs, Switzerland). L-lysine, tris, and sodium lauryl sulfate were obtained from Sigma-Aldrich (London, UK), and Ketofan® capsules were supplied by Amrya Pharmaceuticals (Amrya, Alexandria, Egypt). Empty hard gelatin capsules of size 0 were purchased from Isolab Laborgeräte (GmbH, Am Dillhof, Germany).

2.2. Preparation of Ketoprofen-Excipients Physical and Dispersed Mixtures

2.2.1. Physical Mixtures

Ketoprofen-L-lysine, L-arginine, and tris physical mixtures (PM) were prepared separately by weighing an equivalent molar weight in milligrams. The drug-excipient mixture was then thoroughly mixed in a porcelain dish for 2–3 min using a spatula and sieved through a 125-μm sieve.

2.2.2. Coprecipitated Mixtures of Ketoprofen:L-lysine, Ketoprofen:L-arginine, and Ketoprofen:tris

To prepare coprecipitated mixtures of ketoprofen with L-lysine, L-arginine, and tris, specific weights (in mg) equivalent to the molecular weight of ketoprofen were dissolved in 20 mL of methanol. Accurate weights (in mg) equivalent to the molecular weights of the basic amino acids (L-lysine and L-arginine) and tris were dissolved individually in 10 mL of distilled water. The methanolic solution of ketoprofen and the aqueous solutions of the basic excipients were mixed in a porcelain dish with a 100-mL capacity. The porcelain dish was placed on a hot plate stirrer (LabTech, Daihan, Korea), adjusted to 80 °C, and left until complete evaporation. The resulting powder was ground in a mortar and pestle and passed through a 125 μm sieve.

2.3. Equilibrium Solubility Studies

Excess amounts of ketoprofen were added to various solutions containing different concentrations of the basic excipients (0, 0.1, 0.2, 0.4, 0.5, 1, 2, and 3% *w/v*) of L-arginine, L-lysine, and tris. These mixtures were placed in a thermostatic shaking water bath (Shel Lab water bath, Sheldon Cornelius, OR, USA) at 37 °C ± 0.5 °C, rotating at a speed of 120 strokes per minute. The samples were left for 48 h to attain equilibrium; aliquots (4 mL) were withdrawn, filtered, and measured spectrophotometrically at λ_{max} = 260 nm using a UV-visible spectrophotometer (JENWAY-Model 6305, Chelmsford, UK). The solubility data (μg/mL) were obtained from the standard calibration curve with acceptable linearity (R^2 = 0.9955). The solubility constant (K) was calculated from the slope of the phase solubility diagram obtained from the regression line of solubility (μg/mL) versus concentration (mM) plots [9,15], as shown in the following equation:

$$K = \frac{Slope}{Intercept * (1 - slope)} \quad (1)$$

2.4. Differential Scanning Calorimetry (DSC) and Fourier Transfer Infrared Spectroscopy (FTIR)

Samples of ketoprofen, arginine, lysine, tris, physical mixtures (PM), and coprecipitated mixtures were weighed (2–4 mg) and placed in aluminum pans. The DSC Mettler Toledo Star System (Mettler Toledo, Zürich, Switzerland) was used to gradually increase the temperature from 30 to 300 °C at a rate of 10 °C/min, calibrated with an indium standard, and using nitrogen as a purging gas. A Thermo Scientific Nicole IS 10 FTIR spectrophotometer (Waltham, MA, USA) was used to compress potassium bromide samples into discs using a 10-ton hydraulic press. The samples were scanned 16 times from 400 to 4000 cm^{-1}, and data were collected using Omnic software from Thermo Scientific in Waltham, MA, USA.

2.5. In Vitro Dissolution

In vitro dissolution studies were conducted on two dissolution media. The first dissolution medium consisted of simulated gastric fluid (pH 1.2, 900 mL) containing 1% *w/w* sodium lauryl sulfate (SLS) for the first two hours. Then, in the same flask, the pH of the medium was increased to 6.8 using dibasic sodium phosphate for an additional three hours to simulate intestinal fluid. The dissolution media were agitated using USP apparatus 2 at 50 rpm and a temperature of 37 °C. Ketoprofen powder, PM, and Coppt dispersed mixtures weighing 20 mg (or equivalent to 20 mg of ketoprofen) were filled into hard gelatin capsules of size 0 (Isolab Laborgeräte, GmbH, Am Dillhof, Germany), placed in dissolution sinkers, and transferred to dissolution flasks. A 5 mL sample was withdrawn at specified intervals and replaced with another 5 mL of fresh dissolution medium. The samples were analyzed spectrophotometrically, as previously described in Section 2.3.

2.6. Molecular Docking

Molecular docking studies were performed with the Molecular Operating Environment (MOE) 2014.09 software (Chemical Computing Group, Montreal, QC, Canada) to predict the stability and possible orientation of various bases on the surface of ketoprofen. The 3D structure of ketoprofen was constructed using the builder interface, and its energy was minimized to an RMSD (root mean square deviation) gradient of 0.01 kcal/mol using the QuickPrep tool in the MOE software. Similarly, the 3D structures of arginine, lysine, and tromethamine were built using the MOE builder, and their energies were minimized. The three bases were docked onto the surface of ketoprofen using an induced-fit docking protocol with the Tri-angle Matcher method and dG scoring system for pose ranking. After a visual assessment of the resultant docking poses, those with the highest stability and lowest binding free energy values were selected and reported.

2.7. In Vivo Studies

2.7.1. Writhing Assay

Mice weighing between 25 and 30 g were used in the experiment. The ability of ketoprofen and the prepared coprecipitated mixtures of ketoprofen with the three basic excipients (tris, L-lysine, and L-arginine) to inhibit acetic acid-induced writhing was assessed as previously described [11]. The mice were divided into five groups, as outlined in Table 1. A dose of 50 mg/kg or its equivalent was dispersed in an aqueous solution containing 0.25% carboxymethyl cellulose (CMC) to make the tested solutions (2 mg/mL). An accurate sample (0.5 mL) of the tested solutions was administered orally through a gastric tube. After the dose was administered, 30 µL of diluted acetic acid solution (0.6% v/v) was injected intraperitoneally into the animals. Induced writhes were counted for 20 min.

Table 1. Different groups and treatments received in the writhing assay.

Group	Treatment
I	Solution of 0.25% CMC (Untreated)
II	Ketoprofen (K) suspended in 0.25% CMC
III	K:tris dispersed in 0.25% CMC
IV	K:L-lysine dispersed in 0.25% CMC
V	K:L-arginine dispersed in 0.25% CMC

2.7.2. Indomethacin-Induced Ulcer

Male albino rats were fasted for 24 h and given access to water. They were divided into six groups of five rats each. The positive control group received a single oral dose of indomethacin (30 mg/kg) through a gastric tube, while the control group received saline. The remaining four groups were given a single oral dose of 50 mg/kg of ketoprofen or its equivalent in K:tris, K:lysine, and K:arginine Coppt mixtures. Four hours after dosing, the animals were sacrificed, and their stomachs were dissected, flushed with saline, and opened for inspection of ulcer formation [16].

The ulcers were counted and quantified by pinning the stomach on a piece of flat cork and scoring the ulcers using a dissecting microscope. The area of mucosal damage (ulcer) was expressed as a percentage of the total surface area of the mucosal surface of the stomach [16].

2.8. Histopathological Documentation

The dissected stomachs from the control and treated groups were fixed in 10% formalin-buffered saline for several days, dehydrated, embedded in paraffin blocks, and then sectioned into 5 μm-thick slices. As previously reported, the final sections were stained with H&E stain for microscopic examination and imaging [17,18]. The aggregation of polysaccharides was visualized using periodic acid Schiff (PAS) staining [19].

3. Results and Discussion

3.1. Solubility Studies

The results of the equilibrium solubility of ketoprofen in the presence of increasing concentrations (w/v %) of the three basic excipients (L-lysine, L-arginine, and tris) are shown in Figure 2A. Phase solubility curves of ketoprofen with the three basic excipients were constructed (Figure 2B–D) to determine solubility type. The three basic excipients, tris, L-lysine, and L-arginine, at a concentration of 3% w/v, significantly ($p < 0.05$) improved the solubility of ketoprofen by 4, 4.65, and 6.8-fold, respectively. Arginine showed superior solubilization capacity compared to the other two basic excipients (Figure 2A). This solubility enhancement can be attributed to the electrostatic interaction and alkalinizing effects of the stagnant diffusion layer around dissolved particles of the basic excipients in the solvent, which increased the ionization of the weak acid drug [20]. Arginine (pKa = 12.48) is the strongest basic excipient compared to tris (pKa = 8) and lysine (pKa = 10). Hence, the diffusion layer becomes more alkaline and more ionization occurs, favoring the solubilization of the weak acid ketoprofen. Figure 2B–D shows the phase solubility curves (solubility (mM) against concentrations (mM) of the basic excipients). Tris obtained solely a linear relationship (AL). In contrast, nonlinear relationships were observed with arginine and lysine.

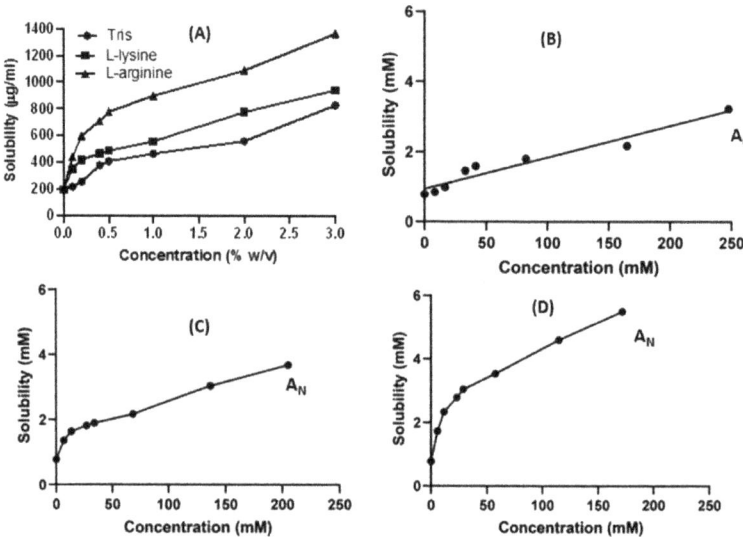

Figure 2. (**A**) Solubility curves μg/mL versus concentration of the three basic excipients (% w/v). Phase solubility curves (mM) versus concentrations of the three basic excipients (mM): (**B**) tris, (**C**) L-lysine, and (**D**) L-arginine.

Similarly, the solubility of ketoprofen in the prepared physical mixtures (PM) and coprecipitated ketoprofen with tris, L-lysine, and L-arginine was enhanced (Figure 3). Ketoprofen's solubility increased significantly ($p < 0.05$), and this increase depended on the type of excipient and the preparation method of the solid dispersion. For example, coprecipitated dispersed mixtures demonstrate superior enhancement in solubility compared to physical mixtures. Coprecipitated mixtures generate drug particles with less particle size due to the solvent effect, in addition to generating more intimate contact and interactions with the basic excipients; hence, higher solubility can be achieved [1].

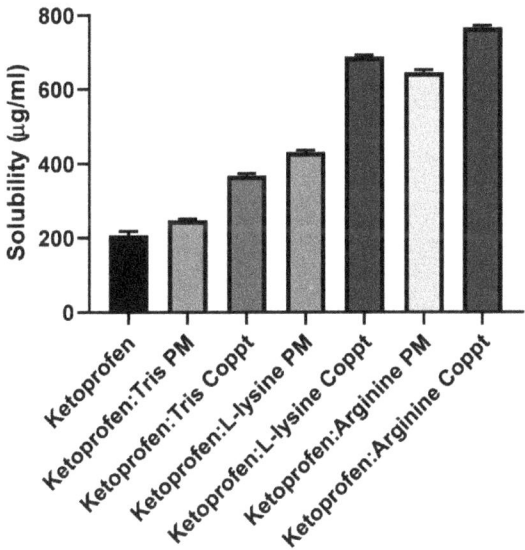

Figure 3. The solubility of ketoprofen in the prepared physical and coprecipitated mixtures.

3.2. FTIR and DSC Studies

FTIR spectroscopy and DSC thermal analysis were used to detect possible physicochemical interactions between ketoprofen and the three basic excipients under investigation. Figure 4A shows the FTIR spectra of ketoprofen, the three basic excipients, and their physical and coprecipitated mixtures. Specific IR absorption bands of pure ketoprofen detected at 1610 cm^{-1} and 1684 cm^{-1} were due to stretching of the ketone group and the carboxylic carbonyl group (C=O), respectively [14]. The characteristic peaks at their assigned wavenumbers were simply additive to the FTIR spectra of the three basic excipients, indicating that no observable physicochemical interactions could be identified with the physical mixtures. In contrast, the vibrational bands of the keto and carbonyl groups of ketoprofen were broadened and shifted for ketoprofen and tris, ketoprofen and L-lysine, and ketoprofen and L-arginine, suggesting hydrogen bonding formation and electrostatic interactions with the basic/cationic excipients [21]. Similarly, DSC analysis revealed the complete disappearance of ketoprofen melting from both physical and coprecipitated ketoprofen mixtures with L-lysine and tris. This indicated the presence of both physicochemical and electrostatic attraction. In contrast, a weak melting transition was found in K:L-arginine PM, but a complete disappearance of K melting was observed in the coprecipitated mixtures.

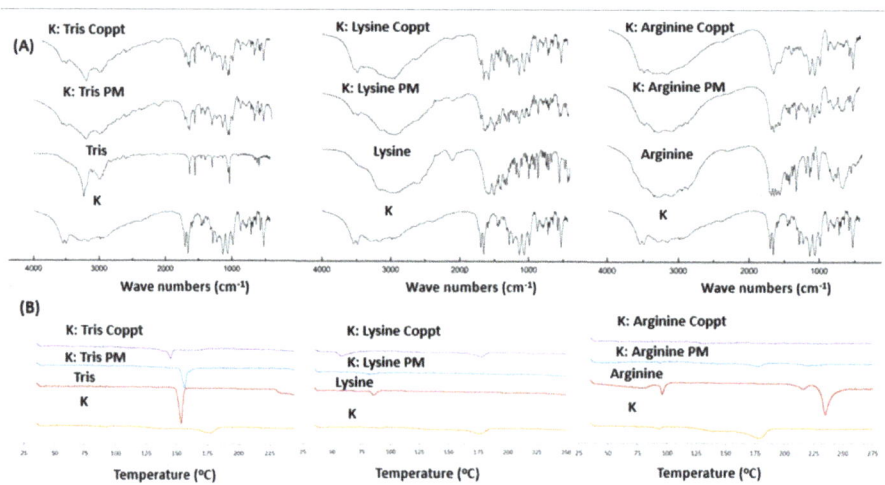

Figure 4. (**A**) FTIR spectra and (**B**) DSC thermograms of ketoprofen (K), basic excipients (tris, lysine, and arginine), physical mixtures (PM), and coprecipitated dispersed mixtures (Coppt).

3.3. Dissolution Studies

For drugs with poor solubility, determined dissolution rates are both a regulatory requirement and essential for distinguishing newly developed formulations. The dissolution medium should mimic physiological fluids and conditions [22]. To determine the exact amount of ketoprofen used for the in vitro dissolution study under sink conditions, equilibrium solubility was measured in different simulated gastric fluids (0.1 M HCl) containing three different concentrations (0.1%, 0.5%, and 1% w/v) of sodium lauryl sulfate as a surfactant. Sodium lauryl sulfate is an anionic surfactant that was selected because it mimics the anionic natural surfactants/bile salts in gastric fluid. To both prevent the surface flotation of drug particles and simulate in vivo performance, it is crucial to wet the dispersed particles prior to dissolution. The surface tension of gastric fluid is considerably lower than that of water, suggesting the presence of surfactants in this region [23]. Ketoprofen solubility was 75, 127.5, 150, and 190 µg/mL for HCl solutions containing SLS of 0.1%, 0.5%, and 1% w/v, respectively. Therefore, an acid dissolution medium with 1% SLS was selected to ensure sink conditions.

This study adopted both acidic gastric conditions and a physiological pH of 6.8 to simulate intestinal pH. The first two hours of dissolution were studied at an acidic pH because the solubility of ketoprofen (a weakly acidic drug with a pKa of 4.4) was very low (0.1 mg/mL), the pH was significantly lower than the pKa of ketoprofen, and the drug was available in a unionized form. In contrast, the solubility of the drug at pH 6.8 (where the drug predominantly exists in ionized forms) was evaluated to determine the capacity of the three basic excipients to improve the dissolution rate under gastric conditions.

Figure 5 shows the dissolution profiles of ketoprofen from the prepared physical and dispersed mixtures, and Table 2 presents three dissolution parameters: the time required for the dissolution of 50% of ketoprofen (T50%) and relative dissolution rates at 60 min and 300 min (RDR_{60} and RDR_{300}, respectively). Slow and incomplete dissolution was recorded for ketoprofen powder over 300 min, with only 50% of the drug dissolving in 240 min. In contrast, Ketofan® capsules showed nearly doubled RDR_{60} and RDR_{300} dissolution parameters. Similarly, physical mixtures of ketoprofen with the three basic excipients enhanced the dissolution parameters by 1.26 to 1.74-fold and shortened the T50% value to 120 and 180 min, respectively, compared to the T50% of 240 min recorded for ketoprofen powder.

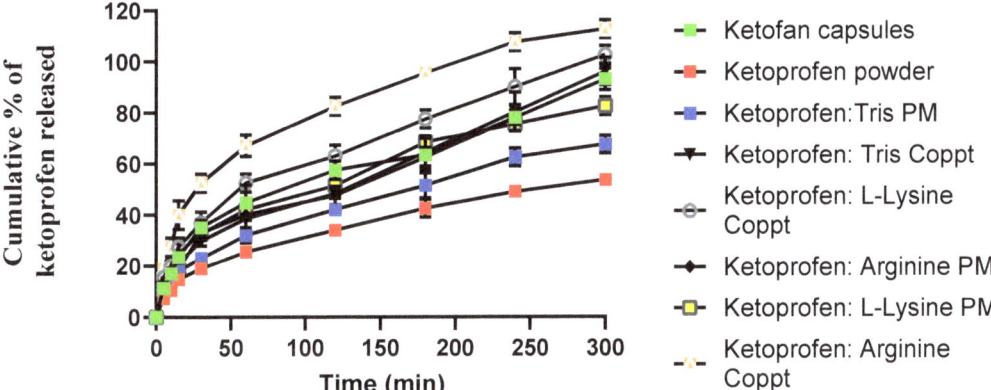

Figure 5. Profiles of in vitro dissolution of ketoprofen powder, commercial capsules, and physical and dispersed mixtures with lysine, arginine, and tris. For the first two hours, simulated gastric fluid (pH = 1.2) was employed, and for the remaining three hours, simulated intestinal fluid (pH = 6.8) was used.

Table 2. Dissolution parameters were measured for ketoprofen, commercial capsules, and ketoprofen with respect to excipient mixtures. * T50% denotes the time required for 50% of the initial amount to be dissolved; ** and *** denote relative dissolution rates of 60 and 300 min, respectively.

Formulation	T50% (min) *	RDR_{60} **	RDR_{300} ***
Ketoprofen powder	240	-	-
Ketofan capsule	120	2	1.75
K:tris PM	180	1.28	1.26
K:tris Coppt	120	1.6	1.8
K:lysine PM	120	1.6	1.5
K:lysine Coppt	60	2.08	1.92
K:arginine PM	120	1.74	1.74
K:arginine Coppt	30	2.68	2.07

Compared to physical mixtures, superior dissolution rates were recorded for coprecipitated mixtures. For example, K:tris, K:lysine, and K:arginine coprecipitates recorded T50% of 120, 60, and 30 min, respectively, compared to 180, 120, and 120 min estimated for K:tris, K:lysine, and K:arginine physical mixtures, respectively. These results indicated that the preparation technique of the dispersed mixtures made a marked difference in dissolution rates.

Furthermore, L-arginine and L-lysine appear superior to tris in terms of their capacity to improve the in vitro dissolution rates of ketoprofen. L-arginine (pKa = 12.48) is the strongest base compared to the other two basic excipients, L-lysine (pKa = 10.79) and tris (pKa = 7.8). The stronger the base, the faster the in vitro dissolution rate can be recorded. This is due to the faster alkalinization of the diffusion layer surrounding the drug particles, as well as the increasing ionization of the acidic drug in this diffusion layer [20]. Additionally, these results correlate well with the solubility studies that demonstrated the following order: L-arginine > L-lysine > tris.

3.4. Molecular Docking

Several methods could be utilized to establish the ability of the three basic excipients to form a salt with ketoprofen. Fundamentally, the difference in acid dissociation constants (pKa (base)–pKa (acid)) for ketoprofen and the three basic excipients is widely used to predict the possibility of cosolvation experiments producing a cocrystal or a salt. A pKa difference greater than 3 suggests a salt formation, while values less than 0 suggest that cocrystal is the predominant form [24–27]. An acidic pKa of 4.39–4.45 [28] for the propionic acid proton of ketoprofen gives a difference of 8, 6.4, and 3.4 with arginine, lysine, and tromethamine, respectively (Figure 1). This supports the previous findings of salt formation between ketoprofen and the three bases.

Additionally, Hirshfeld surface analysis, a tool for visualizing crystal structure interactions (Spackman & Jayatilaka, 2009), of ketoprofen crystals revealed that carboxylic oxygens are the most likely sites for interactions in ketoprofen (shown red areas in Figure 6A). The same conclusion was reached with theoretical docking of the three bases on the surface of ketoprofen using MOE software, suggesting the construction of small stable complexes, as shown in Figure 6B. In the case of arginine, the complexes created showed the proximity of the basic guanidine NH_2 with the highest pKa to the carboxylic group. The stability of such complexes, and their observed proximity, may favor the potential proton transfer between the ketoprofen acidic group and the guanidine amino group of arginine in a salt formation process. Recently, the salt formation between ketoprofen and tromethamine was confirmed [14]. A salt formation between ketoprofen and lysine was also described, substantiating our assumptions [13].

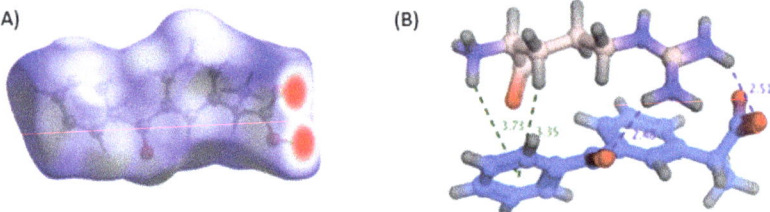

Figure 6. (**A**) Hirshfeld surface analysis of ketoprofen crystals and (**B**) possible interactions formed upon docking arginine onto the ketoprofen surface.

3.5. In Vivo Studies

3.5.1. Writhing Assay

A writhing assay was employed to assess the onset of analgesic activities of the drug alone and the coprecipitated drug mixtures with three basic excipients (tris, L-lysine, and L-arginine) within 20 min. In the current study, both the number of writhes and percentage (%) of writhing inhibition were recorded for the untreated, ketoprofen-, K:tris Coppt-, K:L-lysine Coppt-, and K:L-arginine-treated groups, as illustrated in Figure 7A,B. The number of writhes for the ketoprofen-treated group decreased from 46 to 32, with 30% inhibition. In contrast, the numbers of writhes recorded for the K:tris, K:L-lysine, and K:L-arginine coprecipitated mixture groups were 3, 8, and 10, respectively, with percentage inhibitions of 91%, 82%, and 78%, respectively. These findings suggest that these basic excipients have promising potential to quickly enhance analgesic activity when compared to the drug alone. This is due to their improved solubility and in vitro dissolution rates. Notably, it is worth mentioning that this in vivo study did not significantly correspond with previously mentioned in vitro dissolution studies, where L-arginine showed superior potential for enhancing both solubility and dissolution rates.

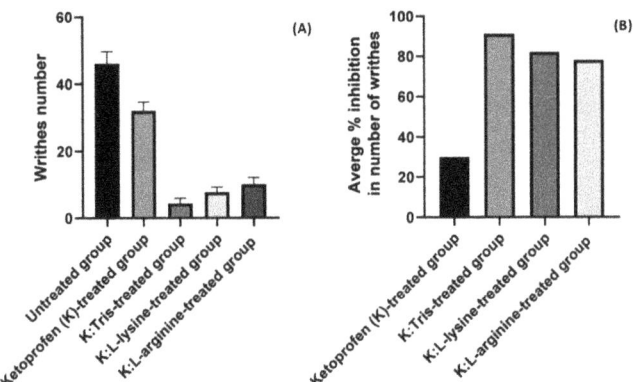

Figure 7. (**A**) The number of writhes and (**B**) average percentage (%) inhibition for ketoprofen and ketoprofen with respect to the three basic excipient coprecipitated mixtures.

K:tris Coppt demonstrated statistically significant inhibition in the number of writhes compared to both K:L-lysine and K:L-arginine Coppt, while the latter two showed significant reductions in the number of writhes (8 and 10, respectively) and percentage inhibition (82% and 79%, respectively). However, no statistically significant differences ($p > 0.05$) were identified for either L-arginine or L-lysine in reducing the number of writhes. Similar results were reported elsewhere for the NSAID drug nimesulide [15]. Nimesulide tris Coppt outperformed the amorphous mixture of nimesulide and PVP K30 in terms of analgesic activity and time to onset of action [15].

In another study, the ketoprofen lysine salt demonstrated a more rapid and complete absorption than the acid form of ketoprofen. Peak plasma concentration for the ketoprofen lysine salt was attained in 15 min, compared to 60 min for the acid form [29]. Additionally, it was reported that the ketoprofen lysine salt demonstrated analgesic activity two times stronger than ketoprofen, as well as a higher LD_{50} [30].

The writhing assay was also used to assess the onset of analgesic activity of nimesulide, a poorly soluble drug. Nimesulide alone inhibited writhing by approximately 22%. In comparison, the more water-soluble form of the drug prepared in an inclusion complex with β-cyclodextrin in a ratio of 1:4 showed a percentage inhibition of 54.5% at 20 min [31]. The nimesulide-tris complex showed a superior reduction in the number of writhes compared to the nimesulide-polyvinylpyrrolidone (PVP) K30 and nimesulide-polyethylene glycol 4000 complexes [15]. Several reports have indicated that, in addition to improving the solubility of poorly soluble drugs, tris can act as a permeability enhancer and alter membrane permeability [32–34].

3.5.2. Indomethacin-Induced Ulcer

NSAIDs cause gastric toxicity, including gastric ulcers. Indomethacin, a commonly used NSAID, is often used as a model drug for inducing gastric ulcers in rats due to its high ulcerogenic index [16,35]. Indomethacin is a potent inhibitor of prostaglandin and can cause significant damage to the gastric mucosa [36]. This study aimed to determine if coprecipitated mixtures of ketoprofen and three basic excipients, which improved solubility and bioavailability, could reduce the gastrointestinal side effects of ketoprofen.

Figure 8 shows stomachs pinned on corkboards to emphasize the location and number of ulcers in the negative and positive (indomethacin) groups, as well as the groups treated with ketoprofen and coprecipitated mixtures of ketoprofen and basic excipients. The indomethacin-treated group (the positive control) had the highest number of ulcers, with nine ulcers recorded. The number of ulcers in the ketoprofen group was reduced to about one-third of that of the indomethacin group, as indomethacin is more potent at causing gastric ulcers [36]. There were no statistically significant ($p > 0.05$) differences in the number of ulcers between the K:tris and ketoprofen groups.

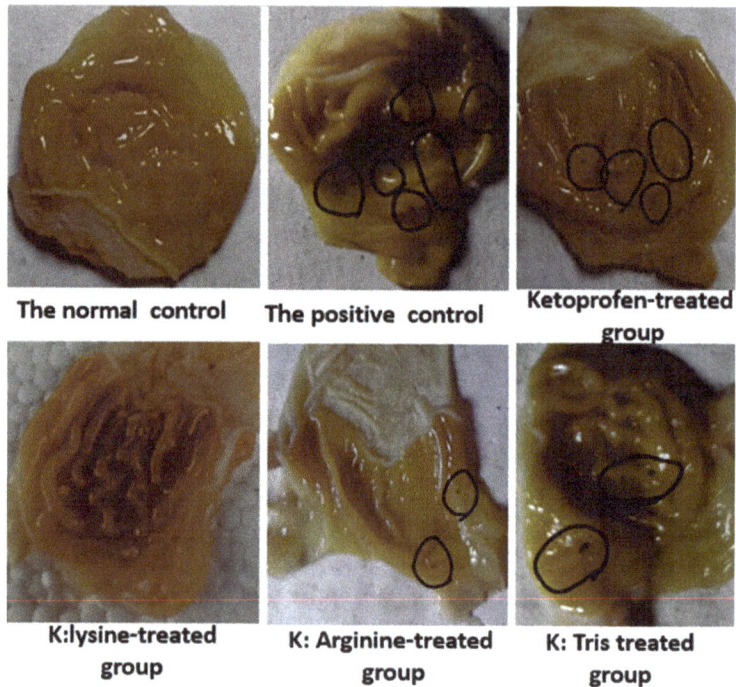

Figure 8. Pinned stomachs on corkboards highlighting the position and number of ulcers (encircled in black lines) for the negative and positive control (indomethacin), ketoprofen (K), K:lysine, K:arginine:K:tris coprecipitated mixtures.

Interestingly, the K:lysine and K:arginine coprecipitated mixtures produced significantly fewer ulcers than ketoprofen alone. These results are consistent with recent reports [5]. Ketoprofen lysine salt has been shown to reduce ulcer side effects compared to the acidic form of ketoprofen [37]. This is likely due to the residual amino groups of L-lysine and L-arginine, which act as carbonyl scavengers; they also offer protection against oxidative damage to the gastric mucosa by providing indirect antioxidant effects and increasing the levels of glutathione S-transferase P at the cellular level in the gastric mucosa [5]. Additionally, L-lysine and L-arginine have been reported to both enhance mucosal integrity and have gastroprotective effects through nitric oxide (NO) donation [37,38].

3.5.3. Histopathological Studies

Figures 9a–e and 10a–e display histopathological documentation of gastric tissues for the control, ketoprofen, ketoprofen:tris coprecipitate, ketoprofen:lysine coprecipitate, and ketoprofen:arginine coprecipitate at low magnification (×100) and high magnification (×400) lenses. The normal control group exhibited intact mucosa (double-headed arrow), healthy surface epithelium (thin black arrow), intact normal gastric glands (white arrows), and normal submucosa (Figure 9a). At higher magnification, the normal control group showed healthy surface epithelium with normal integrity (thin black arrow) and intact normal gastric glands (white arrows) (Figure 10a). In contrast, the ketoprofen-treated group exhibited gastric mucosa (double-headed white arrow) with sporadic superficial degermation and desquamation of the surface epithelium (red arrows). Additionally, degenerative changes and shrinkage of the gastric glands (thick black arrows) were observed (Figure 9b).

Figure 10b shows superficial degermation and desquamation of the surface epithelium (red dotted arrows). Furthermore, degenerative changes and shrinkage of gastric glands (thick black arrows) were recorded for the ketoprofen-treated group (Figure 10b).

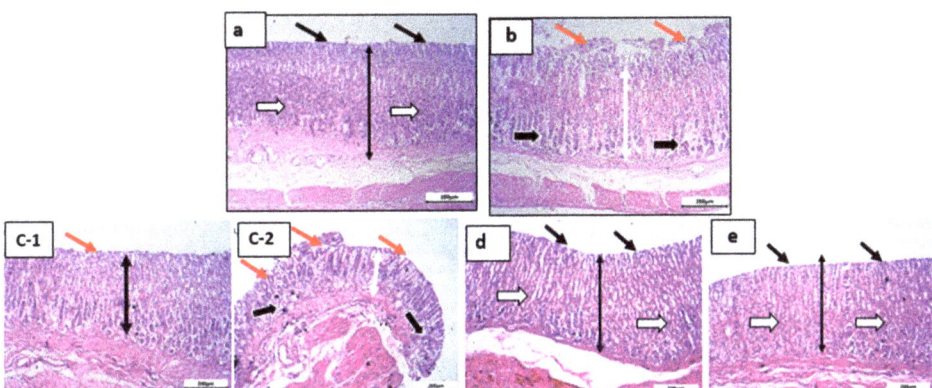

Figure 9. Histological sections from rat stomachs: (**a**) control group, (**b**) ketoprofen-treated group, (**c-1, c-2**) ketoprofen:tris Coppt, (**d**) ketoprofen:L-lysine Coppt, and (**e**) ketoprofen:arginine Coppt stained by H&E and photographed at low power x 100 (bar = 200 μm) and x 400 (bar = 50 μm).

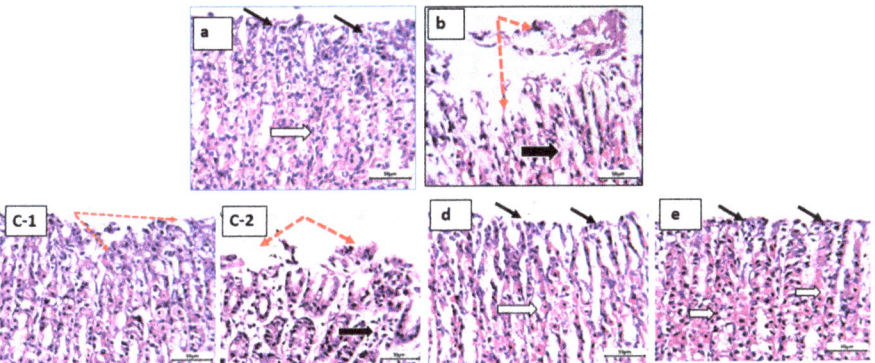

Figure 10. Histological sections from rat stomachs: (**a**) control, (**b**) ketoprofen-treated group, (**c-1, c-2**) ketoprofen:tris Coppt, (**d**) ketoprofen:L-lysine Coppt, and (**e**) ketoprofen:arginine Coppt stained by H&E and photographed at high power x 400 (bar = 50 μm).

Figure 9c-1,-2 shows gastric mucosa (double-headed white arrow) with ulcerated regions (red arrows) and slight degeneration of glands (thick black arrow) in the K:tris-treated group. Ulcerated surface epithelium (red dotted arrows) with slight degeneration and atrophy of gastric glands (thick black arrow) was recorded for the same group and detected at higher magnification in Figure 10c-1,-2.

Figure 9d shows normal, intact mucosa (double-headed arrow), maintained surface epithelial integrity (black arrows), and gastric glands (white arrows) for the K:lysine group. Maintained surface epithelial integrity (black arrows) and intact gastric glands (white arrows) were recorded at higher magnification (Figure 10d).

Figure 9e shows intact, healthy mucosa and possible protection against ketoprofen-induced superficial ulceration (black arrows) for the K:arginine group. In Figure 10e, intact, healthy mucosal surfaces (black arrows) and normal gastric glands (white arrows) were recorded at higher magnification.

These findings correlate significantly with the ulcer indices shown in Table 3, and, in addition to their enhanced solubilization for ketoprofen, confirm the gastroprotective effect and safety benefits of the two basic amino acids L-lysine and L-arginine.

Table 3. Ulcerogenic potential (number of ulcers) and ulcer indices for the positive control (indomethacin), ketoprofen (K), K:lysine, K:arginine:K:tris coprecipitated mixtures.

Test Substance	Ulcer Number	Ulcer Index
Control	0 ± 0.0	0
Indomethacin	8.66 ± 0.88 [a]	7.8 [a]
Ketoprofen	3.33 ± 0.66 [a,b]	3.59 [a,b]
Ketoprofen:tris	2.00 ± 0.0 [b]	1.1 [a,b,c]
Ketoprofen:lysine	1.0 ± 0.33 [b,c]	0.55 [a,b,c]
Ketoprofen:arginine	0.53.00 ± 0.17 [b]	0.33 [a,b,c]

The data are presented as the mean ± SD of six animals. A one-way ANOVA test followed by a Tukey–Kramer post hoc test was used for multiple comparisons. [a] Denotes a significant difference from the control group ($p < 0.05$). [b] Represents a significant difference from the indomethacin group ($p < 0.05$). [c] Indicates a significant difference from the ketoprofen group ($p < 0.05$).

4. Conclusions

This study highlighted the role of three basic excipients (tris, L-lysine, and L-arginine) as potential solubilizers, as well as their capacity to form salts with the non-steroidal anti-inflammatory drug ketoprofen. The three basic excipients were superior in potentiating and advancing analgesic activities due to both their penetration-enhancing activities and their enhanced solubility and dissolution rates of the weak acid drug. However, only L-arginine and L-lysine demonstrated gastric protection against ketoprofen-induced ulcers and erosion of the gastric mucosa. This study recommends L-arginine and L-lysine as promising agents for promoting the analgesic and safety profiles of classical NSAIDs.

Author Contributions: H.A.A.-T., methodology, formal analysis, data curation, and initial draft preparation; M.E.S., methodology, data curation, review, and editing; T.S.M., methodology, data curation, review, and editing; J.A.A.-A., methodology, formal analysis, and writing; H.A., conceptualization, methodology, data curation, review, and editing. All authors have read and agreed to the published version of the manuscript.

Funding: This research was funded by the Deanship of Scientific Research at King Khalid University, which provided funding for this work through the Small Groups Project under Grant No. RGP.1/148/43.

Institutional Review Board Statement: Animal ethical approval number ES28/2020 was granted by the Faculty of Pharmacy at Minia University in Minia, Egypt.

Informed Consent Statement: Not applicable.

Data Availability Statement: Upon request.

Acknowledgments: The authors extend their appreciation to the Deanship of Scientific Research at King Khalid University for funding this work through the Small Groups Project under Grant No. RGP.1/148/43.

Conflicts of Interest: The authors declare no conflict of interest.

References

1. Abdelkader, H.; Fathalla, Z. Investigation into the emerging role of the basic Amino acid L-lysine in enhancing solubility and permeability of BCS Class II and BCS Class IV drugs. *Pharm. Res.* **2018**, *35*, 160–178. [CrossRef]
2. Kalepu, S.; Nekkanti, V. Insoluble drug delivery strategies: Review of recent advances and business prospects. *Acta Pharm. Sin B.* **2015**, *15*, 442–453. [CrossRef]
3. Abou-Taleb, H.; Fathalla, Z.; Abdelkader, H. Comparative studies of the effects of novel excipients amino acids with cyclodextrins on enhancement of dissolution and oral bioavailability of the non-ionizable drug carbamazepine. *Eur. J. Pharm. Sci.* **2020**, *155*, 105562. [CrossRef] [PubMed]

4. Bongioanni, A.; Bueno, M.; Mezzano, B.; Longhi, M.; Garnero, C. Amino acids and its pharmaceutical applications: A mini review. *Int. J. Pharm.* **2022**, *613*, 121375. [CrossRef]
5. Kuczynska, J.; Nieradko-Iwanicka, B. Future prospects of ketoprofen in improving the safety of the gastric mucosa. *Biomed. Pharmacother.* **2021**, *139*, 111608.
6. Granero, G.E.; Ramachandran, C.; Amidon, G.L. Rapid in vivo dissolution of ketoprofen: Implications on the biopharmaceutics classification system. *Pharmazie* **2006**, *61*, 673–676.
7. Yousif, N.; Abdulrasool, A.; Mowafaq, G.; Hussain, S. Solubility and dissolution improvement of ketoprofen by solid dispersion in polymer and surfactant using solvent evaporation method. *Int. J. Pharm. Pharm. Sci.* **2011**, *3*, 431–435.
8. Khoder, M.; Abdelkader, H.; Elshaer, A.; Karam, A.; Najlah, M.; Alany, R. The use of albumin solid dispersion to enhance the solubility of unionisable drugs. *Pharm. Dev. Technol.* **2018**, *23*, 732–738. [CrossRef] [PubMed]
9. Loftsson, T. Drug solubilization by complexation. *Int. J. Pharm.* **2017**, *531*, 276–280. [CrossRef] [PubMed]
10. Zhang, X.; Xing, H.; Zhao, Y.; Ma, Z. Pharmaceutical dispersion techniques for dissolution and bioavailability enhancement of poorly water-soluble drugs. *Pharmaceutics* **2018**, *10*, 74. [CrossRef]
11. Abdelkader, H.; Abdallah, O.Y.; Salem, H.; Alani, A.; Alany, R. Eutectic, monotectic and immiscibility systems of nimesulide with water-soluble carriers: Phase equilibria, solid-state characterisation and in-vivo/pharmacodynamic evaluation. *J. Pharm. Pharmacol.* **2014**, *66*, 439–450. [CrossRef]
12. ElShaer, A.; Hanson, P.; Mohammed, A. A novel concentration dependent amino acid ion pair strategy to mediate drug permeation using indomethacin as a model insoluble drug. *Eur. J. Pharm. Sci.* **2014**, *62*, 124–131. [CrossRef] [PubMed]
13. Aramini, A.; Bianchini, G.; Lillini, S.; Bordignon, S.; Tommasetti, M.; Novelli, R.; Mattioli, S.; Lvova, L.; Paolesse, R.; Chierotti, M.R.; et al. Unexpected Salt/Cocrystal Polymorphism of the Ketoprofen–Lysine System: Discovery of a New Ketoprofen–L-Lysine Salt Polymorph with Different Physicochemical and Pharmacokinetic Properties. *Pharmaceuticals* **2021**, *14*, 555. [CrossRef]
14. Fitriani, L.; Firdaus, W.; Sidadang, W.; Rosaini, H.; Putra, O.; Oyama, H.; Uekusa, H.; Zaini, E. Improved solubility and dissolution rate of ketoprofen by the formation of multicomponent crystals with tromethamine. *Crystals* **2022**, *12*, 275. [CrossRef]
15. Abdelkader, H.; Abdallah, O.Y.; Salem, H. Comparison of the effect of tromethamine and polyvinylpyrrolidone on dissolution properties and analgesic effect of nimesulide. *AAPS PharmSciTech* **2007**, *8*, E1–E8. [CrossRef] [PubMed]
16. El-Moselhy, M.A.; Abdel-Hamid, N.M.; Abdel-Raheim, S.R. Gastroprotective effect of nicorandil in indomethacin and alcohol-induced acute Ulcers. *Appl. Biochem. Biotechnol.* **2009**, *152*, 449–459. [CrossRef]
17. Abdelgawad, M.A.; Labib, M.B.; Ali, W.A.M.; Kamel, G.; Azouz, A.A.; EL-Nahass, E.S. Design, synthesis, analgesic, anti-inflammatory activity of novel pyrazolones possessing aminosulfonyl pharmacophore as inhibitors of COX-2/5-LOX enzymes: Histopathological and docking studies. *Bioorg. Chem.* **2018**, *78*, 103–114. [CrossRef]
18. Abdellatif, K.; Abdelall, E.; Elshemy, H.; Philoppes, J.; Hassanein, E.; Kahk, N. Optimization of pyrazole-based compounds with 1,2,4-triazole-3-thiol moiety as selective COX-2 inhibitors cardioprotective drug candidates: Design, synthesis, cyclooxygenase inhibition, anti-inflammatory, ulcerogenicity, cardiovascular evaluation, and molecular modeling studies. *Bioorg. Chem.* **2021**, *114*, 105122. [PubMed]
19. Harakeh, S.; Saber, S.; Akefe, I.; Shaker, S.; Hussain, M.; Almasaudi, A.; Saleh, S.; Almasaudi, S. Saudi honey alleviates indomethacin-induced gastric ulcer via improving antioxidant and anti-inflammatory responses in male albino rats. *Saudi J. Biol. Sci.* **2022**, *29*, 3040–3050. [CrossRef]
20. Al Fatease, A.; Shoman, M.; Abourehab, M.; Abou-Taleb, H.; Abdelkader, H. A Novel Curcumin Arginine Salt: A Solution for Poor Solubility and Potential Anticancer Activities. *Molecules* **2023**, *28*, 262. [CrossRef]
21. Ishihara, S.; Hattori, Y.; Otsuka, M.; Sasaki, T. Cocrystal formation through solid-state reaction between ibuprofen and nicotinamide revealed using THz and IR spectroscopy with multivariate analysis. *Crystals* **2020**, *10*, 760. [CrossRef]
22. Dahan, A.; Miller, J.M.; Amidon, G.L. Prediction of solubility and permeability class membership: Provisional BCS classification of the world's top oral drugs. *AAPS J.* **2009**, *11*, 740–746. [CrossRef] [PubMed]
23. Saers, E.; Nyström, C.; Aldén, M. Physicochemical aspects of drug release. XVI. The effect of storage on drug dissolution from solid dispersions and the influence of cooling rate and incorporation of surfactant. *Int. J. Pharm.* **1993**, *90*, 105–118. [CrossRef]
24. Bhogala, B.R.; Basavoju, S.; Nangia, A. Tape and layer structures in cocrystals of some di- and tricarboxylic acids with 4,4′-bipyridines and isonicotinamide. *Cryst. Eng. Comm.* **2005**, *7*, 551–562. [CrossRef]
25. Delori, A.; Suresh, E.; Pedireddi, V.R. pKa-directed host- guest assemblies: Rational analysis of molecular adducts of 2,4-diamino-6-methyl-1,3,5-triazine with various aliphatic di- carboxylic acids. *Chem. Eur. J* **2008**, *14*, 6967–6977. [CrossRef]
26. Mohamed, S.; Tocher, D.A.; Vickers, M.; Karamertzanis, P.G.; Price, S.L. Salts or cocrystals? A new series of crystal structures formed from simple pyridines and carboxylic acids. *Cryst. Growth Des.* **2009**, *9*, 2881–2889. [CrossRef]
27. Cheney, M.L.; Weyna, D.; Shan, N.; Hanna, M.; Wojtas, L.; Zaworotko, M. Coformer selection in pharmaceutical cocrystal development: A case study of a meloxicam aspirin cocrystal that exhibits enhanced solubility and pharmacokinetics. *J. Pharm. Sci.* **2011**, *100*, 2172–2181. [CrossRef]
28. Shohin, I.; Kulinich, J.; Ramenskaya, G.; Abrahamsson, B.; Kopp, S.; Langguth, P.; Polli, J.; Shah, V.; Groot, D.; Barends, D.; et al. Biowaiver monographs for immediate release solid oral dosage forms: Ketoprofen. *J. Pharm. Sci.* **2012**, *101*, 3593–3603. [CrossRef]
29. Cerciello, A.; Auriemma, G.; Del Gaudio, P.; Cantarini, M.; Aquino, R.P. Natural polysaccharides platforms for oral controlled release of ketoprofen lysine salt. *Drug Dev. Ind. Pharm.* **2016**, *42*, 2063–2069. [CrossRef] [PubMed]
30. Lee, W.; Kim, J.; Jee, U.; Rhyu, B. Ketoprofen lysinate. *J. Korean Pharm. Sci.* **1982**, *12*, 37–44.

31. Adhage, N.A.; Vavia, P.R. β-Cyclodextrin Inclusion Complexation by Milling. *Pharm. Pharmacol. Commun.* **2000**, *6*, 13–17. [CrossRef]
32. Irvin, R.T.; MacAlister, T.J.; Costerton, J.W. Tris(hydroxymethyl)aminomethane buffer modification of Escherichia coli outer membrane permeability. *J. Bacteriol.* **1981**, *145*, 1397–1403. [CrossRef] [PubMed]
33. Omachi, A.; Macey, R.; Waldeck, J.G. Permeability of cell membranes to amine buffers and their effects on electrolyte transport. *Ann. N. Y. Acad. Sci.* **1961**, *92*, 478–485. [CrossRef] [PubMed]
34. O'Shea, J.; Augustijns, P.; Brandl, M.; Brayden, D.; Brouwers, J.; Griffin, B.; Jacobsen, A.; Lennernäs, H.; Vinarov, Z.; O'Driscoll, C.M. Best practices in current models mimicking drug permeability in the gastrointestinal tract—An UNGAP review. *Eur. J. Pharm. Sci.* **2022**, *170*, 106098. [PubMed]
35. Adinortey, M.B.; Ansah, A.; Galyuon, I.; Nyarko, A. In vivo models used for evaluation of potential antigastroduodenal ulcer agents. *Ulcers* **2013**, *2013*, 1–12. [CrossRef]
36. Suleyman, H.; Abdulmecit, A.; Bilici, M.; Cadirci, E.; Halici, Z. Different mechanisms in formation and prevention of indomethacin-induced gastric ulcers. *Inflammation* **2010**, *33*, 224–233. [CrossRef]
37. Cimini, A.; Brandolini, L.; Gentile, R.; Cristiano, L.; Menghini, P.; Fidoamore, A.; Antonosante, A.; Benedetti, E.; Giordano, A.; Allegretti, M. Gastroprotective effects of L-lysine salification of ketoprofen in ethanol-injured gastric mucosa. *J. Cell Physiol.* **2015**, *230*, 813–820. [CrossRef] [PubMed]
38. Brzozowski, T.; Konturek, S.; Sliwowski, Z.; Drozdowicz, D.; Zaczek, M.; Kedra, D. Role of L-arginine, a substrate for nitric oxide-synthase, in gastroprotection and ulcer healing. *J. Gastroenterol.* **1997**, *32*, 442–452. [CrossRef]

Disclaimer/Publisher's Note: The statements, opinions and data contained in all publications are solely those of the individual author(s) and contributor(s) and not of MDPI and/or the editor(s). MDPI and/or the editor(s) disclaim responsibility for any injury to people or property resulting from any ideas, methods, instructions or products referred to in the content.

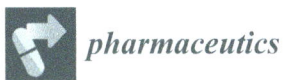

Article

Anti-Alzheimer Activity of Combinations of Cocoa with Vinpocetine or Other Nutraceuticals in Rat Model: Modulation of Wnt3/β-Catenin/GSK-3β/Nrf2/HO-1 and PERK/CHOP/Bcl-2 Pathways

Karema Abu-Elfotuh [1], Amina M. A. Tolba [2], Furqan H. Hussein [3], Ahmed M. E. Hamdan [4,*], Mohamed A. Rabeh [5,*], Saad A. Alshahri [5], Azza A. Ali [6], Sarah M. Mosaad [7], Nihal A. Mahmoud [8], Magdy Y. Elsaeed [9], Ranya M. Abdelglil [10], Rehab R. El-Awady [11], Eman Reda M. Galal [11], Mona M. Kamal [6], Ahmed M. M. Elsisi [12,13], Alshaymaa Darwish [14], Ayah M. H. Gowifel [15] and Yasmen F. Mahran [16]

1. Clinical Pharmacy Department, Faculty of Pharmacy (Girls), Al-Azhar University, Cairo 11651, Egypt; karimasoliman.pharmg@azhar.edu.eg
2. Anatomy Department, Faculty of Medicine, Girls Branch, Al-Azhar University, Cairo 11651, Egypt; amina.tolba65@gmail.com
3. Colleege of Dentistry, University of Alkafeel, Najaf 54001, Iraq; furqan.alshwaily@alkafeel.edu.iq
4. Department of Pharmacy Practice, Faculty of Pharmacy, University of Tabuk, Tabuk 71491, Saudi Arabia
5. Department of Pharmacognosy, College of Pharmacy, King Khalid University, Abha 62521, Saudi Arabia; salshhri@kku.edu.sa
6. Pharmacology and Toxicology Department, Faculty of Pharmacy (Girls), Al-Azhar University, Cairo 11651, Egypt; azzamoro@gmail.com (A.A.A.); mona.kamal@hotmail.com (M.M.K.)
7. Research Unit, Egypt Healthcare Authority, Ismailia Branch, Ismailia 41522, Egypt; sarahmmph822@gmail.com
8. Physiology Department, Faculty of Medicine (Girls), Al-Azhar University, Cairo 11651, Egypt; nehalabdelmonem.medg@azhar.edu.eg
9. Physiology Department, Faculty of Medicine (Boys), Al-Azhar University, Demietta 34517, Egypt; magdyyoussef11175@domazhermedicine.edu.eg
10. Department of Anatomy and Embryology, Faculty of Medicine (Girls), Al-Azhar University, Cairo 11651, Egypt; ranonmohammed2009@gmail.com
11. Biochemistry and Molecular Biology Department, Faculty of Pharmacy (Girls), Al-Azhar University, Cairo 11651, Egypt; r.awady@yahoo.com (R.R.E.-A.); ph.eman.reda@gmail.com (E.R.M.G.)
12. Biochemistry and Molecular Biology Department, Faculty of Pharmacy (Boys), Al-Azhar University, Cairo 11651, Egypt; ahmed.elsisi@nub.edu.eg
13. Biochemistry Department, Faculty of Pharmacy, Nahda University (NUB), Beni-Suef 62521, Egypt
14. Biochemistry Department, Faculty of Pharmacy, Sohag University, Sohag 82524, Egypt; alshaymaa.darwish@pharm.sohag.edu.eg
15. Pharmacology and Toxicology Department, Faculty of Pharmacy, Modern University for Technology and Information (MTI), Cairo 11571, Egypt; ayah.gowifel@pharm.mti.edu.eg
16. Pharmacology & Toxicology Department, Faculty of Pharmacy, Ain Shams University, Cairo 11566, Egypt; jassie_81@hotmail.com
* Correspondence: a_hamdan@ut.edu.sa (A.M.E.H.); mrabeh@kku.edu.sa (M.A.R.)

Abstract: Alzheimer's disease (AD) is a devastating illness with limited therapeutic interventions. The aim of this study is to investigate the pathophysiological mechanisms underlying AD and explore the potential neuroprotective effects of cocoa, either alone or in combination with other nutraceuticals, in an animal model of aluminum-induced AD. Rats were divided into nine groups: control, aluminum chloride (AlCl$_3$) alone, AlCl$_3$ with cocoa alone, AlCl$_3$ with vinpocetine (VIN), AlCl$_3$ with epigallocatechin-3-gallate (EGCG), AlCl$_3$ with coenzyme Q10 (CoQ10), AlCl$_3$ with wheatgrass (WG), AlCl$_3$ with vitamin (Vit) B complex, and AlCl$_3$ with a combination of Vit C, Vit E, and selenium (Se). The animals were treated for five weeks, and we assessed behavioral, histopathological, and biochemical changes, focusing on oxidative stress, inflammation, Wnt/GSK-3β/β-catenin signaling, ER stress, autophagy, and apoptosis. AlCl$_3$ administration induced oxidative stress, as evidenced by elevated levels of malondialdehyde (MDA) and downregulation of cellular antioxidants (Nrf2, HO-1, SOD, and TAC). AlCl3 also upregulated inflammatory biomarkers (TNF-α and IL-1β) and

GSK-3β, leading to increased tau phosphorylation, decreased brain-derived neurotrophic factor (BDNF) expression, and downregulation of the Wnt/β-catenin pathway. Furthermore, AlCl$_3$ intensified C/EBP, p-PERK, GRP-78, and CHOP, indicating sustained ER stress, and decreased Beclin-1 and anti-apoptotic B-cell lymphoma 2 (Bcl-2) expressions. These alterations contributed to the observed behavioral and histological changes in the AlCl$_3$-induced AD model. Administration of cocoa, either alone or in combination with other nutraceuticals, particularly VIN or EGCG, demonstrated remarkable amelioration of all assessed parameters. The combination of cocoa with nutraceuticals attenuated the AD-mediated deterioration by modulating interrelated pathophysiological pathways, including inflammation, antioxidant responses, GSK-3β-Wnt/β-catenin signaling, ER stress, and apoptosis. These findings provide insights into the intricate pathogenesis of AD and highlight the neuroprotective effects of nutraceuticals through multiple signaling pathways.

Keywords: Alzheimer's disease; GSK-3β-Wnt/β-catenin; PERK/CHOP/Bcl-2; oxidative stress; cocoa; vinpocetine

1. Introduction

Alzheimer's is a complex neurological disorder that is progressive. Aβ and tau protein tangles are the key features of AD, found mainly in the entorhinal cortex and hippocampus. The accumulation of Aβ results in impaired cell communication, leading to cell apoptosis. Additionally, an imbalance between Aβ production and clearance strongly correlates with the formation of tau protein tangles [1]. Exposure to aluminum metal is considered the most hazardous risk factor for the etiology of AD [2].

Mounting scientific evidence has firmly linked the onset of AD pathology to oxidative stress. Oxidative stress induces both Aβ accumulation and tau protein phosphorylation, contributing to the pathogenesis of AD [1]. Nuclear factor-erythroid 2-related factor 2 (Nrf2) (Nrf2) reduces oxidative stress by controlling antioxidant proteins such as heme oxygenase-1 (HO-1), decreasing inflammation, and stopping Aβ and tau phosphorylation, which enhances cognitive abilities, learning, and memory. Conversely, a reduction in the transcription factor Nrf2 levels has been observed in AD. Oxidative stress can lead to Nrf2 downregulation and neuroinflammation. Oxidative stress, inflammation, and Nrf2 transcriptional regulation are intertwined. Hence, this highlights that Nrf2 has emerged as a promising novel pharmacological target in the management of AD [3].

It has linked oxidative stress to histopathological changes in AD that increase glycogen synthase kinase-3 beta (GSK-3β) activity. The elevation of GSK-3β leads to the upregulation of phosphorylated tau protein and the dysregulation of wingless-related integration site (Wnt)/β-catenin signaling. Wnt/β-catenin signaling regulates neurogenesis, synaptic plasticity, and Aβ-induced apoptosis [4].

Additionally, endoplasmic reticulum (ER) stress plays a significant role in the pathogenesis of neurodegenerative disorders, including AD. It triggered the expression of C/EBP homologous protein (CHOP), a pro-apoptotic protein, leading to neuronal cell death. ER, stress also impaired autophagy by deregulating the autophagy protein Beclin-1 level. Impaired autophagy has also been found to contribute to the pathological buildup of tau deposition in AD. Clearing abnormal protein aggregation is essential to preventing AD because of its ability to cause neuronal degeneration [5]. Modulating Beclin-1 and Bcl-2 connections regulates autophagy [6].

AD poses a daunting challenge as it lacks any effective therapeutic interventions. Medications can reduce symptoms and slow disease progression, but there may be limited effectiveness and possible side effects with long-term use. However, recent research has identified a promising approach for modifying the overall course of AD by using herbal medicine and nutraceuticals. Notably, herbal medicine and nutraceuticals are safe, affordable, and widely accessible. They offer a diverse range of medical benefits, including powerful antioxidant and anti-inflammatory properties and the ability to inhibit cell death.

These features provide a firm foundation for neuroprotection, ultimately leading to a decline in AD symptoms and an enhancement in overall quality of life [7].

Cocoa is the mature fruit of the cocoa tree (*Theobroma cacao* L.), which possesses potent antioxidants, anti-inflammatory, anti-proliferative, and neuroprotective activities. Cocoa flavonoids are protective against minor cognitive impairment and dementia in AD [8]. Vinpocetine (VIN) is an artificial derivative of the vinca alkaloid. It improves brain metabolism and elevates cognitive power. Therefore, it is used in stroke and other cerebrovascular disorders [9]. EGCG, the principal component of green tea, has been studied for its ability to treat inflammation and neurodegeneration [10]. It is well known for its ability to scavenge the free radicals and for its antioxidant and anti-apoptotic properties [9]. Wheatgrass (WG), an early grass of the wheat plant (*Triticumaestivum*), also possesses potent antioxidant effects because of its abundant chlorophyll, vitamins (A, C, and E), bioflavonoids, and mineral nutrients [11]. Another naturally occurring molecule that resembles a vitamin is coenzyme Q10 (CoQ10), which controls mitochondrial oxidative phosphorylation and, consequently, ATP synthesis [12]. CoQ10 has a potent protective effect against experimental cerebral ischemia/reperfusion injury [13] and AD [14]. In addition, the vitamin B complex group, a combination of eight water-soluble vitamins, has displayed potent protective effects against neurodegenerative diseases such as AD [15]. Clinically, Vit B complex is used to improve neurodegeneration [16]. Moreover, the combination therapy of vitamin C (Vit C), vitamin E (Vit E), and Selenium (Se) acts synergistically to provide valuable antioxidant protection against free radical-triggered cell membrane lipid peroxidation [17]. It has been previously stated that Se, Vit E, and Vit C activities are interconnected. Furthermore, deficiencies in these nutrients can cause various neurodegenerative diseases [18].

Our study builds upon previous research and aims to unravel the complex pathophysiological mechanisms involved in AD. Specifically, we sought to investigate the potential neuroprotective impact of cocoa, either alone or in combination with other nutraceuticals such as VIN, CoQ10, EGCG, WG, a combination of Vit E, Vit C, and Se, or the Vit B complex, using an animal model of aluminum-induced AD. Unlike prior investigations that only examined isolated compounds without comprehensive evaluations of behavioral and histopathological outcomes, our study provides a more comprehensive understanding of both the potential neuroprotective properties of these compounds and the additive effects that may arise from their combination. By evaluating critical pathways involved in AD, including oxidative stress, antioxidants, inflammation, ER stress, autophagy, Wnt3/β-Catenin/GSK-3β, and apoptosis, we can better grasp the underlying pathogenesis of the disease. Additionally, we explore how these nutraceuticals impact the pathways to yield neuroprotective effects.

Overall, our study offers valuable insights into the multifaceted pathogenesis of AD and highlights the potential of various nutraceuticals to exert neuroprotective effects through multiple signaling pathways. These findings could guide the development of novel therapeutic approaches for the treatment and prevention of AD.

2. Materials and Methods

2.1. Ethical Approval

The Animal Care and Use committee of the Faculty of Pharmacy, Al-Azhar University, reviewed and accepted the study protocol with ethical approval number 218/2021. The research complies with the ARRIVE criteria and follows the guidelines outlined in the "Guide for Care and Use of Laboratory Animals", published by the National Institutes of Health (NIH Publications No. 8023, revised 1978).

2.2. Materials

2.2.1. Drugs and Chemicals

Aluminum chloride hydrated (product number: 237078), cocoa extract blend (product number: W584649), CoQ10 (product number: C9538), EGCG (product number: PHL89656), Se (product number: GF59784575), and VIN (product number: V6383) were purchased from Sigma Chemical Co. (St. Louis, MO, USA). Wheatgrass powder was provided by Bioglan Super Foods (Surrey, England, UK). Before oral administration, the WG solution was prepared by suspending it in 1% tween in normal saline. The chemical constituents of WG were previously identified and analyzed in our previous work [19]. To prepare VIN, it was dissolved in distilled water. CoQ10 was dissolved in a 1% aqueous solution of Tween 80. Vit B complex, Vit E, and Vit C were obtained from Kahira Pharmaceutical and Chemicals Ind. Co., Cairo, Egypt. Fresh vitamin E was dissolved in corn oil, and vitamin B complex and vitamin C were dissolved in distilled water. All chemicals used were of the best commercially accessible quality.

2.2.2. Animals

Adult male albino rats ($n = 90$) weighing between 320 and 340 g were provided by Nile Co. for Pharmaceuticals and Chemical Industries, Cairo, Egypt. The rats were purchased and accommodated in cages with three to four rats each under standard laboratory conditions (automatically controlled temperature of 25 °C, humidity, ventilation, and 12-h light/dark cycle). One hour preceding each experiment, rats were taken to experimental locations for acclimatization after food and water were removed from their cages. All studies occurred between the hours of 9 a.m. and 2 p.m.

2.3. Methods

2.3.1. Experimental Design

The animals were divided into nine groups ($n = 10$) and injected daily with either saline for control (group 1) or $AlCl_3$ (70 mg/kg i.p.) for AD model groups for five weeks [20]. The first AD group served as the model control (group 2). While the other groups were administered $AlCl_3$ orally with cocoa (24 mg/kg, group 3) [21], either alone or in combination with EGCG (10 mg/kg, i.p.; Group 4) [22], VIN (20 mg/kg, group 5) [23], CoQ10 (200 mg/kg, group 6) [24], and WG (100 mg/kg, group 7) [19]. Vit B complex (0.2 mg/kg, group 8) [25] was also administered, as was a combination (group 9) of Vit E (100 mg/kg) [26], Vit C (400 mg/kg) [27], and Se (1 mg/kg) [26].

All treatments were administered by gastric gavage, except for $AlCl_3$ and EGCG. Four behavioral experiments were performed: The Y-maze, conditioned avoidance, Morris water maze, and swimming tests. Rats were sacrificed 24 h following the final test, and the brain tissues were then removed and subjected to ice-cold saline washing.

2.3.2. Behavioral Tests

Y Maze Test

After five weeks, the rats were assessed using the Y maze test to measure spatial working memory, evaluating spontaneous alternation behavior expressed as a percentage and calculated as previously described [28]. The Y maze used in this study was made of black wood and comprised three arms (35 cm long, 25 cm high, and 10 cm wide) with an equilateral triangular central area. During an 8-minute session, the rats had unrestricted access to the maze, starting with one arm. They typically alternated visits between the three arms, as they preferred to explore the arm that had not been recently visited. Effective alternation required the rats to use working memory, maintaining a running list of the arms they had most recently visited and updating it frequently. An entry into an arm was considered when the rat's rear paws were entirely inside the arm. An alteration occurred when the animal selected an arm different from the one it had previously visited. Although returning to the first arm was considered an error, it was, in fact, the correct answer. To determine the percentage of alternation, the total number of arm entries and their order were recorded, with the arms labeled as A, B, or C. Spontaneous alternation behavior was defined as entrance into all three arms on sequential choices. For example, if the rat made subsequent arm entrances A-C-B-C-A-B-C-A-C-A-B-C-A, it would have completed thirteen arm entrances, eight of which were actual alternations. Cognitive behavior and working memory were calculated as follows:

% Alternations = (Number of actual alterations made/Total number of arm entries − 2) × 100.

The number of maximal spontaneous alternation behaviors was the total number of arm entries minus two [29].

Conditioned Avoidance Test (CA)

The conditioned avoidance (CA) test was utilized to assess learning and memory after AD induction [30]. Garofalo et al. adopted an adjusted version of the test to evaluate the impact of treatment strategies on learning capacity post-AD induction. The parameters of the CA test were modified, and its application was expanded to assess learning capacity and memory consolidation under highly stressful circumstances.

The device used for the test consists of five interconnected compartments, with four of them equipped with electrified stainless-steel grid floors used to deliver a shock (unconditioned stimulus; 50 volts, 25 pulses/second). The fifth chamber has a glass floor, representing a safe zone. The training involved pairing an auditory stimulus (an electric bell and a conditioned stimulus) for five seconds with an additional 5 s of foot shock. The number of attempts made by each rat to avoid the electric shock and move to the safety area within five seconds of the conditioned stimulus was recorded on the first and second training days, demonstrating their capacity for learning and short-term memory recall.

Morris Water Maze Test

Spatial learning and memory were investigated using the Morris water maze test [31]. Tap water was poured into a circular water tank measuring 150 cm in diameter and 60 cm in height to a depth of 30 cm (25 ± 2 °C), and non-toxic white paint was added to make the water translucent. The pool was virtually divided into four equal quadrants (east, west, north, and south). An escape platform measuring 10 cm in diameter was buried 2 cm beneath the water's surface at a fixed location in the center of one quadrant. During the trial, the platform remained in the same quadrant. A video monitoring camera above the pool captured the rodents' swimming path. Each rat was placed into the water with its back towards the pool wall from a specific location in each quadrant and allowed to swim to the platform. Four trials were performed in each of the training sessions given to the rats each day for three consecutive days. The animals had a maximum of 60 s to locate the hidden platform before being allowed to rest on it for 20 s before the start of the next trial. If it took more than 60 s to find the platform, the rat was placed gently on it and given 20 s to rest. The escape latency, or the time taken to locate the platform, was noted. On the fourth day, a probe test was conducted by removing the platform and allowing the rats to swim freely for 60 s. The time spent in the designated quadrant was recorded.

Swimming Test

The swimming test was conducted using specific and customized methods [32]. The experiment was performed in a glass tank filled with water and maintained at a controlled temperature of 26 ± 2 °C. One end of the glass tank had a ramp, and the swimming activity began from the opposite side. Each rat was positioned in the tank and given three minutes to reach the ramp using its forepaws. Scores were assigned based on the rats' behavior: rats that reached the ramp directly received a score of 4, rats that deviated to the right or left before reaching the ramp received a score of 3, rats that deviated in both right and left directions before reaching the ramp received a score of 2, and rats that deviated in various directions away from the ramp before reaching it received a score of 1.

2.3.3. Tissue Sampling and Preparation

Rats were euthanized 24 h after the last behavioral test, and their brain tissues were then excised and carefully cleaned in isotonic saline. Four brains per group were fixed in 10% neutral buffered formalin overnight for histopathological investigations. Each of the remaining six brains was divided into two parts. The first part was homogenized instantly to produce a 10% homogenate (w/v) using an ice-cold medium containing 50 mM Tris-HCl (pH 7.4) and 300 mM sucrose [33]. For biochemical assays, the homogenate was centrifuged at $1800\times g$ for 10 min at 4 °C, and the supernatant was then stored at -20 °C. The second part was reserved at -80 °C to be used in real-time PCR analysis.

2.3.4. Histopathological Examination of Brain Tissue

After being fixed in 10% formalin for 24 h, samples of brain tissue were rinsed with water and serially diluted with alcohol to cause dehydration. The specimens were divided into 4 μm thick segments using a microtome after being immersed in paraffin. The tissue samples were then gathered on glass slides, deparaffinized, and stained with hematoxylin and eosin to perform a routine histological inspection under a light microscope [34].

2.3.5. Biochemical Measurements

Fluorometric Technique

After the rats were euthanized, levels of brain monoamines were immediately measured, as alterations in the substance's level might occur in a matter of minutes. Fluorometric assays of dopamine (DA), norepinephrine (NA), and serotonin (5-HT) were estimated in brain tissue homogenate according to the Ciarlone method [35].

Colorimetric Technique

The extent of lipid peroxidation in brain homogenate was measured colorimetrically by assessing malondialdehyde (MDA) using the thiobarbituric acid method (Chemie Gmbh, Steinheim, Germany). Nishilimi methods were used to measure the superoxide dismutase (SOD) enzyme activity based on its ability to reduce the nitro blue tetrazolium dye [36]. Lastly, the antioxidants' reactions with exogenously provided hydrogen peroxide (H_2O_2) were used for total antioxidant capacity (TAC) assessment. The residual H_2O_2 was estimated colorimetrically by the enzymatic reaction involving the alteration of 3,5-dichloro-2-hydroxybenzene sulphonate to a colored product.

ELISA Technique

Levels of Aβ, brain-derived neurotrophic factor (BDNF), 78 KDa glucose-regulated protein (GRP-78), phosphorylated PKR-like ER kinase (p-PERK)—C/EBP homologous protein (p-PERK/CHOP), and Beclin-1 were measured in brain tissue homogenate using ELISA kits (catalog numbers MBS702915, MBS494147, MBS807895, MBS251116, MBS3808179, and MBS901662, respectively) provided by My BioSource, Inc., San Diego, USA. Ray Biotech ELISA kits (product numbers ELR-IL1b and RTA00) were used to estimate interleukin-1β (IL-1β) and tumor necrosis factor alpha (TNF-α) levels in brain tissue homogenate, respectively. Rat β-catenin ELISA Kit (K3383, Biovision Inc.) and Wnt Family Member 3A (Wnt3a) (orb555678, Biorbyt Ltd., Cambridge, UK) were used to assess their brain concentrations according to the manufacturer's guidelines. ACHE activity was detected by the ELISA kit (MAK119) provided by Sigma-Aldrich Co. (St. Louis, MO, USA). The quantitative sandwich ELISA method was used consistently with the manufacturer's instructions.

Real-Time Quantitative Polymerase Chain Reaction

The mRNA levels of *Nrf2*, *HO-1*, *GSK-3β*, and *Bcl-2* were assessed using real-time quantitative polymerase chain reaction (RT-qPCR) with the Applied Biosystems Step One Plus apparatus. Total RNA was extracted following the manufacturer's recommendations using the Qiagen tissue extraction kit (Qiagen, Germantown, MD, USA). The isolated mRNA was reverse-transcribed with a sense rapid cDNA synthesis kit (CAT No. BIO-65053) and then amplified using the Maxima SYBR Green qPCR kit (Fermentas, Hanover, MD, USA). The mRNA levels were detected using the ABI Prism 7500 sequence detector system (Applied Biosystems, Foster City, CA, USA). The results were normalized to β-actin expression using the $2^{-\Delta\Delta CT}$ method to calculate the relative expression of the target genes

Nrf2, HO-1, GSK-3β, Bcl-2, and β-actin. The primer sequences for the PCR amplification are shown in Table 1.

Table 1. The sequences of primers employed in real-time RT-PCR analysis.

Gene	Primer Sequence	Accession Number	Product Size (bp)	Annealing Temp. (°C)
Nrf2	F: 5′-CTCTCTGGAGACGGCCATGACT-3′ R: 5′-CTGGGCTGGGGACAGTGGTAGT-3′	NM_031789	149 bp	68.4
HO-1	F: 5′-CACCAGCCACACAGCACTAC-3′ R: 5′-CACCCACCCCTCAAAAGACA-3′	NM_012580	1043 bp	65.3
GSK-3β	F: 5′-AGCCTATATCCATTCCTTGG-3′ R: 5′-CCTCGGACCAGCTGCTTT-3′	NM_032080	701 bp	59.1
Bcl-2	F: 5′-GGATGACTTCTCTCGTCGCTAC-3′ R: 5′-TGACATCTCCCTGTTGACGCT-3′	NM_016993	199 bp	64.9
β-actin	F: 5′-CCGTAAAGACCTCTATGCCA-3′ R: 5′-AAGAAAGGGTGTAAAACGCA-3′	NM_031144	299 bp	61.8

2.4. Statistical Analysis

The one-way ANOVA was employed for multiple comparisons, followed by the Tukey-Kramer test for post-hoc analysis. Results are presented as mean ± SEM, with $p < 0.05$ considered statistically significant. Statistical analysis was conducted using GraphPad Prism software (version 8, ISI®, San Diego, CA, USA), and the graphs were generated using the same software.

3. Results

In this study, we conducted a comprehensive investigation, including seven different normal control groups of rats, each receiving a distinct intervention in addition to the previously studied groups. These interventions involved cocoa alone, a combination of cocoa with EGCG, VIN, WG, CoQ10, and the Vit B complex, or a combination of Vit E, Vit C, and Se. However, despite the variety of interventions, none of the seven groups showed any significant differences in the measured parameters or histopathological findings compared to the normal control group. For the sake of clarity and simplicity in presenting the data, we did not include these findings in the final research paper.

3.1. Behavioral Tests

3.1.1. Y-Maze Test (Percent of Spontaneous Alterations; Assessment of Reference Memory)

As displayed in Figure 1A, the AD group exhibited a substantial but significant reduction (approximately 23%) in the percentage of continuous alternations when compared to the control group. Treatment with cocoa significantly increased, by approximately 8.5%, the percent of spontaneous alternations when compared to the AD group. Conversely, the influence of the combination of cocoa with VIN, or a mixture of Vit E, C, and Se, revealed the maximum improvement in the percent of spontaneous alterations by 1.2-fold compared to the cocoa-treated group.

3.1.2. Conditioned Avoidance Test (CA) (Assessment of Acquired or Learned Response)

As shown in Figure 1B, the AD group displayed a 5-fold increase on the first day compared to the control group, proving very low short-term memory, and no improvement on the second day relative to the control group. Treatment with cocoa caused a diminution in the number of trials on the first day by 38% related to the AD group. The combination of cocoa and VIN exhibited a maximum further reduction in the number of trials by 65% compared to the cocoa-administered group.

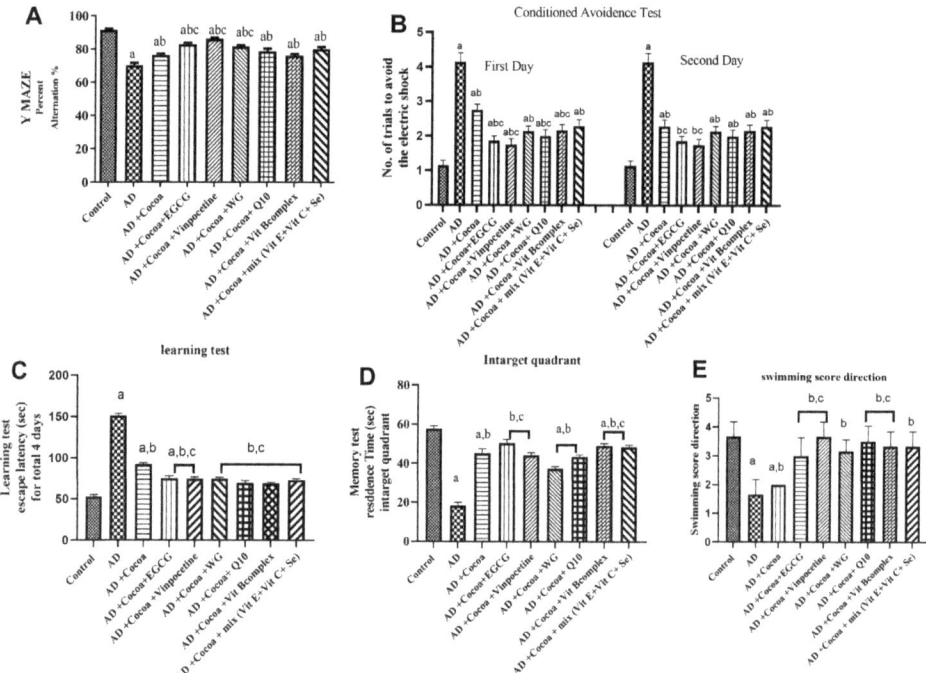

Figure 1. Effect of Cocoa Alone and in Combination with VIN or Other Nutraceuticals on Behavioral Tests in AlCl$_3$-induced AD. EGCG; Epigallocatechin-3-gallate, VIN; vinpocetine, WG; Wheatgrass, Q10; coenzyme Q10, Vit; vitamin. (**A**) Effect of treatments on both the locomotor activity and the % spontaneous alternations in the Y-maze model. (**B**) Influence of interventions on the number of attempts to pass the conditioned avoidance test on the first and second days without receiving an electric shock. (**C**) Influence of treatments on the escape latency in Morris water maze test. (**D**) Effect of treatments on the residence time in target quadrant in Morris water maze test (**E**) Effect of treatments on the swimming score direction. Results are established as mean ± SEM, n = 6. The significance level at $p < 0.05$). ^{a} indicates significant difference from the control group, ^{b} indicates significant difference from AD group, and ^{c} indicates significant difference from (AD + Cocoa) group. AD; Alzheimer's disease.

As revealed in Figure 1C, the average latency over the 4 days of training trials increased by 2.2-fold in the AD group compared to the control animals. Management with cocoa resulted in a 34% decrease in escape latency relative to the AD group. The combination of cocoa and either EGCG or VIN exhibited the maximum reversal effect on the spatial memory impairment by 46% and 47%, respectively, relative to the cocoa-treated group.

Figure 1D displayed a 66.5% reduction in the residence time in the AD group relative to the control group, signifying a strong impairment of memory induced by AlCl$_3$. The cocoa administration increased the residence time by nearly 2.3 times more than the AD group, which markedly enhanced this subpar performance. The combination of cocoa and either EGCG, VIN, or the mixture of Vit E, Vit C, and Se offered the maximum protection and prolonged residence time (2.8, 2.7, and 2.8-fold, respectively) associated with the cocoa-treated AD group. 3.1.4 Swimming test (ST) (used to reflect cognitive function).

Figure 1E revealed that the AlCl$_3$-induced AD group reduced its swimming score direction by 70% compared to the control group. Treatment with cocoa improved the swimming score by 2.6-fold compared with the AD group. Interestingly, co-treatment with cocoa and either EGCG or VIN significantly elevated (3-fold) the swimming score direction compared with the cocoa-treated AD group (adding 60% over the protective effect of cocoa treatment).

3.2. Biochemical Measurements

3.2.1. The Effect of Cocoa Alone and in Combination with VIN or Other Nutraceuticals on Oxidative Stress and Antioxidant Biomarkers in Brain Tissues in $AlCl_3$-Induced AD

As depicted in Figure 2A–C, the administration of $AlCl_3$ significantly reduced the mRNA expression levels of antioxidant Nrf2 and HO-1, as well as the activity of SOD, by 91.6%, 90.5%, and 75%, respectively, compared to the control group. In contrast, treatment with cocoa showed a 4-, 3-, and 2-fold increase in the mRNA expression levels of Nrf2 and HO-1 and the SOD activity, respectively, relative to the AD group.

Notably, co-administration of cocoa with either EGCG or VIN resulted in the most substantial elevation in the mRNA expression levels of both Nrf2 (by 7.6- and 9.6-fold) and HO-1 (by 6.6- and 8.4-fold), as well as the activity of SOD (by 4.7- and 3.6-fold), compared to the AD group. Furthermore, the SOD activity in the cocoa combination with EGCG, VIN, and WG did not show significant differences from the normal group.

Figure 2D demonstrates that the AD group exhibited a significantly reduced TAC (total antioxidant capacity) level of 59.6% compared to the control group. However, administration of cocoa mitigated the $AlCl_3$ effect, leading to a 1.6-fold increase in TAC level compared to the controls. Co-administration of cocoa with either EGCG or VIN exhibited the highest elevation in TAC level by 2.4-fold compared to the AD group. Additionally, the TAC levels in all cocoa combination groups were not significantly different from the normal controls.

As shown in Figure 2E, the administration of $AlCl_3$ resulted in a 14-fold increase in the MDA (malondialdehyde) level compared to the control group. However, cocoa supplementation was able to reverse the $AlCl_3$ effects by reducing the MDA level by 90% compared to the control group. Furthermore, co-administration of cocoa with either EGCG, VIN, or WG exhibited a significant maximum reduction in the MDA level by 96%, 95.5%, and 94.4%, respectively, compared to the AD group. The MDA levels also returned to normal in the cocoa treatment and the combination of cocoa with VIN, WG, and Vit B complex.

3.2.2. Effect of Cocoa Alone and in Combination with VIN or Other Nutraceuticals on the Inflammatory Biomarkers in Brain Tissues

Figure 3A,B exhibited that the levels of IL-1β and TNF-α were considerably augmented in the brain by 4-fold, 14-fold correspondingly in the AD group versus the control group. Treatment with cocoa diminished the $AlCl_3$ mediated inflammatory responses and diminished IL-1β and TNF-α levels significantly by 34% and 46% correspondingly relative to the AD group. Interestingly, co-administration of cocoa with either EGCG, VIN, or WG offered the best downregulation effect on the IL-1β level by 67%, 64.7%, and 57% respectively compared with the AD group. While co-administration of cocoa with either EGCG or VIN could restore the TNF-α brain level and decrease it by 74.5% and 72.8% compared with the AD group.

3.2.3. Effect of Cocoa Alone and in Combination with VIN or Other Nutraceuticals on GSK-3β/BDNF and Wnt/β-catenin Pathways in $AlCl_3$-Induced AD

As shown in Figure 4A,B, the AD group exhibited a significant 12-fold and 11-fold increase in Aβ content and GSK-3β expression levels, respectively, compared to the control group. Treatment with cocoa considerably reduced Aβ content by 70.6% and GSK-3β expression level by 31% compared to the AD group. Interestingly, the combinations of cocoa with either EGCG or VIN further reduced the Aβ levels by 87.6% and 88.7%, respectively, compared to the AD group. Moreover, co-treatment with cocoa and either EGCG or VIN maximally decreased the $AlCl_3$-induced GSK-3β expression by 62% and 68.8%, respectively.

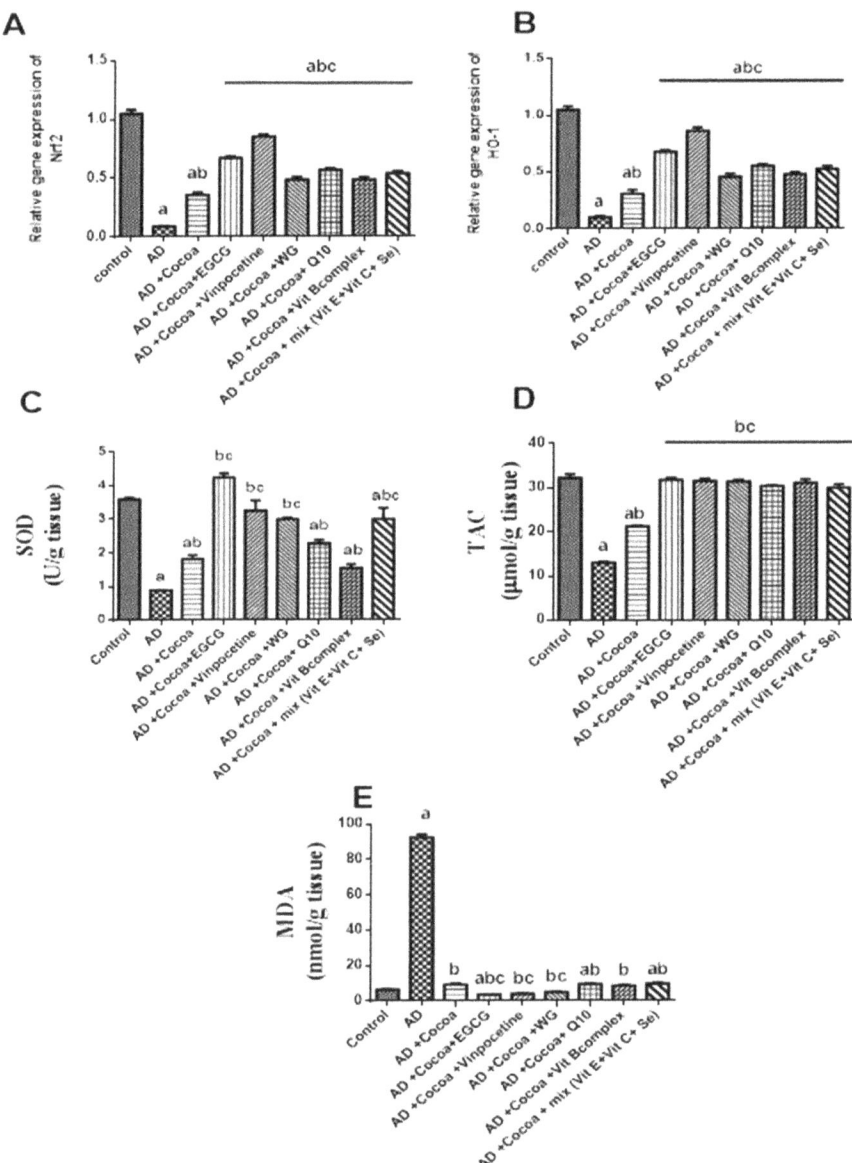

Figure 2. Effect of Cocoa Alone and in Combination with VIN or Other Nutraceuticals on the Oxidative Stress Biomarkers and Antioxidants in Brain Tissue in AlCl$_3$-induced AD. EGCG; Epigallocatechin-3-gallate, VIN; vinpocetine, WG; Wheatgrass, Q10; coenzyme Q10, Vit; vitamin. (**A**) Nrf2 gene expression level, (**B**) HO-1 gene expression level, (**C**) SOD level, (**D**) TAC level, and (**E**) MDA level. Results are proved as mean ± SEM, $n = 6$. The significant level at $p < 0.05$. [a] indicates significant difference from the control group, [b] indicates significant difference from AD group, and [c] indicates significant difference from (AD + Cocoa) group. AD: Alzheimer's disease; Nrf2: erythroid-2 related factor 2; HO-1: Heme oxygenase-1; SOD: Superoxide dismutase; TAC: Total antioxidant capacity; MDA: Malondialdehyde.

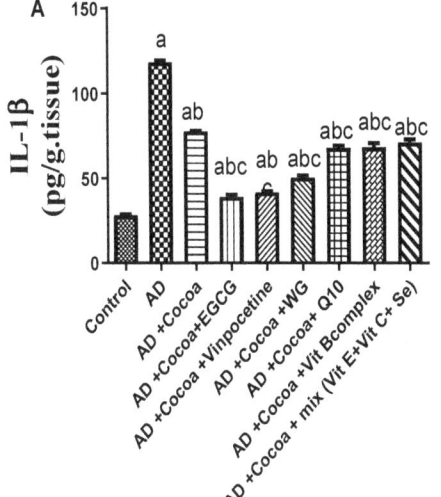 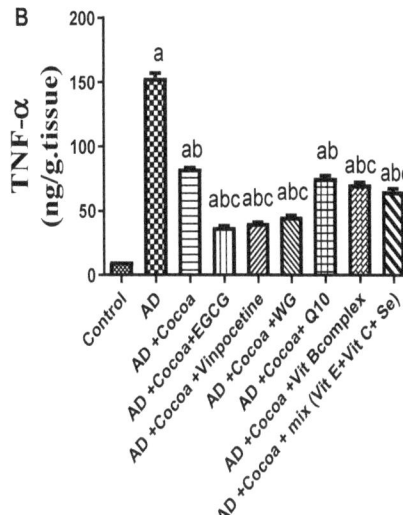

Figure 3. Effect of Cocoa Alone and in Combination with VIN or Other Nutraceuticals on the Brain Inflammatory Mediators. EGCG; Epigallocatechin-3-gallate, VIN; vinpocetine, WG; Wheatgrass, Q10; coenzyme Q10, Vit; vitamin. (**A**) IL-1β level, (**B**) TNF-α level. Results are established as mean ± SEM, $n = 6$. The significant level at $p < 0.05$. [a] indicates significant difference from the control group, [b] indicates significant difference from AD group, and [c] indicates significant difference from (AD + Cocoa) group. AD: Alzheimer's disease; IL-1β: Interlukin-1β; TNF-α: Tumor necrosis factor alpha.

Figure 4C,D demonstrate that administration of $AlCl_3$ resulted in a 7.6-fold and 3.6-fold decrease in Wnt3a and β-catenin levels, respectively, compared to the control group. Treating the rats with cocoa significantly elevated the Wnt3a and β-catenin levels by 20% and 17.5%, respectively, compared to the controls. Co-treatment of cocoa with either EGCG or VIN restored the Wnt3a level in the brain, showing an elevation of 42% and 34%, respectively, compared to the AD group. Similarly, co-treatment with cocoa and either EGCG or VIN augmented the cocoa effect, increasing the β-catenin protein level by 29% and 33%, respectively, compared to the AD group.

As revealed in Figure 4E, the BDNF content was significantly reduced in the AD group by 37.6% compared to the control group. However, treatment with cocoa significantly increased the BDNF content by 1.7-fold compared to the AD group. Interestingly, combinations of cocoa with either EGCG or VIN restored the basal level of BDNF content, showing a 32.8% and 32.7% increase in BDNF content, respectively, compared to the AD group, resulting in maximum cognitive enhancement.

3.2.4. Effect of Cocoa Alone and in Combination with VIN or Other Nutraceuticals on ER Stress, Autophagy, and Apoptotic Markers in $AlCl_3$-Induced AD

As shown in Figure 5A–C, there was a significant elevation in the levels of p-PERK, GRP-78, and CHOP by 99-fold, 390-fold, and 66-fold, respectively, in the AD group compared to the control group. Treatment with cocoa decreased the elevated levels of p-PERK, GRP-78, and CHOP by 25%, 25%, and 34%, respectively, compared to the controls. Moreover, co-treatment with cocoa and either EGCG or VIN further augmented the cocoa's effect, reducing the p-PERK level by 60% and 80%, respectively, compared to the AD group. Additionally, co-administration with cocoa and either EGCG or VIN improved the cocoa's influence, decreasing the GRP-78 level by 75% and 79%, respectively, relative to the AD group. Furthermore, the co-treatment with cocoa and either EGCG or VIN enhanced the cocoa effect, reducing the CHOP level by 68% and 80%, respectively, compared to the AD group.

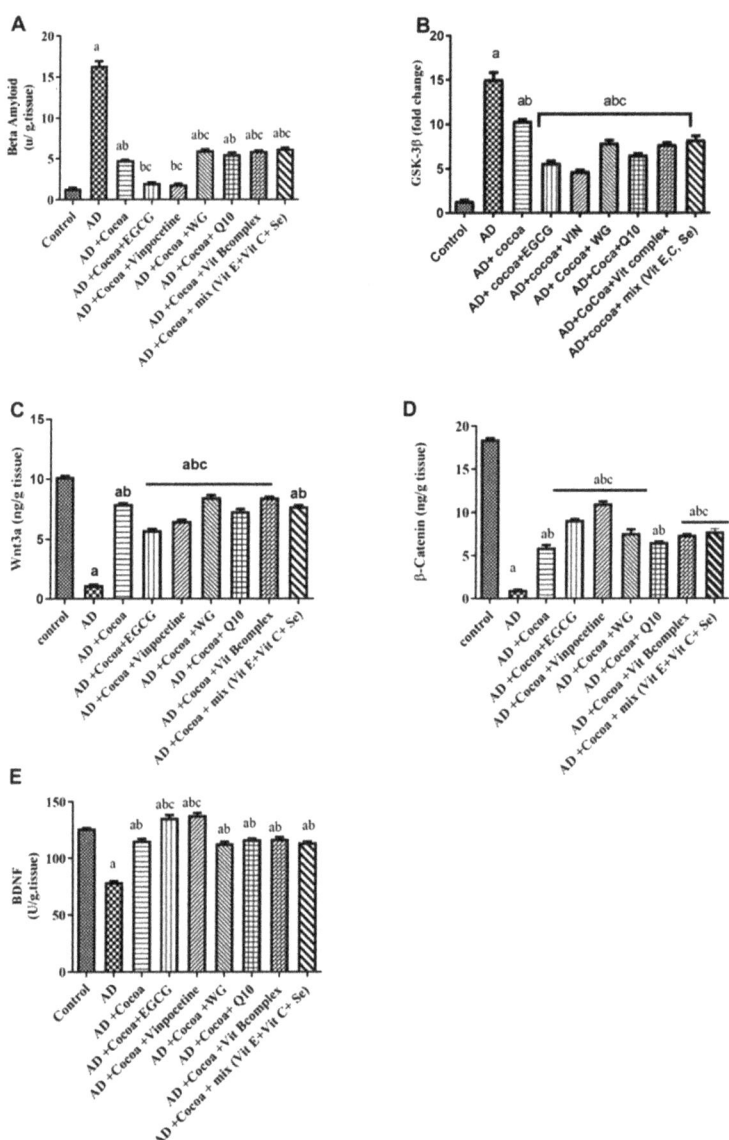

Figure 4. Effect of Cocoa Alone and in Combination with VIN or Other Nutraceuticals on (A) Aβ content and (B) GSK-3β expression level and (C) Wnt3a content (D) β-catenin content (E) BDNF level in AlCl$_3$-induced AD. Results are established as a mean ± SEM, n = 6. The significant level at $p < 0.05$. [a] indicates significant difference from the control group, [b] indicates significant difference from AD group, and [c] indicates significant difference from (AD + cocoa) group. AD: Alzheimer's disease; Aβ: amyloid-beta; Wnt3a: Wnt Family Member 3A; BDNF: Brain-derived neurotrophic factor.

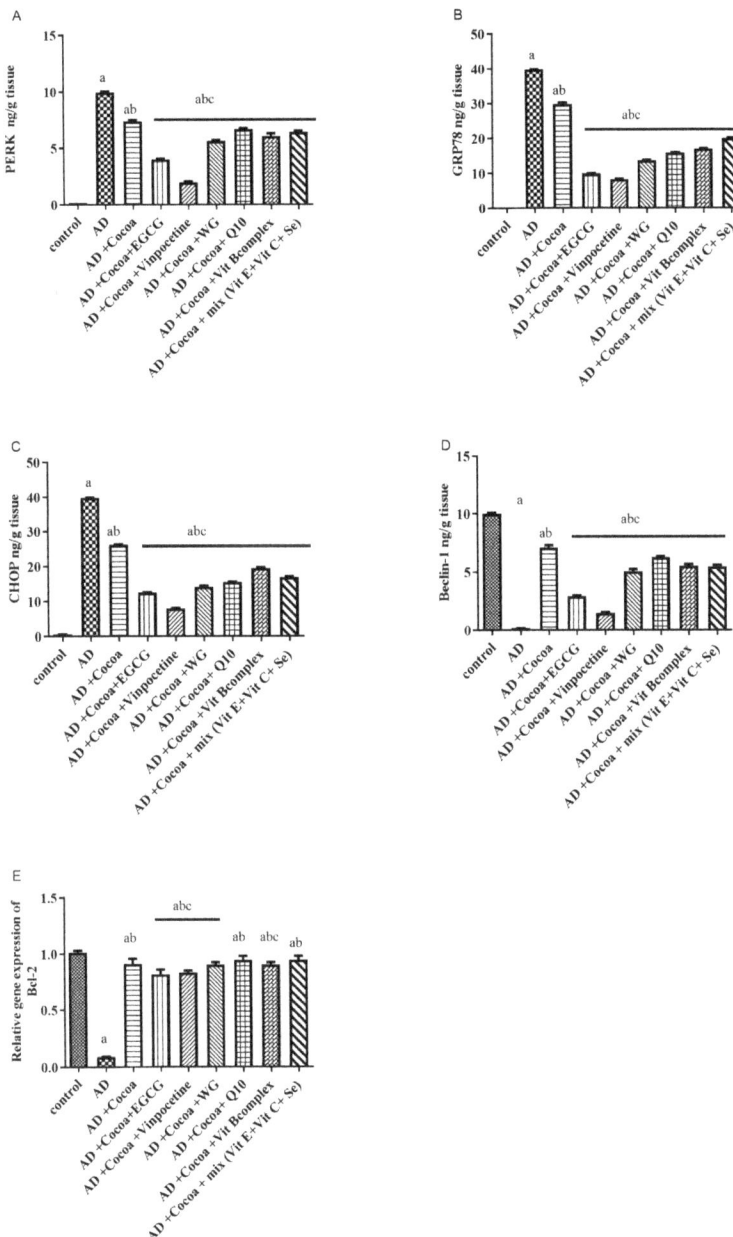

Figure 5. Effect of Cocoa Alone and in Combination with VIN or Other Nutraceuticals on (**A**) p-PERK level (**B**) GRP-78 level (**C**) CHOP level (**D**) Beclin-1 (**E**) *Bcl-2* level, in AlCl$_3$-induced AD. EGCG; Epigallocatechin-3-gallate, VIN; vinpocetine, WG; Wheatgrass, Q10; coenzyme Q10, Vit; vitamin. Results are demonstrated as mean ± SEM, n = 6. The significant level at $p < 0.05$. [a] indicates significant difference from the control group, [b] indicates significant difference from AD group, [c] indicates significant difference from (AD + Cocoa) group. AD: Alzheimer's disease; GRP-78: 78 KDa glucose-regulated protein; p-PERK: phosphorylated PERK; CHOP: C/EBP homologous protein.

Figure 5D,E displayed a substantial decline in the levels of Beclin-1 and the relative gene expression of Bcl-2 by 98% and 92%, respectively, in the AD group compared to the control group. Treatment with cocoa elevated the levels of Beclin-1 and Bcl-2 relative gene expression by 8.9-fold and 9-fold, respectively, compared to the control group. Moreover, co-treatment with cocoa and either EGCG or VIN further augmented the cocoa effect by enhancing the Beclin-1 level by 43-fold and 38-fold, respectively, relative to the AD group. Similarly, co-treatment with cocoa and either EGCG or VIN augmented the cocoa effect and elevated Bcl-2 relative gene expression by 11-fold compared to the AD group.

3.2.5. Effect of Cocoa Alone and in Combination with VIN or Other Nutraceuticals on the Brain Neurotransmitters; Monoamines and ACHE Activity in $AlCl_3$-Induced AD

Figure 6A,B show that the AD group had significantly reduced levels of DA and NE by 67.7% and 65%, respectively, compared to the control group. Administration of cocoa caused a 2-fold and 1.8-fold elevation in dopamine and norepinephrine levels, respectively, relative to the AD group. Consistent with previous results, co-administration of cocoa with either EGCG or VIN displayed the highest increase (2.8- and 3-fold rise) in the DA level compared to the AD group. Moreover, co-administration of cocoa with EGCG, VIN, or WG effectively restored the basal level of NE and caused a 2.5-, 2.5-, and 2.4-fold increase in its level, respectively, compared to the AD group.

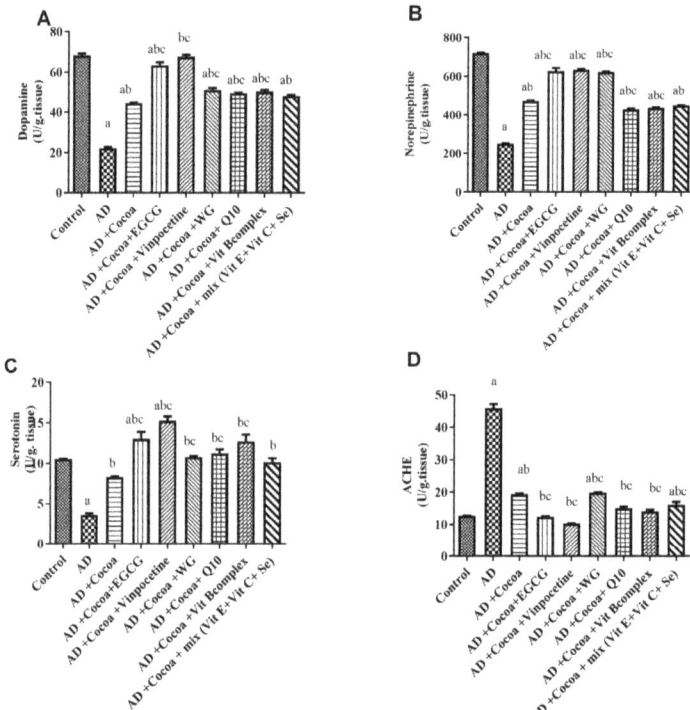

Figure 6. Effect of Cocoa Alone and in Combination with VIN or Other Nutraceuticals on the Brain Monoamine Parameters and ACHE Activity in $AlCl_3$-induced AD. Results of (**A**) Dopamine level, (**B**) Norepinephrine level, (**C**) Serotonin level, (**D**) ACHE activity. Results are established as a mean ± SEM, $n = 6$. The significant level at $p < 0.05$. [a] indicates significant difference from the control group, [b] indicates significant difference from AD group, and [c] indicates significant difference from (AD + cocoa) group. AD: Alzheimer's disease; EGCG: Epigallocatechin-3-gallate; VIN: vinpocetine; WG: Wheatgrass, Q10: coenzyme Q10; Vit: vitamin.

Figure 6C shows the changes in the cerebral level of serotonin. Treatment with $AlCl_3$ revealed a substantial reduction in the level of serotonin by 66% compared to the controls. However, management with cocoa significantly elevated serotonin levels by 2.3-fold compared to the control group. The maximum restoration effect for the serotonin level was observed after treatment with cocoa with either EGCG or VIN, resulting in a 3.6- and 4.2-fold increase in serotonin level, respectively, compared to the AD group.

As displayed in Figure 6D, the administration of $AlCl_3$ (70 mg/kg) in the AD group significantly increased the activity of ACHE by 3.7-fold compared to the controls. However, treatment with cocoa decreased the ACHE activity by 57.7% relative to the AD group. Interestingly, co-treatment of cocoa with VIN exhibited a maximum further reduction in the ACHE activity of 77.5% compared to the AD group.

3.3. Histopathological Alterations of Brain Tissue in Different Regions

As depicted in Figure 7, the picture of brain tissue segments of rodents stained by H&E stain (magnification 40×) exhibited that in the controls, there was no histopathological change, and the normal histological structure of the neurons was exhibited in the cerebral cortex, subiculum, and fascia dentata in the hippocampus, striatum, and cerebellum regions (Inserts a1, a2, a3, a4, a5). Meanwhile, in the AD group, nuclear pyknosis and degeneration were observed in the cerebral cortex, subiculum, and fascia dentata in the hippocampus, besides multiple large-size focal eosinophilic plagues with damage to the neurons detected in the striatum area. Yet, there was no histopathological modification recorded in cerebellum areas (Inserts b1, b2, b3, b4, b5). While in the AD group treated with cocoa, nuclear pyknosis and degeneration were detected in a few neurons of the cerebral cortex and subiculum and fascia dentata of the hippocampus. In addition, no histopathological change and the normal histological structure of the neurons were established in the striatum and cerebellum (Inserts c1, c2, c3, c4, c5). In the AD group managed with cocoa and EGCG, nuclear pyknosis and deterioration were distinguished in all neurons of the cerebral cortex. There was no histopathological change in the subiculum, fascia dentata, or hilus of the hippocampus, striatum, or the cerebellum (Inserts d1, d2, d3, d4, d5). In the AD group that received cocoa and VIN, there was no histopathological change in the cerebral cortex, subiculum, or fascia dentata of the hippocampus or cerebellum. Focal small-size eosinophilic plagues' creation with loss in most of the neurons was recorded in the striatum (Inserts e1, e2, e3, e4, e5). In the AD group treated with cocoa and WG, there was no histopathological modification in the hippocampus's subiculum and cerebellum, but nuclear pyknosis and damage were detected in all the neurons of the cerebral cortex and fascia dentata of the hippocampus. Besides, focal small-size eosinophilic plague formation with nuclear pyknosis in most of the neurons was verified in the striatum area (Inserts f1, f2, f3, f4, f5). In the AD group that received both cocoa and Q10, there was no histopathological modification, as in the cerebral cortex, subiculum of the hippocampus, or cerebellum. Some neurons displayed nuclear pyknosis and degeneration in the fascia dentata of the hippocampus, and there were a few focal eosinophilic small-size plagues produced with nuclear pyknosis in some neurons in the striatum (Inserts g1, g2, g3, g4, g5). In the AD management with both cocoa and the Vit B complex group, there was no histopathological change in the striatum and the cerebellum. However, there was nuclear pyknosis and degeneration in a few neurons of the cerebral cortex, subiculum, and fascia dentata of the hippocampus (Inserts h1, h2, h3, h4, h5). In the AD group administered with cocoa and a mixture of Vit E, Vit C, and Se, there was no histopathological variation in the cerebral cortex, subiculum of the hippocampus, striatum, or cerebellum. Yet, most of the neurons displayed nuclear pyknosis and deterioration in the fascia dentata of the hippocampus (Inserts i1, i2, i3, i4, i5).

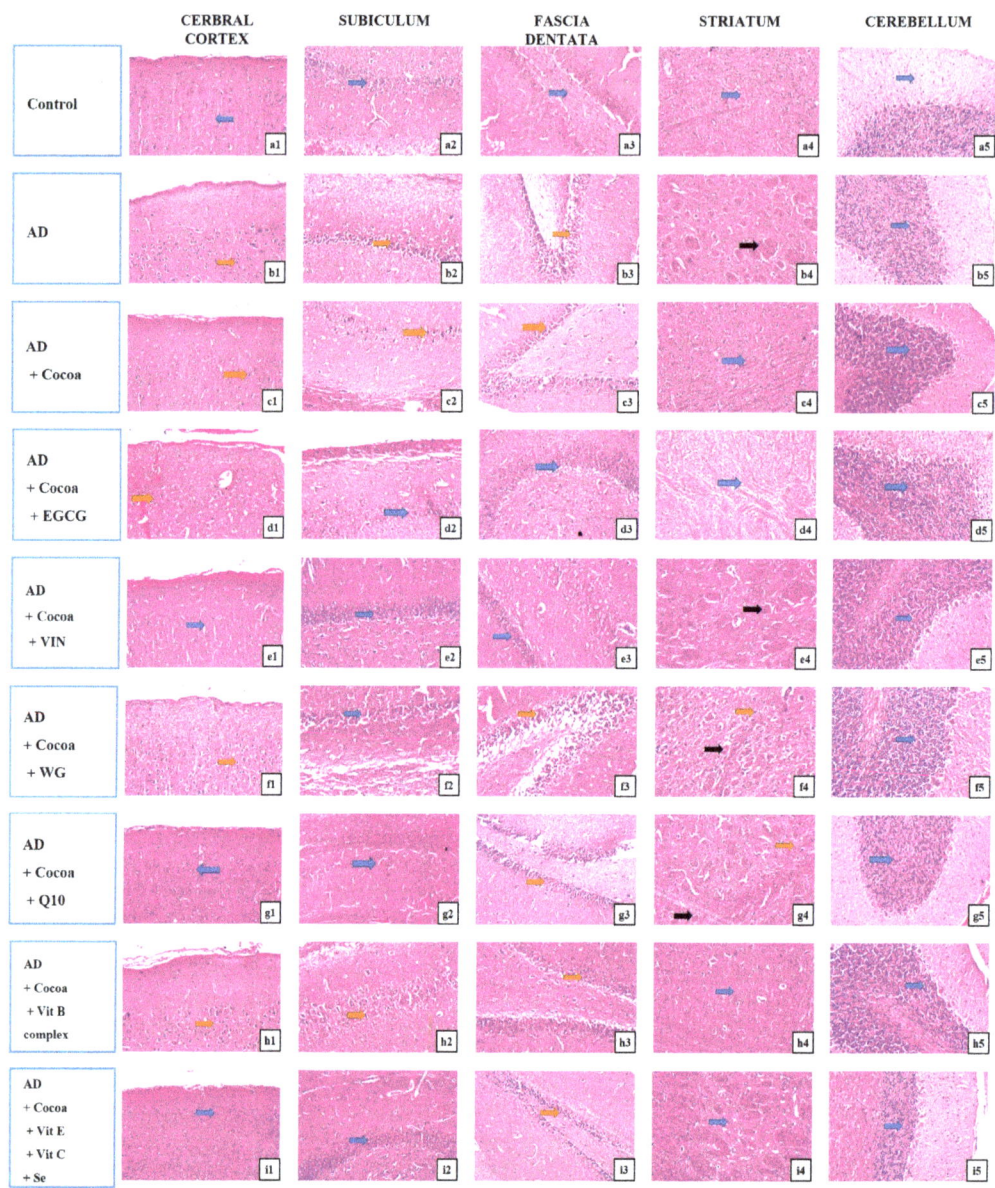

Figure 7. Photomicrographs of brain sections (cerebral cortex, subiculum, and fascia dentata in hippocampus, striatum, and cerebellum areas) stained by hematoxylin and eosin (magnification 40×). AD; Alzheimer disease, EGCG; Epigallocatechin-3-gallate, VIN; vinpocetine, WG; Wheatgrass, Q10; coenzyme Q10, Vit; vitamin. (**a1–a5**): control group, (**b1–b5**): AD group, (**c1–c5**): AD + cocoa group, (**d1–d5**): AD+cocoa+EGCG group, (**e1–e5**): AD + cocoa + VIN group, (**f1–f5**): AD + cocoa + WG group, (**g1–g5**): AD + cocoa + CoQ10 group, (**h1–h5**): AD + cocoa + Vit B complex group, and (**i1–i5**): AD + cocoa + VitE + VitC + Se group. The blue arrow shows no histopathological modification, the orange arrow displays nuclear pyknosis and degeneration, and the black arrow shows focal eosinophilic plagues, the Scare bar was 25μm.

As revealed in Table 2, the maximum neuroprotective effect with the least scores was the AD group treated with cocoa either with EGCG or VIN.

Table 2. The cerebral cortex and hippocampus histopathological score.

Groups' Histopathology		Control	AD Group	AD-Treated with Cocoa	The AD-Induced Group Treated with a Combination of Cocoa with					
					EGCG	VIN	WG	CoQ10	Vit B Complex	Vit E + Vit C + Se
Histopathological Changes	Brain Region									
Nuclear pyknosis and degeneration in the neuronal cells of the of	cerebral cortex	-	+++	+	+	-	+	-	+	-
	the subiculum	-	+++	+	-	-	-	-	+	-
	the fascia dentate of the hippocampus	-	+++	-	-	+	+	+	+	+
Focal eosinophilic plagues in of	the striatum	-	+++	-	-	+	+	+	-	-
Atrophy in the neuronal cells	the cerebellum	-	-	-	-	-	-	-	-	-

AD; Alzheimer disease, EGCG; Epigallocatechin-3-gallate, VIN; vinpocetine, WG; Wheatgrass, Q10; coenzyme Q10, Vit; vitamin. Severe: +++; Mild: +; Nil: -.

4. Discussion

AD is a complex neurodegenerative illness characterized by a progressive deterioration in cognitive abilities, including memory, thinking, and learning. Unfortunately, aluminum (Al), which is widely present in our environment and food sources, poses a significant threat to human health and is considered a potential risk factor for AD [2]. As there is currently no definitive therapy for AD, there is an urgent need for innovative treatment strategies that can halt or reverse the devastating effects of the disease. In this context, natural products, especially those derived from plants, offer a promising avenue for developing safe, effective, and affordable therapies for AD. With their unique chemical structures and diverse pharmacological activities, natural products represent a promising frontier in the search for new approaches to AD therapeutics [7]. Thus, our study aims to deeply understand the pathophysiological mechanisms of AD and to assess and compare the protective benefits of cocoa, either individually or in combination with other nutraceuticals. These nutraceuticals have already demonstrated their neuroprotective effects in prior studies or their significance in ameliorating AD symptoms, particularly in $AlCl_3$-induced AD. While previous studies have focused on the individual influences of these compounds, our current research aims to provide a more comprehensive understanding of their potential combination of neuroprotective effects.

The outcomes of this study unequivocally establish that chronic daily administration of $AlCl_3$ at a dose of 70 mg/kg i.p. for five weeks results in significant neurobehavioral, neurohistopathological, and neurochemical alterations. However, administering cocoa alone or in combination with EGCG, VIN, WG, Q10, the Vit B complex, and a mixture of Vit E, Vit C, and Se was found to be highly effective in providing robust protection against the risks of AD by reversing the adverse effects. These findings have exciting implications for the possible use of these natural compounds in the development of new therapeutic interventions for neurodegenerative illnesses.

In our behavioral study, a significant decline in learning ability and cognitive function was identified, evidenced by an increase in the number of avoidance attempts in the CA test and a decrease in spontaneous alternation in the Y-Maze test among the AD group compared to the control group. These findings suggest a deterioration of learning capability and spatial memory. The declining performance observed in the Morris water maze test supports this. Specifically, the increased escape latency and reduced residence time in the target quadrant among the AD group indicate deficits in learning, memory, and cognitive abilities induced by AlCl$_3$ intoxication. Our results are consistent with the prior research conducted by Gu et al. (2009) [37], who also reported significant spatial working memory deficits using the Y-maze among individuals with AD. Additionally, our findings are supported by previous studies that have established behavioral alterations in AlCl$_3$-treated rats [38,39]. Administering cocoa alone or in combination with other nutraceuticals resulted in a significant improvement in learning and cognitive function in AlCl$_3$-induced AD. In line with our results, previous studies suggested a significant neuromodulator and neuroprotective influence of cocoa flavonoids and their potential for executive ability, behavior, and mental and emotional functions [40]. In addition, the VIN has a neuroprotective influence and can improve learning and memory impairments caused by prolonged cerebral hypoperfusion [9]. EGCG also prevented poor behavioral outcomes associated with AD in rats [19]. Previous studies have revealed that continuous supplementation with Q10, Se, and vitamins (B complex, E, and C) can improve mood and neurotransmitter activity [41].

The observed alterations in behavior in this study were remarkably linked to modifications in underlying histopathological and biochemical parameters. Notably, AD is characterized by severe deterioration of neuronal and synaptic architecture, resulting in the production of Aβ plaques, followed by the buildup of hyperphosphorylated tau protein neurofibrillary tangles in the brain. The extracellular buildup of Aβ and intracellular hyperphosphorylation of the tau protein are the primary culprits of neurons' degeneration. Soluble Aβ oligomers can also accelerate the onset of tau hyperphosphorylation, leading to impaired plasticity of hippocampal synapses and ultimately causing memory dysfunction (Kitagishi et al., 2014) [42]. The progressive buildup of pathological substances, induced by a complex cascade of events, ultimately results in a critical loss of fundamental cholinergic, synaptic, and cognitive functions, which are the hallmarks of AD [43]. Therefore, understanding the intricate interplay between these processes and identifying effective interventions is a pivotal research pursuit with the potential to improve the devastating impact of these debilitating conditions on affected individuals.

AlCl$_3$ induces neuronal oxidative stress [2], resulting in increased expression of free radicals, reactive oxygen species (ROS), and reactive nitrogen species (RNS) [43]. Therefore, oxidative stress triggers destruction in the cellular proteins and nucleic acids, besides lipid peroxidation and raised levels of MDA, a robust biomarker of oxidative stress in the brain [44]. Whereas the Nrf2 transcription factors serve as a critical activators of antioxidant enzymes such as superoxide dismutase-1 (SOD1), HO-1, and CAT to mitigate oxidative stress. Nrf2 also effectively suppresses inflammation mediated by microglia and boosts mitochondrial function. In AD, the Nrf2 pathway undergoes downregulation within the hippocampal neurons because of oxidative stress, leading to a marked reduction in crucial antioxidant enzymes (HO-1, CAT, and SOD1) and a consequent reduction in overall TAC [45,46]. The empirical data corroborate our findings with high consistency and accuracy. However, our drug regimens revealed remarkable antioxidant capabilities, effectively mitigating chronic AlCl$_3$-induced oxidative stress. Markedly, co-administration of cocoa with VIN or EGCG emerged as the most efficacious treatment in our study against AD. Cocoa flavonoids are known for their potent antioxidant activity [47]. In the same scenario, VIN and EGCG have antioxidant potential [48,49]. Similarly, Vit B, Se, and Vit E supplementation decreased oxidative stress markers such as MDA [50]. The combination of Vit E and C is valuable and highly synergistic since Vit C can reactivate Vit E back to its reduced form, making it available as an antioxidant again and protecting the membrane from oxidative stress [51].

The accumulation of ROS and concomitant downregulation of Nrf2 play a crucial role in initiating a cascade of inflammation followed by apoptosis, leading to devastating brain injury in AD [52]. TNF-α has been directly linked to Aβ production in AD, while IL-1β has emerged as one of the most prominent cytokines overexpressed during the initial phase of AD pathogenesis [53]. Subsequently, this inflammation contributes to synapse loss, neuronal damage, and AD development [46]. In the present study, our observations have confirmed the activation of pro-inflammatory cytokines, especially TNF-α and IL-1β, in response to the administration of aluminum chloride, inducing the pathogenesis of AD. On the other side, cocoa with VIN or EGCG had the most potent anti-inflammatory effect against AlCl$_3$-induced inflammation by reducing TNF-α and IL-1β, among other treatments in this work. Like our results, cocoa exhibited anti-inflammatory activity by reducing inflammatory TNF-α in alcohol-induced liver toxicity models in rats [53]. In addition, it was reported previously that VIN and WG inhibited Aβ-induced toxicity by inhibiting TNF-α and IL-1β [54]. Prior research has revealed that EGCG can mitigate amyloid β-induced toxicity by modulating the activity of TNF-α [55]. Earlier studies exhibited the anti-inflammatory activity of coenzyme Q10 in cerebral ischemia [13], the Vit B complex in wound healing [56], and the combination of Vit E, Vit C, and Se in randomized clinical trials of arthritis [57].

In addition, TNF-α directly contributes to the production of Aβ proteins in AD, which are crucial hallmarks of the disease and play a meaningful role in its progression [52]. In our study, a noticeable increase was observed in the dementia marker Aβ in the AD group, which was consistent with prior research [58]. Combined therapy showed better protection against AlCl$_3$ than cocoa alone. This combination resulted in a noteworthy decline in Aβ production. In line with our findings, previous research has shown that cocoa powder administration can reduce Aβ oligomerization [8]. Regarding VIN, its various mechanisms of action are hypothesized to be beneficial in AD [59]. Similarly, EGCG [60] and CoQ10 [61] have been found to reduce Aβ formation in AD transgenic mice. Another study using an in vitro AD model established that Se nanoparticles inhibited Aβ fiber formation [62]. Furthermore, deficiency in vitamins (B complex, E, and C) has been linked to AD patients [63].

The PI3K/AKT/GSK-3β pathway helps promote cell growth and prevent death. This pathway has significant implications for the pathogenesis of various neurological illnesses, including AD. Importantly, it drives the hyperphosphorylation of tau protein, which is a defining hallmark of AD. GSK-3β is the most extensively investigated kinase involved in tau hyperphosphorylation. Furthermore, GSK-3β regulates the neuronal stress response and influences the expression of critical neuropeptides, such as BDNF. These neuropeptides play a vital role in long-term memory and synaptic plasticity. CNS neurons rely on BDNF for survival and differentiation, and its expression is used to measure neurodegenerative changes [64].

GSK-3β is a fascinating multifunctional kinase that is activated by Aβ in AD. It affected multiple signaling pathways, including proinflammatory and proapoptotic [65], and has a critical role in regulating the Wnt/β-catenin pathways. Wnt signaling is an autocrine pathway that has a vital role in brain progress. The elimination of the Wnt3a ligand leads to the disappearance of the hippocampus, underscoring the importance of this pathway in neuronal health [66]. Decreased Wnt activity can intensify the vulnerability of neuronal cells to oxidative insult. Recent research highlights the role of Wnt/β-catenin signaling in inhibiting the production of Aβ and hyperphosphorylation of tau protein in the brain. Consequently, it is involved in the learning and memory processes. Significantly, this pathway is suppressed in the brains of those with AD, pointing towards a potential therapeutic target to mitigate disease progression [66]. GSK-3β is a crucial enzyme responsible for phosphorylating and degrading β-catenin, inhibiting the expression of β-catenin target genes. It has been revealed that the triggering of GSK-3β impedes the Nrf2/HO-1 signaling pathway by augmenting Nrf2 degradation and promoting nuclear factor-κB (NF-kβ) activation, inciting neuroinflammation [67]. Regarding this, it has been established that GSK-3β blockade lowers oxidative injury in a variety of neuronal types [68].

In line with previous findings, our study also revealed the accumulation of Aβ, which triggers the expression of GSK-3β. This leads to the phosphorylation of β-catenin, causing its diminution and the inactivation of Wnt/β-catenin signaling in AD [69]. Consequently, the elevation of GSK-3β reduces the levels of BDNF in the hippocampus, leading to the inhibition of neurogenesis in the brain. Lower BDNF levels have been associated with quicker cognitive decline, poor memory performance, and learning difficulties in AD, as well as other behavioral disturbances in the AD group [70]. However, all our treatment regimens, particularly cocoa alone or in combination with VIN or EGCG, showed improvements in neurogenesis by decreasing GSK-3β activity and consequently activating Wnt/β-catenin signaling, along with increasing BDNF levels. These results align with a previous study that showed cocoa powder's neuroprotective effects by modulating BDNF in an in vitro human AD model [71]. These results align with an early study that showed cocoa powder's neuroprotective effects by modulating BDNF in an in vitro human AD model [64]. Similarly, EGCG has been shown to improve functional outcomes after spinal cord injury by targeting BDNF and reducing the level of GSK-3β [72].

Deposition of Aβ and tau proteins triggers ER stress, which can trigger the initiation and progression of the disease [73]. The Unfolded Protein Response (UPR) is a crucial cellular defense mechanism that acts in response to ER stress. PERK regulates the UPR pathway with two other sensor proteins, all of which are inactive under normal GRP-78 conditions. In ER stress, the releasing of GRP-78 triggers the UPR cascade by dimerization and autophosphorylation of PERK and IRE1α. This also leads to the regulated intramembrane proteolysis of activating transcription factor 6 (ATF6). Once active, ATF6 translocated into the nucleus, where it attached to the promoters of many UPR-associated genes, including CHOP [74]. Once activated, CHOP can elicit a cascade of deleterious effects, which can trigger oxidative damage and ROS, augmented levels of Aβ, interference with iron homeostasis, stimulation of inflammation, DNA damage, and ultimately cell death [75].

ER stress increases the level of GSK-3β and subsequently leads to tau phosphorylation. Excessive ER stress can also impair autophagy, which eliminates damaged or misfolded proteins and cellular organelles resulting from oxidative stress [74]. Thus, autophagy plays a crucial role in cell survival regulation. The essential gene Beclin-1 is involved in regulating autophagy and guides the translocation of other autophagy-associated proteins to the autophagosomes. It is vital for neurodegenerative diseases with protein buildup. Depletion of Beclin-1 has been shown to speed up Aβ aggregation and neurodegeneration [76]. A groundbreaking study by Ho and colleagues showed heightened phosphorylation of p-PERK and GRP-78 in the hippocampal region, suggesting continuous ER stress and ineffective UPR. Maladaptive UPR and sustained ER stress can cause impaired autophagy, severe neuroinflammation, and neuron apoptosis, exacerbating the pathophysiology of AD [74]. Elevated GSK-3β and decreased Beclin-1 cause apoptosis and the loss of dopaminergic neurons [74,75]. Additionally, IL-1β has a pivotal role in inducing mitochondrial apoptosis [77]. AD patients with senile plaques in their brains have been observed to exhibit increased caspase activity and changes in levels of apoptosis-related proteins of the Bcl-2 family. Notably, the Bcl-2 protein family serves a crucial function in the intricate interplay between autophagy and apoptosis [75].

In compliance with the previously mentioned mechanism, our results showed an accumulation of Aβ protein leads to ER stress, as proven by elevated levels of ER stress biomarkers, including GRP-78, p-PERK, and CHOP. Consequently, tau phosphorylation increased, elevated GSK-3β levels, and sustained ER stress, which impairs autophagy and reduces Beclin-1 levels. Furthermore, prolonged ER stress induces neural cell death, or apoptosis. The attenuation of the Bcl-2 protein, a key anti-apoptotic regulator, facilitates this process. Additionally, the upregulation of CHOP stimulates apoptosis. In addition, GSK-3β and IL-1β expression cause neural cell death by accelerating apoptosis.

While cocoa alone or in combination with EGCG, VIN, WG, CoQ10, a complex of Vitamin B, or a mixture of Vitamin E, C, and Se exhibited potential for alleviating Al-induced AD, our findings are consistent with preceding research. Cocoa has been shown to improve ER stress levels and prevent apoptosis by elevating the level of anti-apoptotic Bcl-2 [78]. EGCG has diminished ER stress in AD by decreasing GRP-78 and CHOP, regulating autophagy by elevating Beclin-1, and inhibiting neural apoptosis [79]. CoQ10 has also been revealed to improve ER stress, modulate autophagy, and prevent apoptosis [80]. WG can protect against oxidative stress and apoptosis [81]. Vitamin B supplementation has been shown to restore autophagic flux, lessen ER stress, and repair lysosomal dysfunction caused by hyperhomocysteinemia [82]. Besides, it inhibits DNA damage and neural apoptosis [83]. In addition, it diminishes the apoptosis of cells in the rat hippocampus after polyvinyl chloride exposure [84]. Vitamin C is also useful in modulating oxidative stress, autophagy, and apoptosis in bone marrow stromal cells [85]. Finally, selenium deficiency induces inflammation, autophagy, ER stress, apoptosis, and contraction abnormalities by altering the intestinal flora in the intestinal smooth muscle of mice [86]. These results provide a compelling argument for exploring nutritional interventions to combat AD and other disorders associated with ER stress, impaired autophagy, and apoptosis. The central objective of our investigation was to explore the efficacy of nutritional interventions in ameliorating the deleterious effects of AD, with a particular emphasis on the role of cocoa, either alone or in combination with other nutrients, in fostering a potentiating effect that mitigates the advancement of the disease.

Our study revealed a significant reduction in brain monoamines, suggesting neurological damage in AD patients. Previous research has already shown that AD leads to a decline in noradrenergic and serotonergic neurons in the brain, contributing to various behavioral abnormalities [32]. Consistent with these findings, our results show that behavioral disturbances in the AD group are associated with a significant reduction in these monoamines. Notably, our study highlights the potential of cocoa combined with VIN or EGCG to restore reduced monoamine levels effectively, suggesting these nutraceuticals as agents for neuroprotection. Specifically, VIN has been shown to prevent the decrease in the biosynthesis rate of norepinephrine and serotonin [87]. While EGCG [88], Se supplementations, and CoQ10 [89] have been found to prevent the oxidative deamination reaction of amine neurotransmitters. Additionally, previous studies have reported that vitamins C and E can protect against AD in rat models by modulating brain monoamine levels [90]. Furthermore, the observed increase in BDNF levels and decrease in Aβ levels reported in all treatments may be partially attributed to the elevation of brain monoamines [91]. These findings collectively underscore the role of monoamines in apoptosis-related neurological damage in AD. They also suggest that the consumption of cocoa with VIN or EGCG, along with vitamins C and E, holds potential as neuroprotective interventions by enhancing monoamine levels, promoting BDNF synthesis, and reducing Aβ levels.

The investigation found a notable increase in ACHE activity after $AlCl_3$ exposure. This observation is in harmony with earlier reports suggesting that Al exposure induces an increase in ACHE activity and consequent pathological deterioration in AD etiology [92]. The capability of Al to perturb the blood-brain barrier and modulate cholinergic neurotransmission is posited as the underlying mechanism for these outcomes. This dysregulation may indicate lysosomal malfunctioning, which could worsen the toxic effects of Aβ [93]. These findings warrant further exploration to unravel the intricacies of the pathophysiology of AD. In the present investigation, all treatments elicited a decline in ACHE activity compared to the AD group, with the combination of cocoa and either VIN or EGCG conferring superior neuroprotection. Data on the effect of cocoa on ACHE is limited, so this study provides the first documentation of cocoa's potential neuroprotective effects against ACHE in AD. Prior research has established VIN's ability to attenuate ACHE activity and improve cholinergic function by augmenting acetylcholine levels [9]. Similarly, both EGCG [94] and Q10 [95] administration have been found to mitigate elevated ACHE in streptozotocin-induced dementia models. Moreover, Vit E has been shown to modulate ACHE activity in various brain regions [96]. In the context of Aβ peptide-induced enhancement of ACHE activity, oxidative stress is posited as the underlying mechanism, with Vit E and C successfully abrogating this effect [97,98].

The histopathology analyses confirmed the behavioral and biochemical changes. Nuclear degeneration and pyknosis were found in the cerebral cortex, subiculum, and fascia dentata. These outcomes agree with earlier studies by Abu-Elfotuh et al. and Hamdan et al. [54]. The present study unveils the promising neuroprotective effects of cocoa-based nutraceuticals, either alone or in combination with other dietary supplements, in mitigating the underlying histopathological deterioration. Our study results provide compelling evidence for the potential amelioration effects of the nutraceuticals under investigation, highlighting their therapeutic implications for neurodegenerative disorders. Moreover, our findings suggest that the combination of these compounds potentiates their neuroprotective effects, further emphasizing their potential as a viable treatment option. These promising outcomes pave the way for the development of novel therapeutic strategies that harness the synergistic benefits of these compounds in treating neurodegenerative disorders.

5. Conclusions

Our study provides a comprehensive understanding of the complex pathophysiology underlying Alzheimer's disease, highlighting the interactions between different signaling pathways. By our investigation, we demonstrate the fundamental role of oxidative stress in triggering diminished cellular antioxidants, Aβ and tau protein accumulation, and stimulation of inflammation, sustained ER stress, autophagy, and apoptosis, mediated by pathways such as Wnt/GSK-3β/β-catenin. These alterations lead to neural degeneration, reduced monoamine levels, and changes in brain barrier function and ACHE activity, all of which contribute to the behavioral and histological changes observed in AD.

Our study also highlights the potential of cocoa, either alone or in combination with other nutraceuticals, to ameliorate these biochemical, behavioral, and histological alterations associated with AD, offering a promising avenue for therapeutic intervention to slow cognitive decline. Moreover, the combined intervention of cocoa with VIN or EGCG offers a superior therapeutic effect on behavioral, biochemical, and histological parameters, providing further evidence for the potential of these interventions in the management of Alzheimer's disease. Further cellular studies are warranted to explore the synergistic effects of these combinations in various experimental systems.

Author Contributions: Conceptualization, K.A.-E.; Data curation, K.A.-E., A.M.E.H., A.A.A., A.M.H.G., A.M.A.T., N.A.M., M.Y.E., R.M.A., R.R.E.-A., M.A.R., S.A.A. and S.M.M.; Formal analysis, K.A.-E., A.M.E.H., A.A.A., E.R.M.G., M.M.K., Y.F.M., A.M.H.G., A.D., F.H.H., A.M.M.E., M.A.R., S.A.A. and S.M.M.; Methodology, K.A.-E., A.M.A.T., R.M.A., A.M.E.H., A.A.A., A.M.H.G., N.A.M., M.Y.E., R.R.E.-A., E.R.M.G., M.M.K., A.M.M.E., A.D., S.M.M., Y.F.M. and F.H.H.; Project administration, K.A.-E.; Supervision, K.A.-E. and A.M.E.H.; Validation, K.A.-E., A.A.A. and A.M.E.H.; Visualization, K.A.-E. and A.M.E.H.; Writing—original draft, K.A.-E., A.M.E.H., A.A.A., A.M.H.G., A.D., Y.F.M. and S.M.M.; Writing—review and editing, K.A.-E., A.M.E.H., A.A.A., R.R.E.-A., E.R.M.G., Y.F.M., A.M.H.G., N.A.M., M.Y.E., A.M.A.T., R.M.A., F.H.H., M.M.K., A.M.M.E., A.D., M.A.R., S.A.A. and S.M.M. All authors have read and agreed to the published version of the manuscript.

Funding: Deanship of Scientific Research at King Khalid University.

Institutional Review Board Statement: The Animal Care and Use committee of the Faculty of Pharmacy, Al-Azhar University, reviewed and accepted the study protocol with ethical approval number (218/2021), which complies with the ARRIVE criteria and follows the guidelines outlined in the "Guide for Care and Use of Laboratory Animals", published by the National Institutes of Health (NIH Publications No. 8023, revised 1978).

Informed Consent Statement: Not applicable.

Data Availability Statement: Data will be available on request from the corresponding author.

Acknowledgments: The authors extend their appreciation to the Deanship of Scientific Research at King Khalid University for funding this work via small group Research Project under grant number RGP1/165/44.

Conflicts of Interest: The authors declare no conflict of interest.

References

1. Zhang, H.; Wei, W.; Zhao, M.; Ma, L.; Jiang, X.; Pei, H.; Cao, Y.; Li, H. Interaction between Aβ and Tau in the Pathogenesis of Alzheimer's Disease. *Int. J. Biol. Sci.* **2021**, *17*, 2181–2192. [CrossRef]
2. Kumar, V.; Bal, A.; Gill, K.D. Aluminium-induced oxidative DNA damage recognition and cell-cycle disruption in different regions of rat brain. *Toxicology* **2009**, *264*, 137–144. [CrossRef]
3. Calkins, M.J.; Johnson, D.A.; Townsend, J.A.; Vargas, M.R.; Dowell, J.A.; Williamson, T.P.; Kraft, A.D.; Lee, J.-M.; Li, J.; Johnson, J.A. The Nrf2/ARE Pathway as a Potential Therapeutic Target in Neurodegenerative Disease. *Antioxid. Redox Signal* **2009**, *11*, 497–508. [CrossRef]
4. Hamdan, A.M.E.; Alharthi, F.H.J.; Alanazi, A.H.; El-Emam, S.Z.; Zaghlool, S.S.; Metwally, K.; Albalawi, S.A.; Abdu, Y.S.; Mansour, R.E.-S.; Salem, H.A.; et al. Neuroprotective Effects of Phytochemicals against Aluminum Chloride-Induced Alzheimer's Disease through ApoE4/LRP1, Wnt3/β-Catenin/GSK3β, and TLR4/NLRP3 Pathways with Physical and Mental Activities in a Rat Model. *Pharmaceuticals* **2022**, *15*, 1008. [CrossRef]
5. Zare-shahabadi; Masliah, E.; Johnson, G.V.W.; Rezaei, N. Autophagy in Alzheimer's disease. *Rev. Neurosci.* **2015**, *26*, 385–395. [CrossRef]
6. Hashimoto, S.; Ishii, A.; Kamano, N.; Watamura, N.; Saito, T.; Ohshima, T.; Yokosuka, M.; Saido, T.C. Endoplasmic reticulum stress responses in mouse models of Alzheimer's disease: Overexpression paradigm versus knockin paradigm. *J. Biol. Chem.* **2018**, *293*, 3118–3125. [CrossRef]
7. da Rosa, M.M.; de Amorim, L.C.; de O, J.V.; da Silva, I.F.; da Silva, F.G.; da Silva, M.V.; Santos, M.T.C.D. The promising role of natural products in Alzheimer's disease. *Brain Disord.* **2022**, *7*, 100049. [CrossRef]
8. Wang, J.; Varghese, M.; Ono, K.; Yamada, M.; Levine, S.; Tzavaras, N.; Gong, B.; Hurst, W.J.; Blitzer, R.D.; Pasinetti, G.M. Cocoa Extracts Reduce Oligomerization of Amyloid-β: Implications for Cognitive Improvement in Alzheimer's Disease. *J. Alzheimer's Dis.* **2014**, *41*, 643–650. [CrossRef] [PubMed]
9. Patyar, S.; Prakash, A.; Modi, M.; Medhi, B. Role of vinpocetine in cerebrovascular diseases. *Pharmacol. Rep.* **2011**, *63*, 618–628. [CrossRef] [PubMed]
10. Singh, R.; Akhtar, N.; Haqqi, T.M. Green tea polyphenol epigallocatechi3-gallate: Inflammation and arthritis. *Life Sci.* **2010**, *86*, 907–918. [CrossRef]
11. Ganeshpurkar, A.; Dubey, N.; Bansal, D.; Khan, N. Immunoprophylactic potential of wheat grass extract on benzene-induced leukemia: An in vivo study on murine model. *Indian J. Pharmacol.* **2015**, *47*, 394. [CrossRef] [PubMed]
12. Chen, P.-Y.; Hou, C.-W.; Shibu, M.A.; Day, C.H.; Pai, P.; Liu, Z.-R.; Lin, T.-Y.; Viswanadha, V.P.; Kuo, C.-H.; Huang, C.-Y. Protective effect of Co-enzyme Q10 On doxorubicin-induced cardiomyopathy of rat hearts. *Environ. Toxicol.* **2017**, *32*, 679–689. [CrossRef] [PubMed]
13. El-Aal, S.A.A.; El-Fattah, M.A.A.; El-Abhar, H.S. CoQ10 Augments Rosuvastatin Neuroprotective Effect in a Model of Global Ischemia via Inhibition of NF-κB/JNK3/Bax and Activation of Akt/FOXO3A/Bim Cues. *Front. Pharmacol.* **2017**, *8*, 735. [CrossRef] [PubMed]
14. Yang, X.; Yang, Y.; Li, G.; Wang, J.; Yang, E.S. Coenzyme Q10 Attenuates β-Amyloid Pathology in the Aged Transgenic Mice with Alzheimer Presenilin 1 Mutation. *J. Mol. Neurosci.* **2008**, *34*, 165–171. [CrossRef] [PubMed]
15. Steele, M.; Stuchbury, G.; Münch, G. The molecular basis of the prevention of Alzheimer's disease through healthy nutrition. *Exp. Gerontol.* **2007**, *42*, 28–36. [CrossRef]
16. Jolivalt, C.G.; Mizisin, L.M.; Nelson, A.; Cunha, J.M.; Ramos, K.M.; Bonke, D.; Calcutt, N.A. B vitamins alleviate indices of neuropathic pain in diabetic rats. *Eur. J. Pharmacol.* **2009**, *612*, 41–47. [CrossRef]
17. Rock, C.L.; Jacob, R.A.; Bowen, P.E. Update on the Biological Characteristics of the Antioxidant Micronutrients. *J Am Diet Assoc.* **1996**, *96*, 693–702. [CrossRef]
18. Mark, S.D. Prospective Study of Serum Selenium Levels and Incident Esophageal and Gastric Cancers. *J. Natl. Cancer Inst.* **2000**, *92*, 1753–1763. [CrossRef]
19. MKhalil, G.; Ali, A.A.; Hassanin, S.O.; Al-Najjar, A.H.; Ghosh, S.; Mahmoud, M.O. Comparative study on the effect of EGCG and wheat grass together with mental and physical activities against induction of Alzheimer's disease in both isolated and socialized rats. *Phytomedicine Plus* **2022**, *2*, 100146. [CrossRef]
20. Ali, A.A.; Kamal, M.M.; Khalil, M.G.; Ali, S.A.; Elariny, H.A.; Bekhit, A.; Wahid, A. Behavioral, Biochemical and Histopathological effects of Standardised Pomegranate extract with Vinpocetine, Propolis or Cocoa in a rat model of Parkinson's disease. *Exp. Aging Res.* **2022**, *48*, 191–210. [CrossRef]
21. Bisson, J.-F.; Nejdi, A.; Rozan, P.; Hidalgo, S.; Lalonde, R.; Messaoudi, M. Effects of long-term administration of a cocoa polyphenolic extract (Acticoa powder) on cognitive performances in aged rats. *Br. J. Nutr.* **2008**, *100*, 94–101. [CrossRef] [PubMed]
22. Rasoolijazi, H.; Joghataie, M.T.; Roghani, M.; Nobakht, M. The beneficial effect of (-)-epigallocatechin-3-gallate in an experimental model of Alzheimer's disease in rat: A behavioral analysis. *Iran Biomed. J.* **2007**, *11*, 237–243. Available online: http://www.ncbi.nlm.nih.gov/pubmed/18392085 (accessed on 3 May 2023). [PubMed]
23. Abdel-Salam, O.M.E.; Hamdy, S.M.; Seadawy, S.A.M.; Galal, A.F.; Abouelfadl, D.M.; Atrees, S.S. Effect of piracetam, vincamine, vinpocetine, and donepezil on oxidative stress and neurodegeneration induced by aluminum chloride in rats. *Comp. Clin. Path.* **2016**, *25*, 305–318. [CrossRef]

24. Andreassen, O.A.; Weber, C.; JØrgensen, H.A. Coenzyme Q10 Does Not Prevent Oral Dyskinesias Induced by Long-Term Haloperidol Treatment of Rats. *Pharmacol. Biochem. Behav.* **1999**, *64*, 637–642. [CrossRef]
25. Ahmed, H.H.; Shousha, W.G.; Hussien, R.M.; Farrag, A.R.H. Potential role of some nutraceuticals in the regression of Alzheimer's disease in an experimental animal model. *Turk J. Med. Sci.* **2011**, *41*, 455–466. [CrossRef]
26. Lakshmi, B.V.S.; Sudhakar, M.; Prakash, K.S. Protective Effect of Selenium Against Aluminum Chloride-Induced Alzheimer's Disease: Behavioral and Biochemical Alterations in Rats. *Biol. Trace Elem. Res.* **2015**, *165*, 67–74. [CrossRef]
27. Shivavedi, N.; Tej, G.N.V.C.; Neogi, K.; Nayak, P.K. Ascorbic acid therapy: A potential strategy against comorbid depression-like behavior in streptozotocin-nicotinamide-induced diabetic rats. *Biomed. Pharmacother.* **2019**, *109*, 351–359. [CrossRef]
28. Hritcu, L.; Cioanca, O.; Hancianu, M. Effects of lavender oil inhalation on improving scopolamine-induced spatial memory impairment in laboratory rats. *Phytomedicine* **2012**, *19*, 529–534. [CrossRef] [PubMed]
29. Foyet, H.S.; Hritcu, L.; Ciobica, A.; Stefan, M.; Kamtchouing, P.; Cojocaru, D. Methanolic extract of Hibiscus asper leaves improves spatial memory deficits in the 6-hydroxydopamine-lesion rodent model of Parkinson's disease. *J. Ethnopharmacol.* **2011**, *133*, 773–779. [CrossRef]
30. Garofalo, P.; Colombo, S.; Lanza, M.; Revel, L.; Makovec, F. CR 2249: A New Putative Memory Enhancer. Behavioural Studies on Learning and Memory in Rats and Mice. *J. Pharm. Pharmacol.* **2011**, *48*, 1290–1297. [CrossRef]
31. Morris, R. Developments of a water-maze procedure for studying spatial learning in the rat. *J. Neurosci. Methods.* **1984**, *11*, 47–60. [CrossRef] [PubMed]
32. Ali, A.A.; Khalil, M.G.; Elariny, H.A.; Elfotuh, K.A. Study on Social Isolation as a Risk Factor in Development of Alzheimer's Disease in Rats. *Brain Disord. Ther.* **2017**, *6*, 1000230. [CrossRef]
33. Zanfirescu, A.; Ungurianu, A.; Tsatsakis, A.M.; Ni, G.M.; Kouretas, D.; Veskoukis, A.; Tsoukalas, D.; Engin, A.B.; Aschner, M.; Margină, D. A Review of the Alleged Health Hazards of Monosodium Glutamate. *Compr. Rev. Food Sci. Food Saf.* **2019**, *18*, 1111–1134. [CrossRef] [PubMed]
34. Bancroft, J.D.; Layton, C. The hematoxylins and eosin. In *Bancroft's Theory and Practice of Histological Techniques*; Elsevier: Amsterdam, The Netherlands, 2013; pp. 173–186. [CrossRef]
35. Ciarlone, A.E. Further modification of a fluorometric method for analyzing brain amines. *Microchem. J.* **1978**, *23*, 9–12. [CrossRef]
36. Nishikimi, M.; Rao, N.A.; Yagi, K. The occurrence of superoxide anion in the reaction of reduced phenazine methosulfate and molecular oxygen. *Biochem. Biophys. Res. Commun.* **1972**, *46*, 849–854. [CrossRef]
37. Gu, H.; Long, D.; Song, C.; Li, X. Recombinant human NGF-loaded microspheres promote survival of basal forebrain cholinergic neurons and improve memory impairments of spatial learning in the rat model of Alzheimer's disease with fimbria-fornix lesion. *Neurosci. Lett.* **2009**, *453*, 204–209. [CrossRef] [PubMed]
38. Abdel-Aal, R.A.; Assi, A.-A.A.; Kostandy, B.B. Rivastigmine reverses aluminum-induced behavioral changes in rats. *Eur. J. Pharmacol.* **2011**, *659*, 169–176. [CrossRef]
39. Saba; Khan, S.; Parvez, S.; Chaudhari, B.; Ahmad, F.; Anjum, S.; Raisuddin, S. Ellagic acid attenuates bleomycin and cyclophosphamide-induced pulmonary toxicity in Wistar rats. *Food Chem. Toxicol.* **2013**, *58*, 210–219. [CrossRef]
40. Vauzour, D.; Vafeiadou, K.; Rodriguez-Mateos, A.; Rendeiro, C.; Spencer, J.P.E. The neuroprotective potential of flavonoids: A multiplicity of effects. *Genes Nutr.* **2008**, *3*, 115–126. [CrossRef]
41. Muss, C.; Mosgoeller, W.; Endler, T.; Muss, C. Mood improving Potential of a Vitamin Trace Element Composition-A randomized, double blind, placebo controlled clinical study with healthy volunteers, NEL370116A06. *Neuroendocrinol. Lett.* **2016**, *37*, 26994381.
42. Kitagishi, Y.; Nakanishi, A.; Ogura, Y.; Matsuda, S. Dietary regulation of PI3K/AKT/GSK-3β pathway in Alzheimer's disease. *Alzheimer's Res. Ther.* **2014**, *6*, 35. [CrossRef]
43. Salem, H.A.; Elsherbiny, N.; Alzahrani, S.; Alshareef, H.M.; Elmageed, Z.Y.A.; Ajwah, S.M.; Hamdan, A.M.E.; Abdou, Y.S.; Galal, O.O.; El Azazy, M.K.A.; et al. Neuroprotective Effect of Morin Hydrate against Attention-Deficit/Hyperactivity Disorder (ADHD) Induced by MSG and/or Protein Malnutrition in Rat Pups: Effect on Oxidative/Monoamines/Inflammatory Balance and Apoptosis. *Pharmaceuticals* **2022**, *15*, 1012. [CrossRef]
44. Ngo, V.; Duennwald, M.L. Nrf2 and Oxidative Stress: A General Overview of Mechanisms and Implications in Human Disease. *Antioxidants* **2022**, *11*, 2345. [CrossRef]
45. Saha, S.; Buttari, B.; Profumo, E.; Tucci, P.; Saso, L. A Perspective on Nrf2 Signaling Pathway for Neuroinflammation: A Potential Therapeutic Target in Alzheimer's and Parkinson's Diseases. *Front. Cell Neurosci.* **2022**, *15*, 787258. [CrossRef]
46. Fakhri, S.; Pesce, M.; Patruno, A.; Moradi, S.Z.; Iranpanah, A.; Farzaei, M.H.; Sobarzo-Sánchez, E. Attenuation of Nrf2/Keap1/ARE in Alzheimer's Disease by Plant Secondary Metabolites: A Mechanistic Review. *Molecules* **2020**, *25*, 4926. [CrossRef]
47. Martín, M.Á.; Serrano, A.B.G.; Ramos, S.; Pulido, M.I.; Bravo, L.; Goya, L. Cocoa flavonoids up-regulate antioxidant enzyme activity via the ERK1/2 pathway to protect against oxidative stress-induced apoptosis in HepG2 cells. *J. Nutr. Biochem.* **2010**, *21*, 196–205. [CrossRef]
48. Cheng, Y.-T.; Lu, C.-C.; Yen, G.-C. Phytochemicals enhance antioxidant enzyme expression to protect against NSAID-induced oxidative damage of the gastrointestinal mucosa. *Mol. Nutr. Food Res.* **2017**, *61*, 1600659. [CrossRef]
49. Fattori, V.; Borghi, S.M.; Guazelli, C.F.S.; Giroldo, A.C.; Crespigio, J.; Bussmann, A.J.C.; Coelho-Silva, L.; Ludwig, N.G.; Mazzuco, T.L.; Casagrande, R.; et al. Vinpocetine reduces diclofenac-induced acute kidney injury through inhibition of oxidative stress, apoptosis, cytokine production, and NF-κB activation in mice. *Pharmacol. Res.* **2017**, *120*, 10–22. [CrossRef]

50. Keskes-Ammar, L.; Feki-Chakroun, N.; Rebai, T.; Sahnoun, Z.; Ghozzi, H.; Hammami, S.; Zghal, K.; Fki, H.; Damak, J.; Bahloul, A. Sperm Oxidative Stress and the Effect of an Oral Vitamin E and Selenium Supplement on Semen Quality in Infertile Men. *Arch. Androl.* **2003**, *49*, 83–94. [CrossRef]
51. Packer, L. Oxidants, antioxidant nutrients and the athlete. *J. Sports Sci.* **1997**, *15*, 353–363. [CrossRef] [PubMed]
52. Davies, D.A.; Adlimoghaddam, A.; Albensi, B.C. Role of Nrf2 in Synaptic Plasticity and Memory in Alzheimer's Disease. *Cells* **2021**, *10*, 1884. [CrossRef] [PubMed]
53. McKim, S.E.; Konno, A.; Gäbele, E.; Uesugi, T.; Froh, M.; Sies, H.; Thurman, R.G.; Arteel, G.E. Cocoa extract protects against early alcohol-induced liver injury in the rat. *Arch. Biochem. Biophys.* **2002**, *406*, 40–46. [CrossRef] [PubMed]
54. Abu-Elfotuh, K.; Ragab, G.M.; Salahuddin, A.; Jamil, L.; Al Haleem, E.N.A. Attenuative Effects of Fluoxetine and Triticum aestivum against Aluminum-Induced Alzheimer's Disease in Rats: The Possible Consequences on Hepatotoxicity and Nephrotoxicity. *Molecules* **2021**, *26*, 6752. [CrossRef] [PubMed]
55. Payne; Nahashon, S.; Taka, E.; Adinew, G.M.; Soliman, K.F.A. Epigallocatechin-3-Gallate (EGCG): New Therapeutic Perspectives for Neuroprotection, Aging, and Neuroinflammation for the Modern Age. *Biomolecules* **2022**, *12*, 371. [CrossRef] [PubMed]
56. Neiva, R.F.; Al-Shammari, K.; Nociti, F.H.; Soehren, S.; Wang, H.-L. Effects of Vitamin-B Complex Supplementation on Periodontal Wound Healing. *J. Periodontol.* **2005**, *76*, 1084–1091. [CrossRef]
57. Canter, P.H.; Wider, B.; Ernst, E. The antioxidant vitamins A, C, E and selenium in the treatment of arthritis: A systematic review of randomized clinical trials. *Rheumatology* **2007**, *46*, 1223–1233. [CrossRef]
58. Ma, T.; Klann, E. Amyloid β: Linking synaptic plasticity failure to memory disruption in Alzheimer's disease. *J. Neurochem.* **2012**, *120*, 140–148. [CrossRef]
59. Deshmukh, R.; Sharma, V.; Mehan, S.; Sharma, N.; Bedi, K.L. Amelioration of intracerebroventricular streptozotocin induced cognitive dysfunction and oxidative stress by vinpocetine—A PDE1 inhibitor. *Eur. J. Pharmacol.* **2009**, *620*, 49–56. [CrossRef]
60. Rezai-Zadeh, K.; Shytle, D.; Sun, N.; Mori, T.; Hou, H.; Jeanniton, D.; Ehrhart, J.; Townsend, K.; Zeng, J.; Morgan, D.; et al. Green Tea Epigallocatechin-3-Gallate (EGCG) Modulates Amyloid Precursor Protein Cleavage and Reduces Cerebral Amyloidosis in Alzheimer Transgenic Mice. *J. Neurosci.* **2005**, *25*, 8807–8814. [CrossRef]
61. Dumont, M.; Kipiani, K.; Yu, F.; Wille, E.; Katz, M.; Calingasan, N.Y.; Gouras, G.K.; Lin, M.T.; Beal, M.F. Coenzyme Q10 Decreases Amyloid Pathology and Improves Behavior in a Transgenic Mouse Model of Alzheimer's Disease. *J. Alzheimer's Dis.* **2011**, *27*, 211–223. [CrossRef]
62. Godoi, G.L.; de Oliveira Porciúncula, L.; Schulz, J.F.; Kaufmann, F.N.; da Rocha, J.B.; de Souza, D.O.G.; Ghisleni, G.; de Almeida, H.L. Selenium Compounds Prevent Amyloid β-Peptide Neurotoxicity in Rat Primary Hippocampal Neurons. *Neurochem. Res.* **2013**, *38*, 2359–2363. [CrossRef] [PubMed]
63. Lahiri, D.K.; Maloney, B. The "LEARn" (Latent Early-life Associated Regulation) model integrates environmental risk factors and the developmental basis of Alzheimer's disease, and proposes remedial steps. *Exp Gerontol.* **2010**, *45*, 291–296. [CrossRef] [PubMed]
64. Ahmed, H.I.; Abdel-Sattar, S.A.; Zaky, H.S. Vinpocetine halts ketamine-induced schizophrenia-like deficits in rats: Impact on BDNF and GSK-3β/β-catenin pathway. *Naunyn Schmiedebergs Arch. Pharmacol.* **2018**, *391*, 1327–1338. [CrossRef] [PubMed]
65. Sayas, C.L.; Ávila, J. GSK-3 and Tau: A Key Duet in Alzheimer's Disease. *Cells* **2021**, *10*, 721. [CrossRef]
66. Chen, J.; Long, Z.; Li, Y.; Luo, M.; Luo, S.; He, G. Alteration of the Wnt/GSK3β/β-catenin signalling pathway by rapamycin ameliorates pathology in an Alzheimer's disease model. *Int. J. Mol. Med.* **2019**, *44*, 313–323. [CrossRef]
67. Mousa, H.H.; Sharawy, M.H.; Nader, M.A. Empagliflozin enhances neuroplasticity in rotenone-induced parkinsonism: Role of BDNF, CREB and Npas4. *Life Sci.* **2023**, *312*, 121258. [CrossRef]
68. Shi, S.; Zhao, J.; Yang, L.; Nie, X.; Han, J.; Ma, X.; Wan, C.; Jiang, J. KHSRP Participates in Manganese-Induced Neurotoxicity in Rat Striatum and PC12 Cells. *J. Mol. Neurosci.* **2015**, *55*, 454–465. [CrossRef]
69. Wang, B.; Tian, T.; Kalland, K.-H.; Ke, X.; Qu, Y. Targeting Wnt/β-Catenin Signaling for Cancer Immunotherapy. *Trends Pharmacol. Sci.* **2018**, *39*, 648–658. [CrossRef]
70. Laske, C.; Stellos, K.; Hoffmann, N.; Stransky, E.; Straten, G.; Eschweiler, G.W.; Leyhe, T. Higher BDNF serum levels predict slower cognitive decline in Alzheimer's disease patients. *Int. J. Neuropsychopharmacol.* **2011**, *14*, 399–404. [CrossRef]
71. Cimini, A.; Gentile, R.; D'Angelo, B.; Benedetti, E.; Cristiano, L.; Avantaggiati, M.L.; Giordano, A.; Ferri, C.; Desideri, G. Cocoa powder triggers neuroprotective and preventive effects in a human Alzheimer's disease model by modulating BDNF signaling pathway. *J. Cell. Biochem.* **2013**, *114*, 2209–2220. [CrossRef]
72. Tian, W.; Han, X.-G.; Liu, Y.-J.; Tang, G.-Q.; Liu, B.; Wang, Y.-Q.; Xiao, B.; Xu, Y.-F. Intrathecal Epigallocatechin Gallate Treatment Improves Functional Recovery After Spinal Cord Injury by Upregulating the Expression of BDNF and GDNF. *Neurochem. Res.* **2013**, *38*, 772–779. [CrossRef]
73. Ajoolabady, A.; Lindholm, D.; Ren, J.; Pratico, D. ER stress and UPR in Alzheimer's disease: Mechanisms, pathogenesis, treatments. *Cell Death Dis.* **2022**, *13*, 706. [CrossRef]
74. Ghemrawi, R.; Khair, M. Endoplasmic Reticulum Stress and Unfolded Protein Response in Neurodegenerative Diseases. *Int. J. Mol. Sci.* **2020**, *21*, 6127. [CrossRef]
75. Saha, A.; Saleem, S.; Kumar, P.R.; Biswas, S.C. BH3-only proteins Puma and Beclin1 regulate autophagic death in neurons in response to Amyloid-β. *Cell. Death Discov.* **2021**, *7*, 356. [CrossRef] [PubMed]

76. Bieri, G.; Lucin, K.M.; O'Brien, C.E.; Zhang, H.; Villeda, S.A.; Wyss-Coray, T. Proteolytic cleavage of Beclin 1 exacerbates neurodegeneration. *Mol. Neurodegener.* **2018**, *13*, 68. [CrossRef]
77. Shen, J.; Xu, S.; Zhou, H.; Liu, H.; Jiang, W.; Hao, J.; Hu, Z. IL-1β induces apoptosis and autophagy via mitochondria pathway in human degenerative nucleus pulposus cells. *Sci. Rep.* **2017**, *7*, 41067. [CrossRef] [PubMed]
78. Guan, H.; Lin, Y.; Bai, L.; An, Y.; Shang, J.; Wang, Z.; Zhao, S.; Fan, J.; Liu, E. Dietary Cocoa Powder Improves Hyperlipidemia and Reduces Atherosclerosis in apoE Deficient Mice through the Inhibition of Hepatic Endoplasmic Reticulum Stress. *Mediators Inflamm.* **2016**, *2016*, 1937572. [CrossRef]
79. Zhang, S.; Cao, M.; Fang, F. The Role of Epigallocatechin-3-Gallate in Autophagy and Endoplasmic Reticulum Stress (ERS)-Induced Apoptosis of Human Diseases. *Med. Sci. Monit.* **2020**, *26*, e924558. [CrossRef]
80. Liang, S.; Ping, Z.; Ge, J. Coenzyme Q10 Regulates Antioxidative Stress and Autophagy in Acute Myocardial Ischemia-Reperfusion Injury. *Oxidative Med. Cell. Longev.* **2017**, *2017*, 9863181. [CrossRef]
81. Shyam, C.; Dhawan, D.K.; Chadha, V.D. In Vivo Radioprotective Effects Of Wheatgrass (*Triticum Aestivum*) Extract Against X-Irradaition-Induced Oxidative Stress And Apoptosis In Peripheral Blood Lymphocytes In Rats. *Asian J. Pharm. Clin. Res.* **2018**, *11*, 239. [CrossRef]
82. Tripathi, M.; Zhang, C.W.; Singh, B.K.; Sinha, R.A.; Moe, K.T.; DeSilva, D.A.; Yen, P.M. Hyperhomocysteinemia causes ER stress and impaired autophagy that is reversed by Vitamin B supplementation. *Cell Death Dis.* **2016**, *7*, e2513. [CrossRef] [PubMed]
83. Shamseldeen, A.M.; Hamzawy, M.; Mahmoud, N.A.; Rashed, L.; Kamar, S.S.; Harb, L.A.; Sharawy, N. inhibition of endoplasmic reticulum stress and activation of autophagy-protect intestinal and renal tissues from western diet-induced dysbiosis and abrogate inflammatory response to LPS: Role of vitamin E. *J. Biol. Regul. Homeost. Agents* **2021**, *35*, 457–471.
84. Sadeghi, A.; Ghahari, L. Vitamin E As an Antioxidant Reduces Apoptosis of Cells in Rat Hippocampus Following Exposure to Polyvinyl Chloride. *Ann. Mil. Health Sci. Res.* **2018**, *16*, 257–263. [CrossRef]
85. Sangani, R.; Periyasamy-Thandavan, S.; Pathania, R.; Ahmad, S.; Kutiyanawalla, A.; Kolhe, R.; Bhattacharyya, M.H.; Chutkan, N.; Hunter, M.; Hill, W.D.; et al. The crucial role of vitamin C and its transporter (SVCT2) in bone marrow stromal cell autophagy and apoptosis. *Stem Cell. Res.* **2015**, *15*, 312–321. [CrossRef]
86. Wang, F.; Sun, N.; Zeng, H.; Gao, Y.; Zhang, N.; Zhang, W. Selenium Deficiency Leads to Inflammation, Autophagy, Endoplasmic Reticulum Stress, Apoptosis and Contraction Abnormalities via Affecting Intestinal Flora in Intestinal Smooth Muscle of Mice. *Front. Immunol.* **2022**, *13*, e924558. [CrossRef]
87. Kiss, B.; Szporny, L. On the possible role of central monoaminergic systems in the central nervous system actions of vinpocetine. *Drug Dev. Res.* **1988**, *14*, 263–279. [CrossRef]
88. Lin, S.-M.; Wang, S.-W.; Ho, S.-C.; Tang, Y.-L. Protective effect of green tea (-)-epigallocatechin-3-gallate against the monoamine oxidase B enzyme activity increase in adult rat brains. *Nutrition* **2010**, *26*, 1195–1200. [CrossRef]
89. Mazzio, E.; Harris, N.; Soliman, K. Food Constituents Attenuate Monoamine Oxidase Activity and Peroxide Levels in C6 Astrocyte Cells. *Planta Med.* **1998**, *64*, 603–606. [CrossRef]
90. Ganguly; Guha, D. Alteration of brain monoamines & EEG wave pattern in rat model of Alzheimer's disease & protection by Moringa oleifera. *He Indian J. Med. Res.* **2008**, *128*, 744–751.
91. Brenes, J.C.; Rodríguez, O.; Fornaguera, J. Differential effect of environment enrichment and social isolation on depressive-like behavior, spontaneous activity and serotonin and norepinephrine concentration in prefrontal cortex and ventral striatum. *Pharmacol. Biochem. Behav.* **2008**, *89*, 85–93. [CrossRef]
92. Kaizer, R.R.; Corrêa, M.C.; Gris, L.R.S.; da Rosa, C.S.; Bohrer, D.; Morsch, V.M.; Schetinger, M.R.C. Effect of Long-Term Exposure to Aluminum on the Acetylcholinesterase Activity in the Central Nervous System and Erythrocytes. *Neurochem. Res.* **2008**, *33*, 2294–2301. [CrossRef] [PubMed]
93. Ryter, S.W.; Alam, J.; Choi, A.M.K. Heme Oxygenase-1/Carbon Monoxide: From Basic Science to Therapeutic Applications. *Physiol. Rev.* **2006**, *86*, 583–650. [CrossRef] [PubMed]
94. Biasibetti, R.; Tramontina, A.C.; Costa, A.P.; Dutra, M.F.; Quincozes-Santos, A.; Nardin, P.; Bernardi, C.L.; Wartchow, K.M.; Lunardi, P.S.; Gonçalves, C.-A. Green tea (−)epigallocatechin-3-gallate reverses oxidative stress and reduces acetylcholinesterase activity in a streptozotocin-induced model of dementia. *Behav. Brain Res.* **2013**, *236*, 186–193. [CrossRef] [PubMed]
95. Ishrat, T.; Khan, M.B.; Hoda, M.N.; Yousuf, S.; Ahmad, M.; Ansari, M.A.; Ahmad, A.S.; Islam, F. Coenzyme Q10 modulates cognitive impairment against intracerebroventricular injection of streptozotocin in rats. *Behav. Brain Res.* **2006**, *171*, 9–16. [CrossRef]
96. Mazzanti, C.M.; Spanevello, R.; Ahmed, M.; Pereira, L.B.; Gonçalves, J.F.; Corrêa, M.; Schmatz, R.; Stefanello, N.; Leal, D.B.R.; Mazzanti, A.; et al. Pre-treatment with ebselen and vitamin E modulate acetylcholinesterase activity: Interaction with demyelinating agents. *Int. J. Dev. Neurosci.* **2009**, *27*, 73–80. [CrossRef] [PubMed]

97. Lima, D.D.-D.; Wollinger, L.F.; Casagrande, A.C.M.; Delwing, F.; Cruz, J.G.P.; Wyse, A.T.S. Delwing-Dal Magro, Guanidino compounds inhibit acetylcholinesterase and butyrylcholinesterase activities: Effect neuroprotector of vitamins E plus C. *Int. J. Dev. Neurosci.* **2010**, *28*, 465–473. [CrossRef]
98. Melo, J.B.; Agostinho, P.; Oliveira, C.R. Involvement of oxidative stress in the enhancement of acetylcholinesterase activity induced by amyloid beta-peptide. *Neurosci. Res.* **2003**, *45*, 117–127. [CrossRef]

Disclaimer/Publisher's Note: The statements, opinions and data contained in all publications are solely those of the individual author(s) and contributor(s) and not of MDPI and/or the editor(s). MDPI and/or the editor(s) disclaim responsibility for any injury to people or property resulting from any ideas, methods, instructions or products referred to in the content.

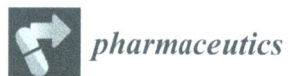

Article

Microwave-Treated Physically Cross-Linked Sodium Alginate and Sodium Carboxymethyl Cellulose Blend Polymer Film for Open Incision Wound Healing in Diabetic Animals—A Novel Perspective for Skin Tissue Regeneration Application

Saima Mahmood [1], Nauman Rahim Khan [1,2,*], Ghulam Razaque [3], Shefaat Ullah Shah [1], Memuna Ghafoor Shahid [4], Hassan A. Albarqi [5], Abdulsalam A. Alqahtani [5], Ali Alasiri [5] and Hafiz Muhammad Basit [6]

[1] Gomal Centre for Pharmaceutical Sciences, Faculty of Pharmacy, Gomal University, DIKhan 29050, Khyber Pakhtunkhwa, Pakistan
[2] Department of Pharmacy, Kohat University of Science and Technology, Kohat 26000, Khyber Pakhtunkhwa, Pakistan
[3] Faculty of Pharmacy, University of Baluchistan, Quetta 87300, Baluchistan, Pakistan
[4] Department of Botany, Government College University, Lahore 54000, Punjab, Pakistan
[5] Department of Pharmaceutics, College of Pharmacy, Najran University, Najran 55461, Saudi Arabia
[6] Akhtar Saeed College of Pharmacy, Bahria Golf City, Rawalpindi 46220, Punjab, Pakistan
* Correspondence: naumanpharma@gmail.com

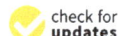

Citation: Mahmood, S.; Khan, N.R.; Razaque, G.; Shah, S.U.; Shahid, M.G.; Albarqi, H.A.; Alqahtani, A.A.; Alasiri, A.; Basit, H.M. Microwave-Treated Physically Cross-Linked Sodium Alginate and Sodium Carboxymethyl Cellulose Blend Polymer Film for Open Incision Wound Healing in Diabetic Animals—A Novel Perspective for Skin Tissue Regeneration Application. *Pharmaceutics* 2023, 15, 418. https://doi.org/10.3390/pharmaceutics15020418

Academic Editor: Giuseppe De Rosa

Received: 4 January 2023
Revised: 20 January 2023
Accepted: 24 January 2023
Published: 27 January 2023

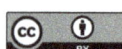

Copyright: © 2023 by the authors. Licensee MDPI, Basel, Switzerland. This article is an open access article distributed under the terms and conditions of the Creative Commons Attribution (CC BY) license (https://creativecommons.org/licenses/by/4.0/).

Abstract: This study aimed at developing the microwave-treated, physically cross-linked polymer blend film, optimizing the microwave treatment time, and testing for physicochemical attributes and wound healing potential in diabetic animals. Microwave-treated and untreated films were prepared by the solution casting method and characterized for various attributes required by a wound healing platform. The optimized formulation was tested for skin regeneration potential in the diabetes-induced open-incision animal model. The results indicated that the optimized polymer film formulation (MB-3) has significantly enhanced physicochemical properties such as high moisture adsorption (154.6 ± 4.23%), decreased the water vapor transmission rate (*WVTR*) value of (53.0 ± 2.8 g/m^2/h) and water vapor permeability (*WVP*) value (1.74 ± 0.08 g mm/h/m^2), delayed erosion (18.69 ± 4.74%), high water uptake, smooth and homogenous surface morphology, higher tensile strength (56.84 ± 1.19 MPa), and increased glass transition temperature and enthalpy (through polymer hydrophilic functional groups depicting efficient cross-linking). The in vivo data on day 16 of post-wounding indicated that the wound healing occurred faster with significantly increased percent re-epithelialization and enhanced collagen deposition with optimized MB-3 film application compared with the untreated group. The study concluded that the microwave-treated polymer blend films have sufficiently enhanced physical properties, making them an effective candidate for ameliorating the diabetic wound healing process and hastening skin tissue regeneration.

Keywords: polymeric film; diabetes mellitus; skin regeneration; wound healing; sodium alginate; sodium carboxy methyl cellulose; microwave; cross-linking

1. Introduction

Skin tissue regeneration following wounds (trauma, severe burns, venous stasis, decubitus/pressure, and diabetic ulcers) has been a challenging task for biomedical scientists, especially the aesthetic outcome [1,2], and a great deal of attention has been concentrated on the research and development of polymer films as wound dressings and drug delivery systems [3,4]. The diabetic wound has been a primary health concern where the normal wound healing process is delayed due to a persistently high blood glucose level, high oxidative stress, and a compromised immune system [5], which makes it imperative to develop scaffolds with properties inculcated that are required by ideal wound dressing materials [1,6].

Wound healing is a cascade of related molecular events that work jointly to reinstate cellular function and tissue integrity [7]. These events efficiently take place in normal, healthy human beings. Still, in certain conditions, such as poor nourishment or diseases such as diabetes, these events are impeded, resulting in chronic or hard-to-heal wounds [8], which are often complicated by secondary bacterial infection, thus not only prolonging the treatment period but also increasing the treatment cost to the patient. Hence adequate blood supply to the wound area, hygiene, the absence of necrotic scraps, sufficient moisture balance, avoidance of microbial infection, and good exudate management are key factors to ensure speedy recovery of the damaged skin tissue [9].

Polymeric films have long been used as a cost-effective strategy to hasten skin tissue regeneration following damage. Hence, various polymers have been used for the purpose, such as cellulose [10], sodium carboxymethyl cellulose [11,12], chitosan [13,14], sodium alginate [3,15,16], gelatin [17], collagen [18], agar [19], pectin [20], dextran [21], carrageenan [22], and hyaluronic acid [23]. The lone use of polymer for film dressing has always been devoid of properties required of an ideal wound healing platform [24], such as efficient moisture adsorption, prevention of trans-epidermal water loss, efficient gaseous exchange between the wound bed and external environment with controlled pore size preventing bacterial infiltration [25,26], enhanced mechanical properties, and delayed degradation [24]. These demerits can be overcome by cross-linking the polymeric films, which not only results in a mechanically strong film but also enables modification of one or more physicochemical properties of the film such as tensile strength, strain, higher temperature performance, cell-matrix interactions, gas permeation reduction, shape memory retention, and resistance to enzymatic and chemical degradation [27].

Crosslinking is described as the generation of physical or chemical linkage between polymer chains, which is generally an easy way to amend the biological, degradation, and mechanical properties of the polymer [28]. This is regarded to happen through functional groups by the generation of additional linkages through either chemical (covalent) or physical bond formation (hydrogen bonds, electrostatic interactions, and/or Vander Waal's forces, etc.) [29]. The majority of materials that undergo no treatment do not hold the required degradation and mechanical properties of the engineered platform; consequently, there is a severe demand to augment those properties by use of smaller molecules named "crosslinking agents" or "crosslinkers" [24]. The prime objective of crosslinking is to enhance the biomechanical properties of the scaffold by creating a compact network in a polymer matrix [30–32]. Ionic cross-linking has been mainly used for this purpose [33,34] by using compounds such as glutaraldehyde, formaldehyde, epoxy compounds, and dialdehyde. It is regarded as a highly versatile method [31]. However, chemical cross-linking is an extremely flexible technique to improve the mechanical properties of polymers, thus offering improved mechanical stability compared with physically cross-linked polymers. Still, these cross-linking compounds are frequently toxic, exhibit undesirable effects, may exert toxic reactions that result in cytotoxicity, can induce unwanted reactions with the scaffold surface, and are not environmentally responsive [24,35,36]. Thus, their complete removal from the reaction mixture makes it prone to induce necrosis in the wound [37,38].

To address the demerits associated with the use of chemical cross-linkers, physical methods of crosslinking were introduced, such as ultraviolet irradiation [39], electron beam irradiation [31], exposing the polymers to X-rays [40], alpha-rays [41], gamma-rays [42,43], and microwaves [44,45]. In physical cross-linking, polymers may be efficiently cross-linked without using any exogenous crosslinking agent, thus reducing the hazard of chemical adulteration or chemically raised harmfulness [35]. Due to the absence of chemical crosslinking agents, biomedical safety is the primary benefit of a physical crosslink, evading possible cytotoxicity from unreacted chemical crosslinkers [46]. Physical crosslinking is through physical interactions such as crystallization, protein interaction, hydrogen bonding, hydrophilic/hydrophobic interaction, stereocomplex formation/complexation, and ionic interactions, which help keep the polymer chains together [36,47].

Microwaves are electromagnetic waves characterized by frequency in the range of 300 MHz to 300 GHz [38] and have long been used for polymerization reactions [48], for the synthesis of an extensive range of polymers [49], for the development of hydrogel scaffolds [50], for the fabrication of hydrogel [51] and nanoparticle gel [52], for improving the mechanical properties of the polymer [53], for polymer modification and composite film formulation [54,55], and for polymeric films [56,57]. Microwave interacts with polar functional groups in a volumetric manner, thereby initiating polymer cross-linking through their polar moieties, with the added merits of excluding the use of catalysts or additives to start the reaction and simplicity of irradiation methods; the crosslinking point may be controlled effortlessly by differing the dose of irradiation [36]. Multiple studies have been performed to evaluate the role of the microwave as a crosslinker which significantly enhanced the physicochemical attributes of the resultant product such as titanium dioxide nanoparticles containing cross-linked chitosan hydrogel scaffold [50], microwave-aided bioactive chitosan scaffold containing gold nanoparticles [58], poly acrylic acid, polyvinyl alcohol, polyacrylamide, hydroxyl ethyl cellulose and polymethyl vinyl-ether-alt-maleic anhydride cross-linked hydrogels without the use of monomers [51], chitosan/polyvinyl alcohol silver nanoparticles gel [52], poly-lactic acid and poly-glycolic acid blend [53], microcrystalline corn-straw cellulose cross-linked film [55], hydroxy propyl methyl cellulose and poly(vinylpyrrolidone) composite films [45], and polyvinyl alcohol and tartaric acid films [56].

Sodium alginate (SA) is a water-solvable hydrocolloid that is obtained from brown seaweed and is composed of (1–4)-linked -d-mannuronic acid and -l-guluronic acid units [59]. The significant abilities of this polymer, such as biocompatibility, non-toxicity, reproducibility, and biodegradation, have directed its usage in several fields, including pharmaceutical additives, tissue engineering materials, food, and biology or enzyme carriers [60]. It has also been investigated for its wound-healing potentials, such as the development of biocompatible povidone-iodine-containing sodium alginate film for enhancement of ulcer healing [16], sodium alginate and gelatin hydrogels as wound dressings [19], and the formation of PVA-sodium alginate hydrogel membrane containing bFGF-entrapped microspheres for enhanced wound healing [61].

Sodium Carboxymethyl cellulose (NaCMC), a biopolymer, is one of the derivatives of cellulose that is developed by substituting the hydroxyl group (-OH) with the carboxymethyl (-COOH2CH-) group, where both units are linked to each other by β 1 and 4 glycosidic linkages [62,63]. It possesses excellent swelling and water-absorbing properties [64] and is biologically inert and biocompatible [65,66]. It also finds widespread applications in reduction, flocculation, detergents, paper, textiles, food, and drug formulation [67]. It also has the added merit of being safe, non-toxic, and non-sensitizing, and hence also finds applications in food, cosmetic, pharmaceutical, and biomedical applications, as well as wound management [68,69]. It also possesses excellent film-forming properties [70] and has been widely studied for wound-healing applications [62,68,71–73].

Both sodium alginate and Na-CMC have been extensively studied from the perspective of wound healing [16,25,62,74–76], but their sole use has been associated with demerits such as high water vapor transmission [77,78], fast erosion due to high hydrophilicity [79], low absorbability [78,80], permeability to bacteria [81], low gaseous exchange between the wound bed and external environment [82,83], and poor mechanical strength [84–87], which necessitates the development of their blends [79].

This project aimed to develop physically cross-linked sodium alginate and NaCMC films through microwave treatment, analyze them for physicochemical attributes, and perform in vivo testing in diabetes-induced animal models for rapid healing following open incision wound infliction. Blended sodium alginate/NaCMC films have been explored as prospective combinations that can be physically crosslinked using the microwave. Their combination was optimized by varying the microwave treatment time while keeping the concentration of both polymers constant. The optimized combination was tested for its ability to regenerate skin tissue in diabetic animals following open incision wound infliction.

2. Materials and Methods

2.1. Materials

Polysorbate 80 (tween-80, purity ~99%), disodium hydrogen orthophosphate (purity ~99%), sodium chloride (purity ~99%), sodium carboxymethyl cellulose (Na-CMC, purity ~99%, molecular weight 262.19 g/mol, high viscosity:1500–3000 centipoise of 1% solution in water at 25 °C), and monobasic potassium phosphate (purity ~98%) were procured from Sigma-Aldrich (St. Louis, MO, USA), while hydrochloric acid (purity ~35%) was purchased from Merck, Darmstat, Germany. Sodium alginate (purity ~99%, molecular weight 216.12 g/mol, viscosity: 15–25 centipoise of 1% solution in water) was bought from Sinopharm Chemical Reagent Co., Ltd., Shanghai, China. Polyethylene glycol-400 (PEG-400, purity ~99%) and glycerol (purity ~99%) were kindly provided by Bio-Labs (Islamabad, Pakistan). All chemicals were used without any further processing or purification.

2.2. Methods

2.2.1. Film Formulation

Bi-polymeric blended films composed of sodium alginate and Na-CMC were developed by solution casting technique as described earlier [33]. Briefly, sodium alginate and Na-CMC were separately dissolved in enough deionized water to prepare (2% w/w) solutions. Both solutions were then added with glycerol (2% w/w), tween 80 (0.1% w/w) and PEG-400 (0.05% w/w) and thoroughly mixed to ensure homogeneity. Both polymer solutions were mixed in a ratio of 60:40 (60 parts sodium alginate and 40 parts Na-CMC) and subjected to microwave treatment for different time intervals (1 and 3 min) at fixed power of 500 watts and a fixed frequency of 2450 MHz, utilizing a commercially available microwave oven (LG, MS2022D, Beijing, China). Following microwave treatment, a total of 50 g of bubble-free polymer mixture was transferred into petri dishes (Ø 34.30 mm) and dried in a convection oven (SH SCIENTIFIC, Model: SH- DO-100NG, Sejong, Korea) at 40 °C for 72 h or until complete dryness.

The dried polymeric films were detached from petri dishes and kept in a desiccator until they were subjected to several physicochemical characterization tests. The untreated blend films were developed similarly for comparison. The formulation ingredients and microwave treatment conditions are depicted in Table 1.

Table 1. Composition of modified blended sodium alginate and sodium CMC film formulations.

Formulations	Microwave Treatment Time (min)	Sodium Alginate (w/w) g	Na-CMC (w/w) g	Tween 80 (w/w) G	PEG-400 (w/w) G	Glycerol (w/w) g	Water (w/w) G
Untreated blend (UB)	—	2	2	0.1	0.05	2	93.85
MB-1	1	2	2	0.1	0.05	2	93.85
MB-3	3	2	2	0.1	0.05	2	93.85

2.2.2. Moisture Adsorption

An already-reported method [88] was used to determine moisture adsorption. Concisely, the film was sliced into 2.5 × 3 cm pieces and accurately weighed. The film pieces were dehydrated in a desiccator with anhydrous calcium sulfate ($CaSO_4$) at virtual relative humidity (RH) of 0% for 48 h. Following complete desiccation, the dried film pieces were weighed again and incubated again with a saturated solution of potassium sulfate in a desiccator at 25 ± 2 °C with relative humidity maintained at 97 ± 2% for an additional 48 h to allow the films to become fully hydrated and were weighed again. The percent (%) moisture adsorption was determined using the following equation.

$$MA\ (\%) = (Wt - Wi)/Wi \times 100 \tag{1}$$

Wt = Final weight after rehydration, and Wi = Initial weight after dehydration.
The test was repeated three times and results were averaged with ± standard deviation.

2.2.3. Water Vapor Transmission Rate (*WVTR*) and Water Vapor Permeability (*WVP*)

The water vapor transmission rate (*WVTR*) through the polymeric film was assessed by the ASTM method with some modifications using a plastic bottle with its mouth area determined [89]. The film was cut in size according to the mouth of the bottle. The bottle was filled with a 30 mL saturated potassium chloride solution, and the film was tied onto its mouth with an adhesive. The whole system was initially weighed and then placed in a desiccator containing calcium chloride at room temperature with RH maintained at 1.5%. The system's weight was determined hourly for up to 8 h. The loss in weight is considered equal to the amount of water transmitted across the film, which was absorbed by desiccant material ($CaCl_2$). The thickness of the films was determined using a micrometer screw gauge. The values were placed in equations to determine the WVT, which was estimated by dividing the slope of a linear regression of weight loss vs. time by *film area*, and the *WVP* (gm/m^2 s Pa) was determined by using an equation.

$$WVTR = \frac{Slope}{Film\ area} \tag{2}$$

The *slope* is the slope of the graph calculated from the weight loss vs. time curve, and the *film area* was 0.000903 m^2.

$$WVP = \frac{WVTR \times T}{\Delta P} \tag{3}$$

T is the mean film thickness (mm) and ΔP is the partial water vapor pressure difference (mmHg) through two sides of the film sample (the partial vapor pressure of water at 25 °C = 23.73 mmHg).

The experiment was repeated three times, and results averaged with ± SD.

2.2.4. Erosion and Water Uptake

Briefly, film pieces were cut, each having a 3 × 2.5 cm dimension. Then dry film pieces were weighed and placed in 20 mL PBS of pH 7.4 in a petri dish. After that, it was incubated at 37 ± 3 °C in a convection oven (SH SCIENTIFIC, Model: SH- DO-100NG, Sejong-si, Republic of Korea). The film pieces were taken from the petri dish at a specific time interval (every 5 min), blotted dry, and weighed again. The same was repeated for the entire incubation time of over 20 min. After 20 min, the buffer solution was discarded, and the same film pieces were dried in an oven at 40 ± 2 °C for 5 days. After 5 days, the oven-dried weight was taken, and the following relations were used to calculate percent erosion (*E%*) and percent water uptake (*WU%*). The test was executed in triplicate, and the results were averaged with standard deviation.

$$E\ (\%) = \frac{Wi - Wt(d)}{Wi} \times 100 \tag{4}$$

$$WU\ (\%) = \frac{Wt - Wt(d)}{Wt(d)} \times 100 \tag{5}$$

Wi = weight of film before immersion, $Wt\ (d)$ = dry weight of film taken at time t, and Wt = wet weight of film at time t.

2.2.5. Morphology

Scanning electron microscopy was used to analyze the film's surface morphology using an ultra-high-resolution field-emission scanning electron microscope (UHR-FESEM, MERLIN/344999-9001-030, Zeiss, Aalen, Germany). Each film was sliced into a 3 × 3 mm piece, which was then attached to a stub via double-sided adhesive carbon tape. The samples were then placed in the microscope chamber after being subjected to a 5-min gold sputter coating procedure (QUORUM Sputter Coater Q150R S, Quorum, Lewes, UK), followed by SEM examination at a 10-KV accelerating voltage. Using the smartTiff tool, the photographs of corresponding parts were taken at magnification powers of 100, 500, 1000, 2000, and 3000× [34].

2.2.6. Tensile Strength

Using a universal testing device (Testometrics, Rochdale, UK), the polymeric films' ultimate tensile strength was assessed at 25 ± 1 °C. The polymeric film's tensile strength was measured employing a texture analyzer after being trimmed into rectangular-shaped strips. For each film sample, three rectangular-shaped strips of 7.5 cm in length and 3.5 cm in width were trimmed, and they were then fastened between the machine's grips. The initial grip distance was set to 50 mm, and the crosshead speed was set to 5 mm/min. The sample was pulled with a 50 N load [34]. The most significant breaking force was noted. The results were averaged across three replicated tests.

2.2.7. Differential Scanning Calorimetry (DSC)

The films' thermal characteristics were assessed using differential scanning calorimetry (DSC; PerkinElmer Thermal Analysis, USA) [89]. A 5–7 mg film sample was taken in the sample pan. The reference pan was left empty. Melting transition temperatures (T) of various films were recorded while continuously purging with N_2 gas with a 40 mL/min flow rate and a heating scan rate of 10 °C/min from 0–400 °C. Each film peak's transition temperature and enthalpy (ΔH) values were calculated in triplicate, and the results were averaged.

2.2.8. Vibrational Spectroscopic Analysis

An ATR-FTIR spectrophotometer (UATR TWO, Perkin Elmer, Beaconsfield, UK) [89] captured the dried polymeric films' distinctive peaks. Each film was laid on the diamond crystal's surface and secured to guarantee close contact and great sensitivity. All samples were scanned with a 2 min acquisition time spanning the 400 to 4000 cm^{-1} wavenumber range. Results were averaged after three analyses of each sample.

2.2.9. In Vivo Wound Healing

Healthy male Sprague–Dawley rats with a weight range of 200–250 g were procured and acclimatized/adjusted for 14 days with an easy approach to water and food at a temperature of 19 to 23 °C with a 12-h dark-light cycle. Before the diabetes induction, the rats abstained from eating for 24 h with free access to water. They were weighed, and their fasting blood sugar levels were determined using a glucometer (CodeFree, SD Biosensor, Korea). A single dose of freshly prepared streptozotocin solution was intraperitoneally injected in rats at a dosage of 50 mg/kg body weight of the animal. The blood sugar levels of the animals were monitored starting on day 3 of the streptozotocin injection [90], and rats were considered people with diabetes when their blood sugar levels were >250 mg/dL [91]. Following the diabetes induction, the diabetic rats were divided randomly into two groups (n = 8 for each group), i.e., untreated and polymeric film groups. The rats were anesthetized by I/P injection of a mixture of xylazine (10 mg/kg) and ketamine (100 mg/kg), and the back hair of the rats was shaved. An open incision wound was inflicted on a mid-dorsal thoracic section of the rats with the help of sterilized forceps and surgical scissors. Following the infliction of the wound, the treatments were applied to the injured part, covered with sterile gauze, and adhered with 3M adhesive tape. The untreated group received only the gauze application, while the polymeric film group received only the (3 × 3 dimensional) film piece. The treatments were applied daily until complete wound healing was observed. The institutional Ethical Review Board approved the animal study protocol, vide reference number: 502/QEC/GU, dated: 29 March 2019, Gomal University Pakistan.

The photographs of wounds were taken by a Canon D5200 camera (Tokyo, Japan) on days 0, 3, 7, 14, and 16 post-administration to record the surface morphology of the wound. The wound size was investigated by Image J software (version 1.53K, US National Institutes of Health, Bethesda, MD, USA). The % re-epithelization was then estimated using the following relation.

$$Re-epithelialization\ (\%) = \frac{Wound\ size\ at\ time\ 0 - Wound\ size\ at\ time\ t}{Wound\ size\ at\ time\ 0} \times 100 \quad (6)$$

2.2.10. Physicochemical Characterization of Skin Samples
Thermal Analysis

To estimate changes produced in the lipid and protein regions of skin with film treatment compared with the control group, the skin samples with wounds were also exposed to thermal analysis employing DSC (Perkin Elmer, Thermal Analysis, Boston, MA, USA). In a nutshell, a precisely measured 3 mg of full-thickness skin-containing wound was trimmed/cut with great care and enclosed in a standard aluminum pan before being subjected to thermal analysis at temperatures ranging between 30–180 °C at a heating rate of 10 °C/min, under constant pulses of nitrogen gas at a 40 mL/min flow rate. For the lipidic and protein regions, the melting temperature and enthalpy were noted. Results were averaged after at least three separate analyses of each sample.

Tensile Strength

The tensile strength of the excised skin samples was measured after they were cut into strips of 5 cm in length and 2.5 cm in width (Testometric M-500, Rochdale, UK). The strips were fastened between the lower and upper jaws of the tensiometer and perpendicularly pulled/strained with loads of 30 kg at test speeds of 5 mm/s and 10 mm/s, respectively. The greatest power necessary to rupture the skin sample and the breaking point were noted. Test of every skin specimen was performed thrice, and results were averaged.

Vibrational Spectroscopy

ATR-FTIR (UATR TWO, Perkin Elmer, Buckinghamshire, UK) was used to record the vibrational spectra of the dermal layer of skin samples from treated and untreated animal groups with a resolution of 16 cm^{-1} and acquisition/exposure duration of 2 min. The corresponding ATR-FTIR spectra were compared to determine the degree of collagen deposition. The amide-I and amide-II absorbances, which come from the skin's protein composition, were measured for this purpose. The degree of collagen deposition was estimated using this unique technique that compared the absorbance of the treatment group with the control group. The results from three analyses of each sample were averaged.

Histology

Animals were killed by cervical dislocation when needed, and the skin-containing wound was surgically removed, cleaned with normal saline, and stored at −20 °C until further usage. Histological testing was conducted on the newly repaired skin tissue that covered the incision. The stored skin samples were thawed at room temperature for 3 h, then fixed in a 10% aqueous solution of formalin for three days at ambient temperatures. The skin samples were then prepped by cutting, washing with regular saline, and dehydrating in ethanol. The samples of desiccated skin were cleaned with xylene before being fixed in paraffin wax. Using a microtome (HM-340E, Microm Inc., Boise, ID, USA), 5 µm thick sections were created. They were then processed separately by Masson's trichrome and

H&E (hematoxylin and eosin) stains. The slides were observed, and relevant portions were photographed employing an inverted microscope equipped with a camera (HDCCE—X5N).

2.3. Statistical Analysis

At a minimum, three data replicates were used to calculate the mean and standard deviation. The significance level was established at $p < 0.05$, and the analysis of variance (ANOVA) followed by post hoc analysis or a Student's t-test was employed for analysis.

3. Results and Discussion

3.1. Moisture Adsorption

An ideal wound-healing platform requires a hydrophilic extracellular matrix that can remove wound exudate and keep the wound bed moist for rapid regeneration [79,92,93]. To check a material's capacity to hold sufficient moisture in the wound bed, various methods, such as water contact angle and water retention, can be used [9]. The moisture adsorption test results indicated that the percentage moisture adsorption of blended films ranged from 131 ± 6.6% to 154.6 ± 4.23%. The moisture adsorption ability was found to increase significantly with an increase in microwave treatment time, as shown in Figure 1. The increase in water adsorption ability of polymer blend film following microwave treatment can be attributed to free OH functional groups shifting to the surface area, thereby promoting the water attacking ability of the film [94].

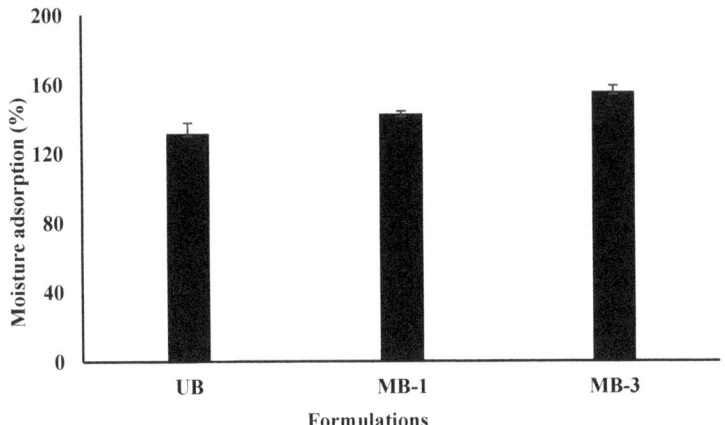

Figure 1. Percentage moisture adsorption of blended film formulations.

Furthermore, microwave treatment is envisaged to increase the crosslinking density between the polymers and other film ingredients such as glycerol, which has been reported to immobilize between polymer chains, resulting in increased water absorbency and enhanced water moisture adsorption ability of the film [88]. Microwaves are polarphilic electromagnetic waves that interact with a polymer's polar regions in a volumetric manner [95]. Following microwave treatment, the polar functional groups of sodium alginate and sodium carboxymethyl cellulose (i.e., OH, amide-I, and amide-II) may interact via hydrogen bonding [96], forming a compact structure. Moreover, the strong interlinks between the polymer chains cause the polymer fibers to arrange themselves in a uniform/even manner during drying, resulting in voids forming between polymer chains and leading to distinct pore sizes throughout the polymer matrix [97]. Reduced pore size renders maximum moisture absorption at the wound surface [98]. It may decrease the penetration of bacteria into the wound bed, thus preventing complications in the wound [99].

3.2. Water Vapor Transmission Rate (WVTR) and Water Vapor Permeability (WVP)

The *WVTR* of a wound healing platform determines its efficiency in reducing the transepidermal water loss and facilitating the easy exchange of oxygen and carbon dioxide between the wound bed and external environment [100], which is inversely proportional to a wound dressing's ability to retain moisture, implying that a dressing having a low *WVTR* will be capable of retaining more moisture at the wound surface since dry wounds take longer time to heal [101]. The results of *WVTR* are shown in Figure 2a, where though the difference between all formulations was insignificant (Student's *t*-test, $p > 0.05$), microwave-treated blends tend to have lower *WVTR* compared with the UB formulation, where MB-3 was found to have significantly lower *WVTR* compared with UB (Table 2). Similarly, the *WVP* was highest for UB compared with MB-1 and MB-3 (Figure 2b). More water prevention ability by microwave-treated films could be attributed to specifically engineered pore size due to the arrangement of polymer layers/fibers in a specific geometric manner, probably allowing gaseous passage (O_2 and CO_2) through but preventing water molecules passage due to large molecular size [89], which was reported earlier to be due to the initiation of strong interactions between the film moieties following microwave treatment, probably in the form of strong hydrogen bonds [94]. Additionally, microwave irradiation of polymers is also reported to enhance the inter-polymer cross-linking, resulting in enhanced intermolecular forces that arrange the polymers into a better orientation [57]. Furthermore, this phenomenon is envisaged to prevent bacterial infiltration, thereby reducing the chances of secondary bacterial infection by opportunistic bacteria [102].

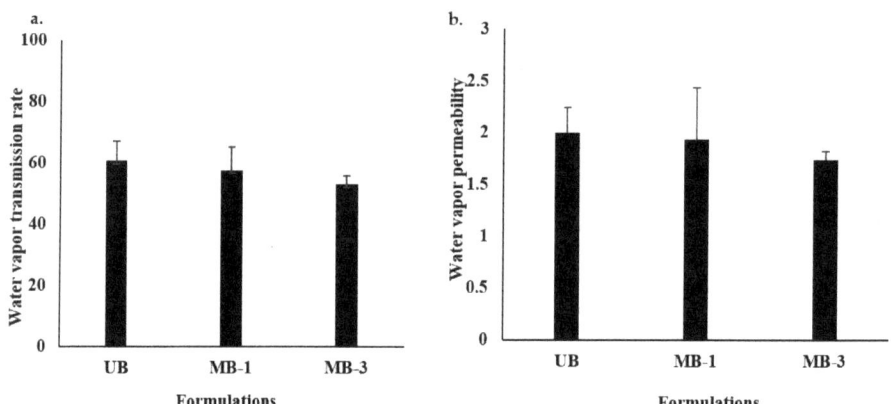

Figure 2. (a) Water vapor transmission rate; (b) water vapor permeability across various film formulations.

Table 2. *WVTR* and *WVP* along with standard deviation of blend films.

Sodium Alginate and NaCMC Blend Films			
Formulation	*WVTR* (g/m^2/h)	*WVP* (g mm/h/m^2)	The Thickness of the Film (mm)
UB	60.7 ± 6.2	2.00 ± 0.24	0.78 ± 0.01
MB-1	57.5 ± 7.7	1.93 ± 0.51	0.80 ± 0.01
MB-3	53.0 ± 2.8	1.74 ± 0.08	5.12 ± 0.03

3.3. Erosion and Water Uptake

The water uptake capacity regulates the film formulation's swelling, degradability, functionality, and stability [103], which are governed by pH, type, and ions at the wound bed. Delayed erosion and high water uptake are deemed favorable from the perspective of skin regeneration, where delayed erosion translates into better patient compliance and a long duration of action. In contrast, water uptake ability reflects the ability of the film formulation to remove exudates from the wound bed [73]. The percentage erosion results of all formulations are shown in Figure 3a, while water uptake is shown in Figure 3b. The results indicated that the UB formulation degraded up to 21.87 ± 6.62%, while microwave treatment reduced the percent erosion ability up to 18.69 ± 4.74%, though the difference was statistically insignificant (Student's *t*-test, $p > 0.05$). In the case of UB, which was composed of untreated sodium alginate and Na-CMC blend, it is more likely to expose more hydrophilic surface groups due to loosening structure formation as a result of relaxed polymer chains, allowing the easy penetration of erosion media into the matrix, resulting in hastened solubility and hence quick erosion [104]. Conversely, following microwave treatment, a densely cross-linked structure might have been formed, resulting in egg box formation between sodium alginate and Na-CMC polar functional groups [105], thereby offering higher resistance to water penetration into a polymer matrix and delaying matrix damage [89].

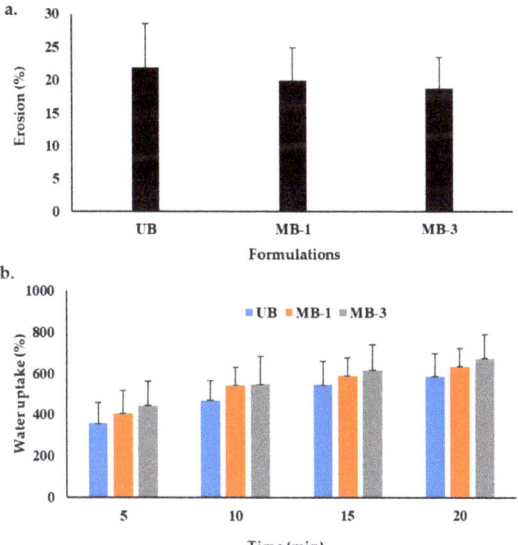

Figure 3. (**a**) Percentage erosion, and (**b**) Water uptake ability of various film formulations.

The water uptake results indicated that an increase in microwave irradiation time resulted in a higher water uptake capacity with time compared with the untreated blend. However, the difference was insignificant (ANOVA, $p > 0.05$). It is believed that due to the affinity of microwaves towards polar functional groups of the polymers and/or other formulation ingredients, hydrophilic as well as hydrophobic interactions might have resulted in surface shifting of OH/NH, amide, and ester functional groups, enabling more attraction of water molecules, translating into higher water uptake [89], which is envisaged to effectively remove wound exudate and enable faster skin regeneration.

3.4. Morphology

The surface morphology pictographs of untreated and microwave-treated blend films are shown in Figure 4. The results indicated that the untreated (UB) had a rough/granular appearance, which could be attributed to removing some of the formulation ingredients from the matrix and accumulating on the surface of the mixture as the two polymers were not wholly homogenous and there was minimal separation of the ingredients due to the loose structure of the polymer film. In contrast, the microwave treatment resulted in a more homogenous surface appearance of the film following drying, advocating proper mixing of all formulation ingredients with no phase separation at the interface owing to the microwave's ability to affect the polymer arrangement [106]. The role of the microwave as an efficient crosslinking agent is augmented by Sun et al. (2018), who described that without microwave treatment, the corn di-starch phosphate/corn straw cellulose film had a rough appearance with a loose structure when viewed cross-sectionally [57]. After microwave/ultrasonic treatment, the surface of the film became homogenous and smooth, with a dense and compact arrangement of polymer chains having no phase separation at the interface. All this happened due to efficient crosslinking between the polymers due to microwave/ultrasonic treatment. Wang et al. (2014) also advocated the role of the microwave as an excellent physical crosslinking method to create the smooth and homogenous appearance of blend films [107].

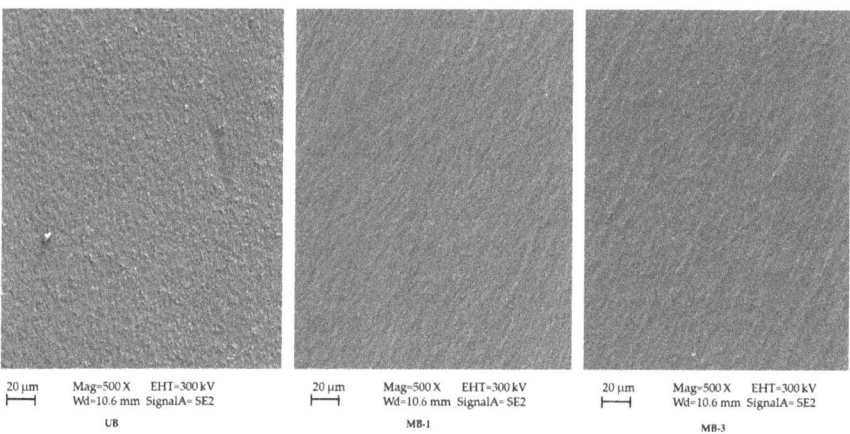

Figure 4. SEM of different blend film formulations.

3.5. Tensile Strength

The mechanical strength of a polymeric film reflects its ability to withstand friction and stress during handling and/or application at the wound site [108]. The tensile strength results of all formulations are shown in Table 3. The results indicated that the untreated blend tends to have significantly lower tensile strength than microwave-treated blends (Student's t-test, $p < 0.05$). The tensile strength tends to increase with microwave treatment time; significantly higher (Student's t-test, $p < 0.05$) tensile strength was observed when the blend was subjected to 3 min of microwave treatment. Higher tensile strength is believed to appear due to higher cross-linking density, which shall be optimized as higher cross-linking density translates into a reduction in percent elongation, which may make the film non-elastic [36]. Microwaves affect the physical attributes of polymers such as particle shape, size, distribution, packing style, and diameter, ultimately influencing the substance's mechanical properties [109]. In a study, microwave-treated soy protein isolate/titanium dioxide film exposed to 500-watt microwave power for 15 min showed maximum tensile strength due to the microwave, which reducing particle size and increased surface area. Increasing the surface area provides an improved opportunity for the particles to interact. Thus, a more stable film is created, which leads to better tensile strength [107]. Sun et al. (2018) showed the same results of improved mechanical strength of corn di-starch phosphate/corn straw cellulose film due to irradiating the film solution with microwaves [57]. They concluded that the increased tensile strength is due to the improved integration of the polymer blend due to enhanced intermolecular force, which amends the molecular structure of the polymer network.

Table 3. Tensile strength values of different blend film formulations.

Formulation	Tensile Strength (MPa)	Elongation at Break (%)	Elastic Modulus (MPa)
UB	40.54 ± 1.02	65.34 ± 2.53	57.12 ± 10.76
MB-1	48.06 ± 1.30	69.13 ± 2.87	65.88 ± 9.87
MB-3	56.84 ± 1.19	77.54 ± 1.59	79.26 ± 7.68

3.6. Thermal Analysis

Thermal analysis, such as DSC, depicts the films' behavior as a function of temperature and interprets the degradation process, thermal transition, and thermal stability of the films [11]. The DSC thermograms of the blended polymeric films were obtained to describe the thermal properties of films and estimate the effect of microwave treatment on the thermal properties of polymers. The effect of microwaves on the cross-linking ability between sodium alginate and Na-CMC was evaluated by subjecting all formulations to thermal analysis. The DSC thermograms of all formulations are shown in Figure 5. The results indicated that microwave treatment significantly increased the corresponding melting transition temperatures and enthalpies of sodium alginate and Na-CMC moieties. In the case of UB, two transitions were observed, i.e., at 111.36 ± 0.08 °C and 191.62 ± 0.06 °C, with corresponding ΔH values of 0.49 ± 0.05 J/g and 1.11 ± 0.03 J/g, respectively, where the former was attributed to sodium alginate and the latter to Na-CMC moieties. In the absence of microwave treatment, polymer chains become flexible due to surfactant/plasticizer incorporation, due to which molecules move easily, and so less heat is required to reach the glass transition temperature [88]. With the introduction of microwave treatment, the melting transition, as well as corresponding enthalpies, tend to increase. A significant (Student's t-test, $p < 0.05$) rise in the melting transition temperature as well as corresponding enthalpies was observed for MB-3, where the sodium alginate moiety showed ΔT value of 199.23 ± 2.08 °C and ΔH value of 2.35 ± 0.02 J/g. In comparison, for Na-CMC, the ΔT value of 260.32 ± 0.58 °C and ΔH value of 1.48 ± 0.06 J/g were observed. A significant rise in melting transition, as well as the energy required to induce transition, during the thermal analysis of the microwave-treated blend film depicted that microwave treatment enabled the formation of additional interactive forces between both polymer moieties, i.e., electrostatic and/or hydrogen bonding, through both polymer polar functional groups [11,110], thereby requiring higher temperature and energy to induce transition.

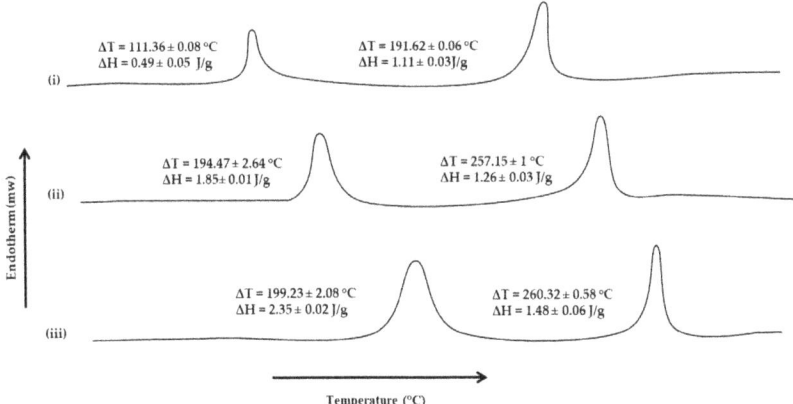

Figure 5. DSC thermograms of (i) UB, (ii) MB-1, and (iii) MB-3.

3.7. Vibrational Spectroscopic Analysis

All the film formulations were subjected to vibrational spectroscopic analysis using an ATR-FTIR to elucidate the extent of hydrophilic and hydrophobic interactions between the polymers and/or polymers and excipients following microwave treatment. The results are shown in Figure 6. The UB film showed characteristic hydrophilic (OH/NH, C=O) and hydrophobic bands (asymmetric CH), which tend to show significant shifts when subjected to microwave treatment. In the case of MB-3, a significant decrease in hydrophilic moieties (OH/NH, 3306–3315 cm^{-1}) and a significant increase in hydrophobic moieties (asymmetric CH, 2925–2930 cm^{-1}) were observed, depicting rigidification of hydrophilic domains of the film and fluidization/elasticity of hydrophobic domains occurred when films were treated with a microwave for 3 min. The rigidification of hydrophilic moieties of the polymeric blend film could be attributed to the formation of additional linkages between the polar functional groups of both polymers and/or polymers and excipients, which is envisaged to translate into a delay in erosion ability. In contrast, fluidization of hydrophobic domains is predicted to increase the elasticity of the matrix, translating into higher mechanical strength when the polymer blend was treated with microwaves for 3 min.

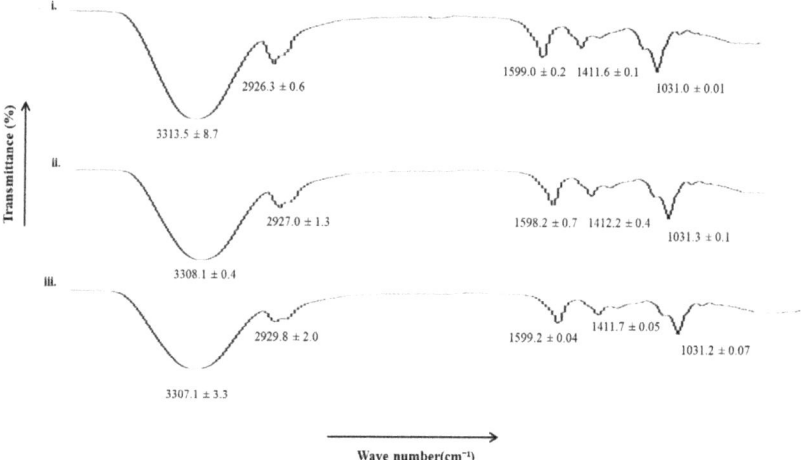

Figure 6. FTIR spectra of (i) UB, (ii) MB-1, and (iii) MB-3.

3.8. Wound Morphology

The in vivo wound healing ability of the microwave-treated polymer film group and the untreated control group was tested in the diabetic rat model. The pictographs of wound morphology are shown in Figure 7, and wound size and percent re-epithelialization results are in Figure 8a,b. The in vivo evaluation of wounds indicated that the untreated control group did not heal entirely for up to 16 days. Only 58% re-epithelialization was observed, while the polymeric film group showed a prominently high percentage of re-epithelialization (89.7%). The polymeric film group significantly hastened the skin tissue regeneration in diabetic animals in comparison to the untreated/control group with a significantly reduced wound size (ANOVA, $p < 0.05$, Figure 8a), where almost near-complete wound healing (90%) was achieved within 16 days of the experiment with nearly no scar. The absence of scarring can be attributed to the *WVP* of the film scaffold. As stated earlier, the sodium alginate-sodium CMC film scaffold showed an optimal range of *WVP*; thus, wound therapy in a wet environment positively influenced re-epithelialization; hence, it encourages healing with no scar development [111]. The polymeric film group resulted in 89.7% re-epithelialization on day 16, which was significantly higher (ANOVA, $p < 0.05$) as compared with that found for the untreated control group (58%). Among both test groups, the polymeric film proved significantly efficient in healing diabetic wounds.

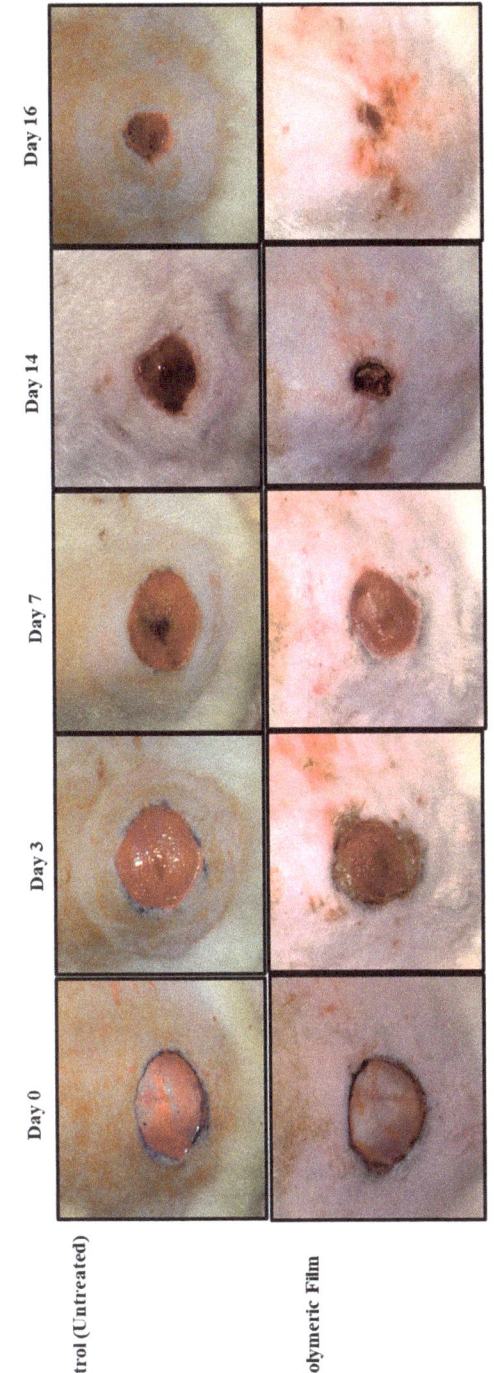

Figure 7. Photographs of skin wound morphology with and without film treatment in diabetic rats.

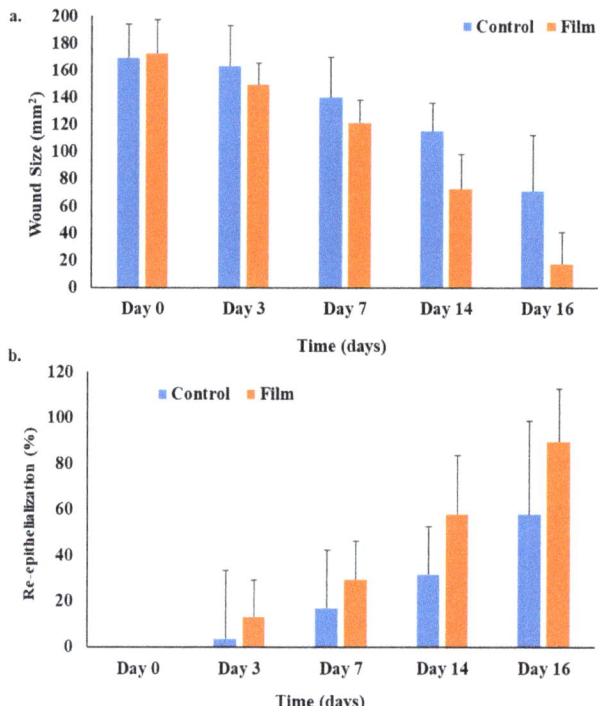

Figure 8. (**a**) Wound sizes (mm^2) and (**b**) percentage re-epithelialization in the diabetic rats.

Re-epithelialization, a characteristic hallmark of cutaneous wound contraction, is governed by the restoration of skin tissues to form a granulation barricade on the open wound [112]. The wound healing in terms of contraction and percent re-epithelialization presented promising results in the polymeric film group, which encouraged the process of wound contraction in less time than the control/untreated group. The polymeric film group also supported wound healing better, with 89.7% re-epithelialization, due to the inherent wound-healing nature of films constituting polymers (alginate and CMC) [113]. In wound healing, increased division and migration of epithelial cells along with keratinocytes occur from the periphery of the wound towards the wound site, both of which depend upon the interaction of keratinocytes with the extracellular matrix at the wound surface [114].

3.9. Physicochemical Characterization Tests Results of Skin Samples

3.9.1. Thermal Analysis

The thermal analysis results of skin samples harvested on the 14th day of post-wounding from both animal groups are presented in Figure 9. Thermal analysis was performed to investigate the extent of collagen deposition during the healing process, which is envisaged to either increase or decrease in the transition melting temperature and enthalpy of the proteinous domains in the skin samples. The results indicated that in both group samples, the melting transition, as well as corresponding enthalpies, did not differ significantly (Student's *t*-test, $p > 0.05$), where the untreated skin samples showed $\Delta T = 66.86 \pm 1.08\,°C$, with corresponding $\Delta H = 0.89 \pm 0.4$ J/g, while in the film-treated group, it appeared to be $69.32 \pm 1.20\,°C$, with corresponding enthalpy $\Delta H = 1.25 \pm 0.2$ J/g. In contrast, in the case of proteinous domains, a significant increase in the melting transition temperatures and enthalpies was observed in samples harvested from the film-treated group compared with the untreated group. The transition temperature significantly increased from 159.54 ± 1.78 °C to 176.42 ± 1.18 °C (Student's *t*-test, $p < 0.05$), with a significant rise in enthalpy (Student's *t*-test, $p < 0.05$, ΔH = 120.55 ± 4.03 J/g to 222.48 ± 3.16 J/g). The rise in melting transition and enthalpies of skin protein domains in the film-treated group advocates forming a compact and cross-linked protein structure at the wound site. Sodium alginate and Na-CMC are already reported to possess wound-healing properties [11,62,86]. Microwave treatment might have enabled controlled pore size formation in the polymer matrix, which facilitated skin regeneration by accelerating the process of collagen deposition, which is envisaged to promote rapid wound closure.

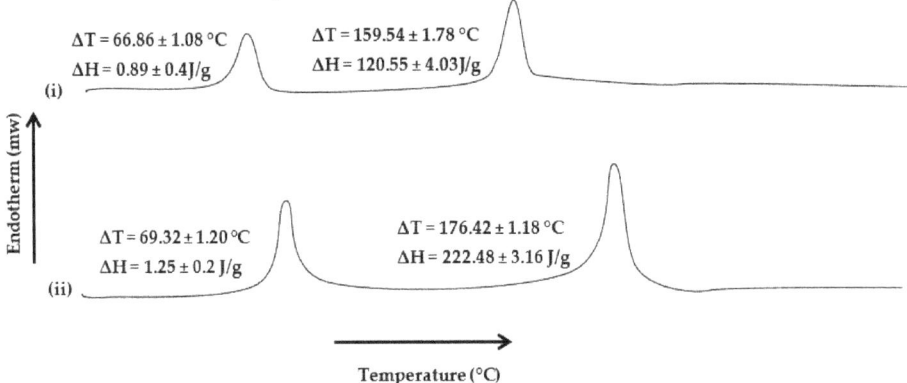

Figure 9. DSC thermograms of rat's skin without (i, ii) with polymeric film treatment.

3.9.2. Tensile Strength

Uniform and greater extents of collagen deposition are expected to significantly increase the mechanical strength of the newly regenerated skin tissue at the wound site. Therefore, the skin samples harvested on the 14th day of wounding were subjected to tensile strength analysis, and the results are shown in Table 4. The results indicated that the film-treated group showed a significant increase in the tensile strength and percent elongation break compared with the untreated animal group (Student's *t*-test, $p < 0.05$). The increased tensile strength indicates a compact and dense arrangement of collagen protein in skin structure due to the rigidification of the dermal layer's hydrophilic moieties (NH/OH, C=O, C-N), depicting the development of a more dense skin structure [97,115].

Table 4. Tensile strength of skin in various treatment groups.

Tested Groups	Tensile Strength (MPa)	Elongation at Break (%)	Elastic Modulus (MPa)
Untreated	7.43 ± 1.13	11.09 ± 0.32	1.49 ± 1.71
Polymeric film	12.4 ± 1.02	16.71 ± 0.21	3.84 ± 1.32

3.9.3. Vibrational Spectroscopy

The ATR-FTIR spectra of the dermal layer of skin samples from the untreated control group and polymeric film-treated animal groups are demonstrated in Figure 10. The ATR-FTIR analysis was performed to cement the results obtained with the thermal and tensile strength analyses. For this purpose, the wavenumbers with the corresponding absorbance ratios of the OH/NH, amide-I, and amide-II bands were investigated. The amide-I region in the skin is reported to be associated with collagen protein (1650 cm^{-1}, C=O stretching in O=C–N–H), while amide-II bands (1550 cm^{-1}, N–H bending in O=C–N–H) have been reported to arise from peptide linkages of collagen [116,117]. As shown in Figure 10, the OH/NH absorbance band underwent significant rigidification in the film group (Student's *t*-test, $p < 0.05$, 3344.3 cm^{-1} to 3327.5 cm^{-1}) compared with the untreated control group (Figure 10a). Similarly, the amide-I experienced significant rigidification (Student's t-test, $p < 0.05$), where the absorbance band underwent a significant shift to a lower wavenumber region of 1638.8 from 1643.1 cm^{-1}, with similar changes observed with the amide-II (Student's t-test, $p < 0.05$, 1556.6 to 1553.5 cm^{-1}). To further strengthen this claim, a ratio of absorbance values of corresponding bands of untreated to film-treated skin was calculated, which was found to be significantly higher for film-treated groups (Student's t-test, $p < 0.05$, amide-I to amide-II = 1.98 ± 0.02), showing more rigidity of hydrophilic moieties in the dermis compared with the untreated group (1.20 ± 0.04). The high wavenumbers and absorbance ratios indicated the rigidity of hydrophilic OH/NH parts of the dermal layer, describing the development of a denser skin structure [97] and a greater extent of protein deposition at the wound site [118].

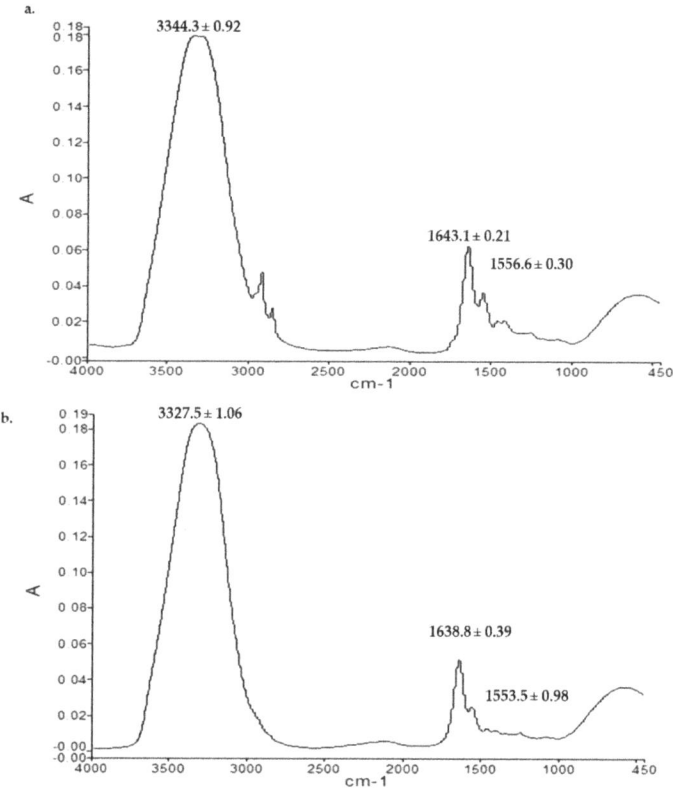

Figure 10. ATR-FTIR spectra of the dermis of (**a**) untreated skin and (**b**) film-treated skin.

3.9.4. Skin Histology

Histological analysis results of the H&E and Masson trichrome staining are shown in Figure 11. The H&E was performed to visually analyze the inflammatory phase of both animal group samples, while Masson trichrome was employed to investigate the extent and pattern of collagen deposition. As shown in Figure 11, the untreated H&E staining revealed significant inflammation yet on day 14, which was evident from signs of ulceration, edema with loose dermal layer crust, low epithelization, and an abundance of mononuclear cell infiltration compared with film-treated skin samples, with a lesser extent and nonuniform collagen deposition. In contrast, the film-treated samples showed a diverse level of granulation tissue formation, epithelium migration over the dermis, dermal remodeling, lesser edema, ulceration, and a fair quantity of granulation where signs of healed skin structure with fine-shaped were observed with close to normal epidermis, adnexa restoration, and extensive and uniform collagen fiber deposition. The animals treated with the film group presented almost complete wound re-epithelialization, together with well-formed and distinguished epithelium and substantially augmented accumulation of connective tissue and collagen within the dermis.

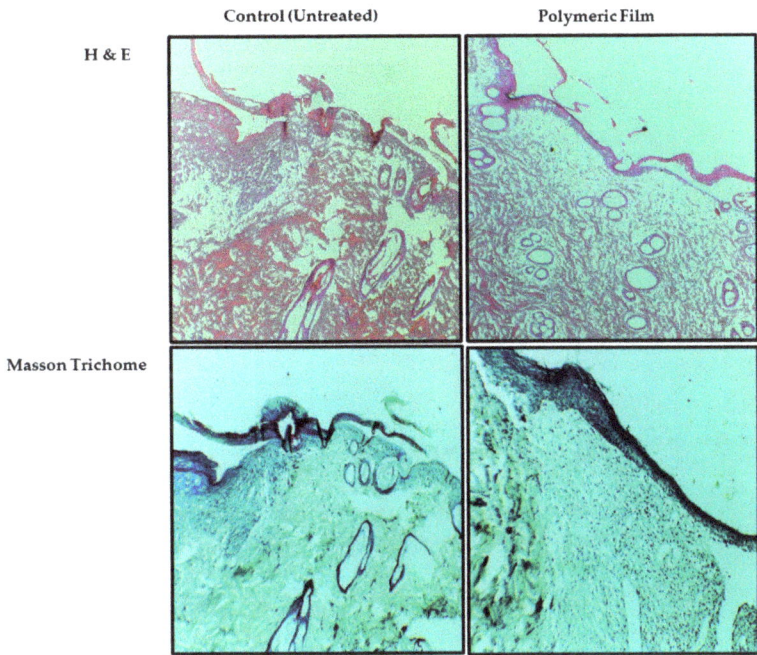

Figure 11. Photomicrographs showing the histological analysis of wound healing at day 14 after H&E and Masson trichrome staining at ×10 magnification.

Similarly, as evident in the results of Masson trichrome, film-treated samples showed a higher amount of collagen accumulation along with proper orientation at the wound site [118]. Wound contraction and healing occur due to inflammatory markers principally activating the keratinocytes and fibroblast cells to hasten the development of the collagen and extracellular matrix, forming the skin tissue's stroma [119].

4. Conclusions

The present study investigated the effectiveness of microwaves in physically cross-linking two natural polymer blends to improve the resulting film's physicochemical properties from the perspective of wound healing application. The results demonstrated that treating sodium alginate and Na-CMC blend with a fixed frequency of 2450 MHz microwave at a fixed power for 3 min improved the physicochemical properties of individual polymers, thus customizing polymer properties in the form of increased moisture adsorption, low water vapor permeability and water vapor transmission rate, delayed erosion, high water uptake, increased mechanical strength, and homogeneous and uniform surface morphology. These properties were achieved due to tailored pore size and enhanced interaction and compatibility between polymers, facilitating the exchange of oxygen and carbon dioxide between the wound bed and the external environment, preventing enhanced water loss from the wound, which is envisaged to promote healing. Moreover, in the in vivo study, the microwave-modified (MB-3) blend film hastened the skin tissue regeneration, with rapid wound closure, increased collagen deposition, and higher percent re-epithelization compared with the untreated group. Combining sodium alginate and sodium CMC with microwave treatment in film formulation may open new horizons in skin tissue regeneration applications in diabetic wound treatment.

Author Contributions: All authors equally contributed to the finalization of this article. Conceptualization, N.R.K.; methodology, S.M., N.R.K. and S.U.S.; software, S.M., N.R.K., G.R., H.M.B. and M.G.S.; validation, N.R.K., H.A.A., A.A.A. and A.A; formal analysis, S.M., N.R.K. and S.U.S.; investigation, S.M. and N.R.K.; resources, N.R.K., H.A.A., A.A.A. and A.A.; data curation, S.M. and N.R.K.; writing—original draft preparation, S.M., N.R.K. and H.M.B.; writing—review and editing, N.R.K., S.U.S., H.A.A., M.G.S. and H.M.B.; visualization, N.R.K.; supervision, N.R.K.; project administration, N.R.K.; funding acquisition, N.R.K. All authors have read and agreed to the published version of the manuscript.

Funding: This research was funded by the Higher Education Commission of Pakistan, grant number 7493.

Institutional Review Board Statement: The Institutional Ethical Review Board approved the animal study protocol (502/QEC/GU, dated: 29/03/2019, Gomal University Pakistan).

Informed Consent Statement: Not applicable.

Data Availability Statement: All data about this project has been presented in this manuscript.

Conflicts of Interest: The authors declare no conflict of interest.

References

1. Singer, A.J.; Dagum, A.B. Current Management of Acute Cutaneous Wounds. *N. Engl. J. Med.* **2008**, *359*, 1037–1046. [CrossRef]
2. Vig, K.; Chaudhari, A.; Tripathi, S.; Dixit, S.; Sahu, R.; Pillai, S.; Dennis, V.A.; Singh, S.R. Advances in Skin Regeneration Using Tissue Engineering. *Int. J. Mol. Sci.* **2017**, *18*, 789. [CrossRef]
3. Kamoun, E.A.; Kenawy, E.-R.S.; Tamer, T.M.; El-Meligy, M.A.; Eldin, M.S.M. Poly (vinyl alcohol)-alginate physically crosslinked hydrogel membranes for wound dressing applications: Characterization and bio-evaluation. *Arab. J. Chem.* **2015**, *8*, 38–47. [CrossRef]
4. Piaggesi, A.; Baccetti, F.; Rizzo, L.; Romanelli, M.; Navalesi, R.; Benzi, L. Sodium carboxyl-methyl-cellulose dressings in the management of deep ulcerations of diabetic foot. *Diabet. Med.* **2001**, *18*, 320–324. [CrossRef]
5. Kant, V.; Gopal, A.; Pathak, N.N.; Kumar, P.; Tandan, S.K.; Kumar, D. Antioxidant and anti-inflammatory potential of curcumin accelerated the cutaneous wound healing in streptozotocin-induced diabetic rats. *Int. Immunopharmacol.* **2014**, *20*, 322–330. [CrossRef]
6. Abdelrahman, T.; Newton, H. Wound dressings: Principles and practice. *Surgery* **2011**, *29*, 491–495. [CrossRef]
7. Telser, A.G.; Young, J.K.; Baldwin, K.M. *Elsevier's Integrated Histology*, 1st ed.; Elsevier: Amsterdam, The Netherlands, 2007.
8. Sarheed, O.; Ahmed, A.; Shouqair, D.; Boateng, J. Antimicrobial Dressings for Improving Wound Healing. In *Wound Healing—New Insights into Ancient Challenges*; Intechopen: London, UK, 2016; pp. 373–398.
9. Maver, T.; Hribernik, S.; Mohan, T.; Smrke, D.M.; Maver, U.; Stana-Kleinschek, K. Functional wound dressing materials with highly tunable drug release properties. *RSC Adv.* **2015**, *5*, 77873–77884. [CrossRef]
10. Bajpai, M.; Bajpai, S.K.; Gautam, D. Investigation of Regenerated Cellulose/Poly (acrylic acid) Composite Films for Potential Wound Healing Applications: A Preliminary Study. *J. Appl. Chem.* **2014**, *2014*, 1–9. [CrossRef]
11. Basu, P.; Narendrakumar, U.; Arunachalam, R.; Devi, S.; Manjubala, I. Characterization and Evaluation of Carboxymethyl Cellulose-Based Films for Healing of Full-Thickness Wounds in Normal and Diabetic Rats. *ACS Omega* **2018**, *3*, 12622–12632. [CrossRef]
12. Vinklárková, L.; Masteiková, R.; Vetchý, D.; Doležel, P.; Bernatonienė, J. Formulation of Novel Layered Sodium Carboxymethylcellulose Film Wound Dressings with Ibuprofen for Alleviating Wound Pain. *BioMed Res. Int.* **2015**, *2015*, 1–11. [CrossRef]
13. Ahmed, S.; Ikram, S. Chitosan Based Scaffolds and Their Applications in Wound Healing. *Achiev. Life Sci.* **2016**, *10*, 27–37. [CrossRef]
14. Dai, M.; Zheng, X.; Xu, X.; Kong, X.; Li, X.; Guo, G.; Luo, F.; Zhao, X.; Wei, Y.Q.; Qian, Z. Chitosan-Alginate Sponge: Preparation and Application in Curcumin Delivery for Dermal Wound Healing in Rat. *J. Biomed. Biotechnol.* **2009**, *2009*, 1–8. [CrossRef]
15. Li, S.; Li, L.; Guo, C.; Qin, H.; Yu, X. A promising wound dressing material with excellent cytocompatibility and proangiogenesis action for wound healing: Strontium loaded Silk fibroin/Sodium alginate (SF/SA) blend films. *Int. J. Biol. Macromol.* **2017**, *104*, 969–978. [CrossRef] [PubMed]
16. Summa, M.; Russo, D.; Penna, I.; Margaroli, N.; Bayer, I.S.; Bandiera, T.; Athanassiou, A.; Bertorelli, R. A biocompatible sodium alginate/povidone iodine film enhances wound healing. *Eur. J. Pharm. Biopharm.* **2018**, *122*, 17–24. [CrossRef] [PubMed]
17. Adhirajan, N.; Shanmugasundaram, N.; Shanmuganathan, S.; Babu, M. Functionally modified gelatin microspheres impregnated collagen scaffold as novel wound dressing to attenuate the proteases and bacterial growth. *Eur. J. Pharm. Sci.* **2009**, *36*, 235–245. [CrossRef]

18. Xie, H.; Chen, X.; Shen, X.; He, Y.; Chen, W.; Luo, Q.; Ge, W.; Yuan, W.; Tang, X.; Hou, D.; et al. Preparation of chitosan-collagen-alginate composite dressing and its promoting effects on wound healing. *Int. J. Biol. Macromol.* **2018**, *107*, 93–104. [CrossRef]
19. Saarai, A.; Kasparkova, V.; Sedlacek, T.; Saha, P. A Comparative Study of Crosslinked Sodium Alginate/Gelatin Hydrogels for Wound Dressing. *Recent Res. Geogr. Geol. Energy Environ. Biomed.* **2011**, 384–389.
20. Gohil, R.M. Synergistic blends of natural polymers, pectin and sodium alginate. *J. Appl. Polym. Sci.* **2010**, *120*, 2324–2336. [CrossRef]
21. Sun, G.; Zhang, X.; Shen, Y.-I.; Sebastian, R.; Dickinson, L.E.; Fox-Talbot, K.; Reinblatt, M.; Steenbergen, C.; Harmon, J.W.; Gerecht, S. Dextran hydrogel scaffolds enhance angiogenic responses and promote complete skin regeneration during burn wound healing. *Proc. Natl. Acad. Sci. USA* **2011**, *108*, 20976–20981. [CrossRef]
22. Boateng, J.S.; Pawar, H.V.; Tetteh, J. Polyox and carrageenan based composite film dressing containing anti-microbial and anti-inflammatory drugs for effective wound healing. *Int. J. Pharm.* **2013**, *441*, 181–191. [CrossRef]
23. Price, R.D.; Myers, S.; Leigh, I.M.; Navsaria, H.A. The role of hyaluronic acid in wound healing: Assessment of clinical evidence. *Am. J. Clin. Dermatol.* **2005**, *6*, 393–402. [CrossRef] [PubMed]
24. Oryan, A.; Kamali, A.; Moshiri, A.; Baharvand, H.; Daemi, H. Chemical crosslinking of biopolymeric scaffolds: Current knowledge and future directions of crosslinked engineered bone scaffolds. *Int. J. Biol. Macromol.* **2018**, *107*, 678–688. [CrossRef] [PubMed]
25. Mayet, N.; Choonara, Y.E.; Kumar, P.; Tomar, L.K.; Tyagi, C.; Du Toit, L.C.; Pillay, V. A Comprehensive Review of Advanced Biopolymeric Wound Healing Systems. *J. Pharm. Sci.* **2014**, *103*, 2211–2230. [CrossRef]
26. Abrigo, M.; McArthur, S.L.; Kingshott, P. Electrospun Nanofibers as Dressings for Chronic Wound Care: Advances, Challenges, and Future Prospects. *Macromol. Biosci.* **2014**, *14*, 772–792. [CrossRef] [PubMed]
27. Chaterji, S.; Kwon, I.K.; Park, K. Smart polymeric gels: Redefining the limits of biomedical devices. *Prog. Polym. Sci.* **2007**, *32*, 1083–1122. [CrossRef]
28. Reddy, N.; Li, Y.; Yang, Y. Alkali-catalyzed low temperature wet crosslinking of plant proteins using carboxylic acids. *Biotechnol. Prog.* **2009**, *25*, 139–146. [CrossRef]
29. Daemi, H.; Rajabi-Zeleti, S.; Sardon, H.; Barikani, M.; Khademhosseini, A.; Baharvand, H. A robust super-tough biodegradable elastomer engineered by supramolecular ionic interactions. *Biomaterials* **2016**, *84*, 54–63. [CrossRef]
30. Daemi, H.; Barikani, M. Synthesis and characterization of calcium alginate nanoparticles, sodium homopolymannuronate salt and its calcium nanoparticles. *Sci. Iran.* **2012**, *19*, 2023–2028. [CrossRef]
31. Maitra, J.; Shukla, V.K. Cross-linking in Hydrogels—A Review. *Am. J. Polym. Sci.* **2014**, *4*, 25–31.
32. Song, Y.; Wang, L.; Gyanda, R.; Sakhuja, R.; Cavallaro, M.; Jackson, D.C.; Meher, N.K.; Ciamitaro, D.A.; Bedford, C.D.; Katritzky, A.R.; et al. Effect of the crosslink functionality on the mechanical properties of crosslinked 1,2,3-triazole polymers as potential binders for rocket propellants. *J. Appl. Polym. Sci.* **2010**, *117*, 473–478. [CrossRef]
33. Han, Y.; Wang, L. Sodium alginate/carboxymethyl cellulose films containing pyrogallic acid: Physical and antibacterial properties. *J. Sci. Food Agric.* **2016**, *97*, 1295–1301. [CrossRef] [PubMed]
34. Rezvanian, M.; Amin, M.C.I.M.; Ng, S.-F. Development and physicochemical characterization of alginate composite film loaded with simvastatin as a potential wound dressing. *Carbohydr. Polym.* **2016**, *137*, 295–304. [CrossRef] [PubMed]
35. Hennink, W.E.; van Nostrum, C.F. Novel crosslinking methods to design hydrogels. *Adv. Drug Deliv. Rev.* **2002**, *54*, 13–36. [CrossRef]
36. Saini, K. Preparation method, Properties and Crosslinking of hydrogel: A review. *PharmaTutor* **2017**, *5*, 27–36.
37. Moshnikova, A.B.; Moshnikov, S.A.; Afanasyev, V.N.; Krotova, K.E.; Sadovnikov, V.B.; Beletsky, I.P. Cell death induced by chemical homobifunctional cross-linkers Cross-linker induced apoptosis. *Int. J. Biochem. Cell Biol.* **2001**, *33*, 1160–1171. [CrossRef]
38. Kuang, T.K.; Kang, Y.-B.; Segarra, I.; Kanwal, U.; Ahsan, M.; Bukhari, N.I. Microwave-assisted Preparation of Cross-linked Gelatin-Paracetamol Matrices: Optimization Using the D-optimal Design. *Turk. J. Pharm. Sci.* **2021**, *18*, 167–175. [CrossRef]
39. Davidenko, N.; Bax, D.V.; Schuster, C.F.; Farndale, R.W.; Hamaia, S.W.; Best, S.M.; Cameron, R.E. Optimisation of UV irradiation as a binding site conserving method for crosslinking collagen-based scaffolds. *J. Mater. Sci. Mater. Med.* **2015**, *27*, 1–17. [CrossRef] [PubMed]
40. Gupta, T.; Strelcov, E.; Holland, G.; Schumacher, J.; Yang, Y.; Esch, M.; Aksyuk, V.; Zeller, P.; Amati, M.; Gregoratti, L.; et al. Focused Electron and X-ray Beam Crosslinking in Liquids for Nanoscale Hydrogels 3D Printing and Encapsulation. *arXiv* **2019**, arXiv:1904.01652.
41. Itzhaki, R.F.; Alexander, P. The Effect of Polonium Alpha Rays on the Physical Properties of Polyethylene and of Polymethyl Methacrylate. *Radiat. Res.* **1961**, *15*, 553. [CrossRef]
42. Ibrahim, S.M.; El Salmawi, K.M. Preparation and Properties of Carboxymethyl Cellulose (CMC)/Sodium alginate (SA) Blends Induced by Gamma Irradiation. *J. Polym. Environ.* **2013**, *21*, 520–527. [CrossRef]
43. Jeong, J.-O.; Park, J.-S.; Kim, Y.-A.; Yang, S.-J.; Jeong, S.-I.; Lee, J.-Y.; Lim, Y.-M. Gamma Ray-Induced Polymerization and Cross-Linking for Optimization of PPy/PVP Hydrogel as Biomaterial. *Polymers* **2020**, *12*, 111. [CrossRef]
44. Xing, -Y.; Xue, -Y.; Qin, -D.; Zhao, -P.; Li, P. Microwave-induced ultrafast crosslinking of Poly (vinyl alcohol) blended with nanoparticles as wave absorber for pervaporation desalination. *J. Membr. Sci. Lett.* **2022**, *2*, 100021. [CrossRef]

45. Somashekarappa, H.; Prakash, Y.; Dasaiah, M.; Demappa, T.; Rudrappa, S. Effect of microwave radiation on hydroxy propyl methyl cellulose polymer films and HPMC/poly (vinylpyrrolidone) polymer blend films using the wide-angle X-ray technique. *Radiat. Eff. Defects Solids Inc. Plasma Sci. Plasma Technol.* **2013**, *168*, 1–12. [CrossRef]
46. Berger, J.; Reist, M.; Mayer, J.; Felt, O.; Gurny, R. Structure and interactions in chitosan hydrogels formed by complexation or aggregation for biomedical applications. *Eur. J. Pharm. Biopharm.* **2003**, *57*, 35–52. [CrossRef] [PubMed]
47. Ermis, M.; Calamak, S.; Kocal, G.C.; Guven, S.; Durmus, N.G.; Rizvi, I.; Hasan, T.; Hasirci, N.; Hasirci, V.; Demirci, U. Hydrogels as a New Platform to Recapitulate the Tumor Microenvironment. In *Handbook of Nanomaterials for Cancer Theranostics*; Elsevier: Amsterdam, The Netherlands, 2018; pp. 463–494. [CrossRef]
48. Iwamura, T.; Ashizawa, K.; Adachi, K.; Takasaki, M. Anionic hydrogen-transfer polymerization of N-isopropylacrylamide under microwave irradiation. *J. Polym. Sci. Part A Polym. Chem.* **2019**, *57*, 2415–2419. [CrossRef]
49. Ebner, C.; Bodner, T.; Stelzer, F.; Wiesbrock, F. One Decade of Microwave-Assisted Polymerizations: Quo vadis? *Macromol. Rapid Commun.* **2011**, *32*, 254–288. [CrossRef]
50. Radwan-Pragłowska, J.; Piątkowski, M.; Janus, Ł.; Bogdał, D.; Matysek, D.; Čablik, V. Microwave-assisted synthesis and characterization of antibacterial O-crosslinked chitosan hydrogels doped with TiO_2 nanoparticles for skin regeneration. *Int. J. Polym. Mater. Polym. Biomater.* **2019**, *68*, 881–890. [CrossRef]
51. Cook, J.P.; Goodall, G.W.; Khutoryanskaya, O.V.; Khutoryanskiy, V.V. Microwave-Assisted Hydrogel Synthesis: A New Method for Crosslinking Polymers in Aqueous Solutions. *Macromol. Rapid Commun.* **2012**, *33*, 332–336. [CrossRef] [PubMed]
52. Hiep, N.T.; Khon, H.C.; Niem VV, T.; Toi, V.V.; Quyen, T.N.; Hai, N.D.; Anh MN, T. Microwave-Assisted Synthesis of Chitosan/Polyvinyl Alcohol Silver Nanoparticles Gel for Wound Dressing Applications. *Int. J. Polym. Sci.* **2016**, *2016*, 1–11. [CrossRef]
53. Pandey, A.; Pandey, G.C.; Aswath, P.B. Synthesis of polylactic acid–polyglycolic acid blends using microwave radiation. *J. Mech. Behav. Biomed. Mater.* **2008**, *1*, 227–233. [CrossRef]
54. Rivero, I.E.; Balsamo, V.; Müller, A.J. Microwave-assisted modification of starch for compatibilizing LLDPE/starch blends. *Carbohydr. Polym.* **2009**, *75*, 343–350. [CrossRef]
55. Shao, X.; Sun, H.; Jiang, R.; Qin, T.; Ma, Z. Mechanical and moisture barrier properties of corn distarch phosphate film influenced by modified microcrystalline corn straw cellulose. *J. Sci. Food Agric.* **2018**, *98*, 5639–5646. [CrossRef]
56. Sonker, A.K.; Verma, V. Influence of crosslinking methods toward poly(vinyl alcohol) properties: Microwave irradiation and conventional heating. *J. Appl. Polym. Sci.* **2017**, *135*, 46125. [CrossRef]
57. Sun, H.; Shao, X.; Jiang, R.; Ma, Z.; Wang, H. Effects of ultrasonic/microwave-assisted treatment on the properties of corn distarch phosphate/corn straw cellulose films and structure characterization. *J. Food Sci. Technol.* **2018**, *55*, 1467–1477. [CrossRef]
58. Radwan-Pragłowska, J.; Piątkowski, M.; Kitala, D.; Janus, Ł.; Klama-baryła, A.; Łabuś, W.; Tomanek, E.; Glik, J.; Matysek, D.; Bogdał, D.; et al. Microwave-assisted synthesis and characterization of bioactive chitosan scaffolds doped with Au nanoparticles for mesenchymal stem cells culture. *Int. J. Polym. Mater. Polym. Biomater.* **2019**, *68*, 351–359. [CrossRef]
59. Norajit, K.; Kim, K.M.; Ryu, G.H. Comparative studies on the characterization and antioxidant properties of biodegradable alginate films containing ginseng extract. *J. Food Eng.* **2010**, *98*, 377–384. [CrossRef]
60. Yang, L.; Liang, G.; Zhang, Z.; He, S.; Wang, J. Sodium Alginate/Na+-rectorite Composite Films: Preparation, Characterization, and Properties. *J. Appl. Polym. Sci.* **2009**, *114*, 1235–1240. [CrossRef]
61. Bahadoran, M.; Shamloo, A.; Nokoorani, Y.D. Development of a polyvinyl alcohol/sodium alginate hydrogel-based scaffold incorporating bFGF-encapsulated microspheres for accelerated wound healing. *Sci. Rep.* **2020**, *10*, 1–18. [CrossRef] [PubMed]
62. Karami, M.Y.; Zekavat, O.R.; Amanat, A. Excisional wound healing activity of Carboxymethyle cellulose in diabetic rat. *J. Jahrom Univ. Med. Sci.* **2012**, *9*, 48–57.
63. Muppalla, S.R.; Kanatt, S.R.; Chawla, S.; Sharma, A. Carboxymethyl cellulose–polyvinyl alcohol films with clove oil for active packaging of ground chicken meat. *Food Packag. Shelf Life* **2014**, *2*, 51–58. [CrossRef]
64. Barbucci, R.; Magnani, A.; Consumi, M. Swelling Behavior of Carboxymethylcellulose Hydrogels in Relation to Cross-Linking, pH, and Charge Density. *Macromolecules* **2000**, *33*, 7475–7480. [CrossRef]
65. Ludwig, A. The use of mucoadhesive polymers in ocular drug delivery. *Adv. Drug Deliv. Rev.* **2005**, *57*, 1595–1639. [CrossRef] [PubMed]
66. Ng, S.-F.; Jumaat, N. Carboxymethyl cellulose wafers containing antimicrobials: A modern drug delivery system for wound infections. *Eur. J. Pharm. Sci.* **2013**, *51*, 173–179. [CrossRef]
67. Yadav, M.; Rhee, K.Y.; Park, S. Synthesis and characterization of graphene oxide/carboxymethylcellulose/alginate composite blend films. *Carbohydr. Polym.* **2014**, *110*, 18–25. [CrossRef] [PubMed]
68. Rowe, R.C.; Sheskey, P.J.; Quinn, M.E. *Handbook of Pharmaceutical Excipients*, 6th ed.; Pharmaceutical Press: London, UK, 2009.
69. Tongdeesoontorn, W.; Mauer, L.J.; Wongruong, S.; Sriburi, P.; Rachtanapun, P. Effect of carboxymethyl cellulose concentration on physical properties of biodegradable cassava starch-based films. *Chem. Cent. J.* **2011**, *5*, 6. [CrossRef] [PubMed]
70. Paunonen, S. Strength and Barrier Enhancements of Cellophane and Cellulose Derivative Films: A Review. *Bioresources* **2013**, *8*, 3098–3121. [CrossRef]
71. Garrett, Q.; Simmons, P.A.; Xu, S.; Vehige, J.; Zhao, Z.; Ehrmann, K.; Willcox, M. Carboxymethylcellulose Binds to Human Corneal Epithelial Cells and Is a Modulator of Corneal Epithelial Wound Healing. *Investig. Ophthalmol. Vis. Sci.* **2007**, *48*, 1559–1567. [CrossRef]

72. Ramli, N.A.; Wong, T.W. Sodium carboxymethylcellulose scaffolds and their physicochemical effects on partial thickness wound healing. *Int. J. Pharm.* **2011**, *403*, 73–82. [CrossRef] [PubMed]
73. Sweeney, I.R.; Miraftab, M.; Collyer, G. A critical review of modern and emerging absorbent dressings used to treat exuding wounds. *Int. Wound J.* **2012**, *9*, 601–612. [CrossRef]
74. Draget, K.I.; Moe, S.T.; Skjak-Bræk, G.; Smidsrød, O. *Food Polysaccharides and Their Applications*, 2nd ed.; Taylor & Francis Group: Boca Raton, FL, USA, 2006.
75. Wong, T.W.; Ramli, N.A. Carboxymethylcellulose film for bacterial wound infection control and healing. *Carbohydr. Polym.* **2014**, *112*, 367–375. [CrossRef]
76. Qing, Z.; Jiachao, X.; Xin, G.; Xiaoting, F. Optimized water vapor permeability of sodium alginate films using response surface methodology. *Chin. J. Oceanol. Limnol.* **2013**, *31*, 1196–1203.
77. Rhim, J.-W. Physical and mechanical properties of water resistant sodium alginate films. *LWT Food Sci. Technol.* **2004**, *37*, 323–330. [CrossRef]
78. Trevisol, T.C.; Fritz, A.R.M.; De Souza, S.M.A.G.U.; Bierhalz, A.; Valle, J.A.B. Alginate and carboxymethyl cellulose in monolayer and bilayer films as wound dressings: Effect of the polymer ratio. *J. Appl. Polym. Sci.* **2018**, *136*, 46941. [CrossRef]
79. Yue, Y.; Wang, X.; Han, J.; Yu, L.; Chen, J.; Wu, Q.; Jiang, J. Effects of nanocellulose on sodium alginate/polyacrylamide hydrogel: Mechanical properties and adsorption-desorption capacities. *Carbohydr. Polym.* **2018**, *206*, 289–301. [CrossRef] [PubMed]
80. Horst, B.; Moiemen, N.S.; Grover, L.M. 6—Natural polymers: Biomaterials for skin scaffolds. In *Biomaterials for Skin Repair and Regeneration*; Elsevier Ltd.: Amsterdam, The Netherlands, 2019; pp. 151–192.
81. Bora, A.; Mishra, P. Characterization of casein and casein-silver conjugated nanoparticle containing multifunctional (pectin—sodium alginate/casein) bilayer film. *J. Food Sci. Technol.* **2016**, *53*, 3704–3714. [CrossRef]
82. Wang, Z.; Hu, S.; Wang, H. Scale-Up Preparation and Characterization of Collagen/Sodium Alginate Blend Films. *J. Food Qual.* **2017**, *2017*, 1–10. [CrossRef]
83. Sirviö, J.A.; Kolehmainen, A.; Liimatainen, H.; Niinimäki, J.; Hormi, O.E. Biocomposite cellulose-alginate films: Promising packaging materials. *Food Chem.* **2014**, *151*, 343–351. [CrossRef]
84. Wu, Y.; Qi, H.; Shi, C.; Ma, R.; Liu, S.; Huang, Z. Preparation and adsorption behaviors of sodium alginate-based adsorbent-immobilized β-cyclodextrin and graphene oxide. *RSC Adv.* **2017**, *7*, 31549–31557. [CrossRef]
85. Fan, L.; Du, Y.; Zhang, B.; Yang, J.; Zhou, J.; Kennedy, J.F. Preparation and properties of alginate/carboxymethyl chitosan blend fibers. *Carbohydr. Polym.* **2006**, *65*, 447–452. [CrossRef]
86. Riyajan, S.-A.; Nuim, J. Interaction of Green Polymer Blend of Modified Sodium Alginate and Carboxylmethyl Cellulose Encapsulation of Turmeric Extract. *Int. J. Polym. Sci.* **2013**, *2013*, 1–10. [CrossRef]
87. Ghanbarzadeh, B.; Almasi, H. Physical properties of edible emulsified films based on carboxymethyl cellulose and oleic acid. *Int. J. Biol. Macromol.* **2011**, *48*, 44–49. [CrossRef] [PubMed]
88. Ali, M.; Khan, N.R.; Basit, H.M.; Mahmood, S. Physico-chemical based mechanistic insight into surfactant modulated sodium Carboxymethylcellulose film for skin tissue regeneration applications. *J. Polym. Res.* **2019**, *27*, 20. [CrossRef]
89. Yoon, D.S.; Lee, Y.; Ryu, H.A.; Jang, Y.; Lee, K.-M.; Choi, Y.; Choi, W.J.; Lee, M.; Park, K.M.; Park, K.D.; et al. Cell recruiting chemokine-loaded sprayable gelatin hydrogel dressings for diabetic wound healing. *Acta Biomater.* **2016**, *38*, 59–68. [CrossRef] [PubMed]
90. Sharma, M.; Sahu, K.; Singh, S.P.; Jain, B. Wound healing activity of curcumin conjugated to hyaluronic acid: In vitro and in vivo evaluation. *Artif. Cells Nanomed. Biotechnol.* **2018**, *46*, 1009–1017. [CrossRef] [PubMed]
91. Widgerow, A.D. Chronic wound fluid-thinking outside the box. *Wound Repair Regen.* **2011**, *19*, 287–291. [CrossRef]
92. Kim, H.S.; Sun, X.; Lee, J.-H.; Kim, H.-W.; Fu, X.; Leong, K.W. Advanced drug delivery systems and artificial skin grafts for skin wound healing. *Adv. Drug Deliv. Rev.* **2018**, *146*, 209–239. [CrossRef]
93. Wang, Z.; Zhou, J.; Wang, X.; Zhang, N.; Sun, X.; Ma, Z. The effects of ultrasonic/microwave assisted treatment on the water vapor barrier properties of soybean protein isolate-based oleic acid/stearic acid blend edible films. *Food Hydrocoll.* **2014**, *35*, 51–58. [CrossRef]
94. Wang, Z.; Zhao, Z.; Khan, N.; Hua, Z.; Huo, J.; Li, Y. Microwave assisted chitosan-polyethylene glycol hydrogel membrane synthesis of curcumin for open incision wound healing. *Pharmazie* **2020**, *75*, 118–123.
95. Gonçalves, V.; Gurikov, P.; Poejo, J.; Matias, A.; Heinrich, S.; Duarte, C.; Smirnova, I. Alginate-based hybrid aerogel microparticles for mucosal drug delivery. *Eur. J. Pharm. Biopharm.* **2016**, *107*, 160–170. [CrossRef]
96. Basit, H.M.; Ali, M.; Shah, M.M.; Shah, S.U.; Wahab, A.; Albarqi, H.A.; Alqahtani, A.A.; Walbi, I.A.; Khan, N.R. Microwave Enabled Physically Cross Linked Sodium Alginate and Pectin Film and Their Application in Combination with Modified Chitosan-Curcumin Nanoparticles. A Novel Strategy for 2nd Degree Burns Wound Healing in Animals. *Polymers* **2021**, *13*, 2716. [CrossRef]
97. Namuiriyachote, N.; Lipipun, V.; Althhatuattananglzul, Y.; Charoonrut, P.; Ritthidej, G.C. Development of polyurethane foam dressing containing silver and asiaticoside for healing of dermal wound. *Asian J. Pharm. Sci.* **2019**, *14*, 63–77. [CrossRef]
98. Hiro, M.E.; Pierpont, Y.N.; Ko, F.; Wright, T.E.; Robson, M.C.; Payne, W.G. Comparative Evaluation of Silver-Containing Antimicrobial Dressings on In Vitro and In Vivo Processes of Wound Healing. *Eplasty* **2012**, *12*, e48.
99. Ahmed, A.S.; Mandal, U.K.; Taher, M.; Susanti, D.; Jaffri, J.M. PVA-PEG physically cross-linked hydrogel film as a wound dressing: Experimental design and optimization. *Pharm. Dev. Technol.* **2017**, *23*, 751–760. [CrossRef] [PubMed]

100. Febriyenti, F.; Noor, A.M.; Bin Bai, S. Mechanical properties and water vapour permeability of film from Haruan (Channa striatus) and fusidic acid spray for wound dressing and wound healing. *Pak. J. Pharm. Sci.* **2010**, *23*, 155–159. [PubMed]
101. Gonçalves, M.M.; Carneiro, J.; Justus, B.; Espinoza, J.T.; Budel, J.M.; Farago, P.V.; de Paula, J.P. Preparation and characterization of a novel antimicrobial film dressing for wound healing application. *Braz. J. Pharm. Sci.* **2020**, *56*, 1–11. [CrossRef]
102. Farzanian, K.; Ghahremaninezhad, A. On the Effect of Chemical Composition on the Desorption of Superabsorbent Hydrogels in Contact with a Porous Cementitious Material. *Gels* **2018**, *4*, 70. [CrossRef]
103. Peles, Z.; Zilberman, M. Novel soy protein wound dressings with controlled antibiotic release: Mechanical and physical properties. *Acta Biomater.* **2012**, *8*, 209–217. [CrossRef]
104. Cabrera, J.C.; Boland, A.; Messiaen, J.; Cambier, P.; Van Cutsem, P. Egg box conformation of oligogalacturonides: The time-dependent stabilization of the elicitor-active conformation increases its biological activity. *Glycobiology* **2008**, *18*, 473–482. [CrossRef] [PubMed]
105. Wang, Z.; Sun, X.; Lian, Z.; Wang, X.; Zhou, J.; Ma, Z. The effects of ultrasonic/microwave assisted treatment on the properties of soy protein isolate/microcrystalline wheat-bran cellulose film. *J. Food Eng.* **2013**, *114*, 183–191. [CrossRef]
106. Wang, Z.; Zhang, N.; Wang, H.; Sui, S.; Sun, X.; Ma, Z. The effects of ultrasonic/microwave assisted treatment on the properties of soy protein isolate/titanium dioxide films. *LWT Food Sci. Technol.* **2014**, *57*, 548–555. [CrossRef]
107. Croisier, F.; Jérôme, C. Chitosan-based biomaterials for tissue engineering. *Eur. Polym. J.* **2013**, *49*, 780–792. [CrossRef]
108. Li, H.; Liu, E.-T.; Chan, F.Y.; Lu, Z.; Chen, R. Fabrication of ordered flower-like ZnO nanostructures by a microwave and ultrasonic combined technique and their enhanced photocatalytic activity. *Mater. Lett.* **2011**, *65*, 3440–3443. [CrossRef]
109. Gupta, B.; Agarwal, R.; Alam, M.S. Preparation and characterization of polyvinyl alcohol-polyethylene oxide-carboxymethyl cellulose blend membranes. *J. Appl. Polym. Sci.* **2012**, *127*, 1301–1308. [CrossRef]
110. Gomaa, S.F.; Madkour, T.M.; Moghannem, S.; El-Sherbiny, I.M. New polylactic acid/cellulose acetate-based antimicrobial interactive single dose nanofibrous wound dressing mats. *Int. J. Biol. Macromol.* **2017**, *105*, 1148–1160. [CrossRef] [PubMed]
111. Banerjee, K.; Madhyastha, H.; Sandur, V.R.; Manikandanath, N.T.; Thiagarajan, N.; Thiagarajan, P. Anti-inflammatory and wound healing potential of a clove oil emulsion. *Colloids Surf. B Biointerfaces* **2020**, *193*, 1–9. [CrossRef] [PubMed]
112. Del Gaudio, P.; Amante, C. In situ gelling alginate-pectin blend particles loaded with Ac2-26: A new weapon to improve wound care armamentarium. *Carbohydr. Polym.* **2020**, *227*, 115305. [CrossRef]
113. Evans, N.D.; Oreffo RO, C.; Healy, E.; Thurner, P.J.; Man, Y.H. Epithelial mechanobiology, skin wound healing, and the stem cell niche. *J. Mech. Behav. Biomed. Mater.* **2013**, *28*, 397–409. [CrossRef]
114. Panchatcharam, M.; Miriyala, S.; Gayathri, V.S.; Suguna, L. Curcumin improves wound healing by modulating collagen and decreasing reactive oxygen species. *Mol. Cell. Biochem.* **2006**, *290*, 87–96. [CrossRef]
115. Lucassen, G.W.; Van Veen, G.N.A.; Jansen, J.A.J. Band Analysis of Hydrated Human Skin Stratum Corneum Attenuated Total Reflectance Fourier Transform Infrared Spectra In Vivo. *J. Biomed. Opt.* **1998**, *3*, 267–280. [CrossRef]
116. Rabotyagova, O.S.; Cebe, P.; Kaplan, D.L. Collagen structural hierarchy and susceptibility to degradation by ultraviolet radiation. *Mater. Sci. Eng. C* **2008**, *28*, 1420–1429. [CrossRef] [PubMed]
117. Cheheltani, R.; McGoverin, C.M.; Rao, J.; Vorp, D.A.; Kiani, M.F.; Pleshko, N. Fourier transform infrared spectroscopy to quantify collagen and elastin in an in vitro model of extracellular matrix degradation in aorta. *Analyst* **2014**, *139*, 3039–3047. [CrossRef] [PubMed]
118. Lai, H.Y.; Lim, Y.Y.; Kim, K.H. Potential dermal wound healing agent in Blechnum orientale Linn. *BMC Complement. Altern. Med.* **2011**, *11*, 62. [CrossRef] [PubMed]
119. Harishkumar, M.; Masatoshi, Y.; Hiroshi, S.; Tsuyomu, I.; Masugi, M. Revealing the Mechanism of In Vitro Wound Healing Properties of *Citrus tamurana* Extract. *BioMed Res. Int.* **2013**, *2013*, 1–8. [CrossRef] [PubMed]

Disclaimer/Publisher's Note: The statements, opinions and data contained in all publications are solely those of the individual author(s) and contributor(s) and not of MDPI and/or the editor(s). MDPI and/or the editor(s) disclaim responsibility for any injury to people or property resulting from any ideas, methods, instructions or products referred to in the content.

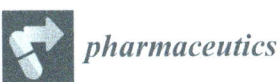

Article

The Combined Anti-Tumor Efficacy of Bioactive Hydroxyapatite Nanoparticles Loaded with Altretamine

Yahia Alghazwani [1], Krishnaraju Venkatesan [1], Kousalya Prabahar [2], Mohamed El-Sherbiny [3,4,*], Nehal Elsherbiny [5,6] and Mona Qushawy [7,8]

[1] Department of Pharmacology, College of Pharmacy, King Khalid University, Abha 62529, Saudi Arabia
[2] Department of Pharmacy Practice, Faculty of Pharmacy, University of Tabuk, Tabuk 71491, Saudi Arabia
[3] Department of Basic Medical Sciences, College of Medicine, AlMaarefa University, Riyadh 13713, Saudi Arabia
[4] Department of Anatomy and Embryology, Faculty of Medicine, Mansoura University, Mansoura 35516, Egypt
[5] Department of Pharmaceutical Chemistry, Faculty of Pharmacy, University of Tabuk, Tabuk 71491, Saudi Arabia
[6] Department of Biochemistry, Faculty of Pharmacy, Mansoura University, Mansoura 35516, Egypt
[7] Department of Pharmaceutics, Faculty of Pharmacy, University of Tabuk, Tabuk 71491, Saudi Arabia
[8] Department of Pharmaceutics, Faculty of Pharmacy, Sinai University, Alarish 45511, Egypt
* Correspondence: msharbini@mcst.edu.sa

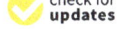

Citation: Alghazwani, Y.; Venkatesan, K.; Prabahar, K.; El-Sherbiny, M.; Elsherbiny, N.; Qushawy, M. The Combined Anti-Tumor Efficacy of Bioactive Hydroxyapatite Nanoparticles Loaded with Altretamine. *Pharmaceutics* 2023, 15, 302. https://doi.org/10.3390/pharmaceutics15010302

Academic Editor: Jingyuan Wen

Received: 17 November 2022
Revised: 29 December 2022
Accepted: 10 January 2023
Published: 16 January 2023

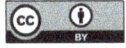

Copyright: © 2023 by the authors. Licensee MDPI, Basel, Switzerland. This article is an open access article distributed under the terms and conditions of the Creative Commons Attribution (CC BY) license (https://creativecommons.org/licenses/by/4.0/).

Abstract: In the current study, the combined anti-tumor efficacy of bioactive hydroxyapatite nanoparticles (HA-NPs) loaded with altretamine (ALT) was evaluated. The well-known fact that HA has great biological compatibility was confirmed through the findings of the hemolytic experiments and a maximum IC_{50} value seen in the MTT testing. The preparation of HA-NPs was performed using the chemical precipitation process. An in vitro release investigation was conducted, and the results demonstrated the sustained drug release of the altretamine-loaded hydroxyapatite nanoparticles (ALT-HA-NPs). Studies using the JURKAT E6.1 cell lines MTT assay, and cell uptake, as well as in vivo pharmacokinetic tests using Wistar rats demonstrated that the ALT-HA-NPs were easily absorbed by the cells. A putative synergism between the action of the Ca^{2+} ions and the anticancer drug obtained from the carrier was indicated by the fact that the ALT-HA-NPs displayed cytotoxicity comparable to the free ALT at 1/10th of the ALT concentration. It has been suggested that a rise in intracellular Ca^{2+} ions causes cells to undergo apoptosis. Ehrlich's ascites model in Balb/c mice showed comparable synergistic efficacy in a tumor regression trial. While the ALT-HA-NPs were able to shrink the tumor size by six times, the free ALT was only able to reduce the tumor volume by half.

Keywords: altretamine; cancer therapy; sustained delivery; hydroxyapatite nanoparticles; chemical precipitation method

1. Introduction

Apoptosis is a fundamental biological process that multicellular organisms use to replace aging, damaged, or unhealthy cells. Caspases (protein-digesting enzymes) are activated by an extrinsic or intrinsic mechanism, initiating a tightly controlled process that ultimately results in cell death. TNF-α, and Fas are examples of extracellular ligands that begin the extrinsic pathway, whereas stress-induced intracellular signals start the intrinsic pathway [1]. One of the mechanisms that stimulate intracellular apoptotic signaling is increased intracellular calcium ion (Ca^{2+}) concentrations. Cancerous cells are currently being treated with chemotherapy employing substances that interfere with the calcium ion homeostasis in cells. Kim et al. examined the effects of panaxydol, which was extracted from Panax Ginseng roots, on MCF-7 (human breast cancer) cells. They discovered that the substance might cause cell death and raise intracellular Ca^{2+} ion concentrations [2]. Nagoor Meeran et al. investigated the effects of carvacrol, a phenol-derived (monoterpenoid) from origanum vulgare, on human glioblastoma cells. Carvacrol had a raised intracellular Ca^{2+} ion concentration, promotes Ca^{2+} release from the ER store, is phospholipase C-dependent, and results in cell death [3]. Apoptosis has also been shown to be induced via a similar method by other substances of natural sources, such as Cryptotanshinone (a tanshinone isolated from the root of *Salvia miltiorrhiza*) and Diospyrin (a naphthoquinone isolated from the stem bark of Diospyrosmontana). Apoptosis is known to be induced similarly by synthetic substances including Auranofin, Vismodegib, and GaQ(3) (KP46), a new gallium complex. The testing of these substances is still in its early stages. The significant expenses involved with their production/isolation further restrict their medicinal value. Utilizing the NPs of calcium phosphates and hydroxyapatite (HA) is one of the practical options for increasing the Ca^{2+} content of the interior part of the cell [4]. HA is a substance that is abundant in nature and is biologically active, particularly in the calcified tissue of vertebrates. It has been utilized as a transporter when creating delivery systems for medicinal agents such as medicines, enzymes, antigens, DNA, and other proteins. Additionally, it has been discovered that hydroxyapatite nanoparticles have a proapoptotic and antiproliferative effects on malignant cells [5,6]. In their study of the anticancer inhibitory impact of HA, Zhang et al. found that the treatment with HA significantly inhibited cancer cells when compared to normal cells [7]. Similar research was conducted by Tang et al., who concluded that the increased intracellular calcium ion concentration may be the cause of the inhibitory effect of HA [8].

This investigation proposes the usage of altretamine (ALT)-loaded HA-NPs for synergistic anticancer action based on the above explanation. Once in the cell, the HA-NPs will progressively break down, releasing the medication over time while also raising the Ca^{2+} concentration there. The methyl melamine class of these compounds includes the synthetic alkylating agent known as altretamine (ALT). The alkylating chemicals work by altering and cross-linking DNA, which prevents the production of DNA, RNA, proteins, and results in the cell death of rapidly proliferating cells [9]. To evaluate the synergistic anticancer potential of this combination, acute T cell leukemia cells, JURKAT E6-1 cells, in vivo pharmacokinetic experiments in Wistar rats, and tumor regression studies in Balb/c mice utilizing the Ehrlich's ascites model were also employed.

Calcium levels are controlled at 400–600 mM in lysosomes and 200–400 nM in the cytosol. In cellular metabolism, even small variations in intracellular calcium concentration have a significant impact. The pH of lysosomes and endosomes will rise as the amounts of calcium and phosphate ions increase [10]. The compartment will become Ca^{2+} supersaturated, which will prevent HA-NPs from dissolving further. This may be the reason why altretamine-loaded hydroxyapatite nanoparticles (ALT-HA-NPs) are additionally effective after 72 h of treatment, owing to the comparatively slow dissolution of HA-NPs, which results in an improved penetration and retention effect. High endosomal or lysosomal calcium ions allow HA-NPs to bypass the phagocytic route and move directly into the cell nucleus where they can infect it. An increase in calcium ions up-regulates the movement of particles through nuclear pores and their escape from phagocytic pathways. The rate of programmed cell death is accelerated by the intracellular Ca^{2+} concentration [11]. DNA had expurgated by calcium-dependent endonucleases when Ca^{2+} is present. Intracellular calcium ions promote the permeabilization of the mitochondrial sheath and the release of proapoptotic mitochondrial protein, i.e., cytochrome C. The endoplasmic reticulum releases more calcium ions, which in turn releases more cytochrome C from the mitochondria. This is the result of the original release of cytochrome C. The Apoptosome was formed by further combining Cytochrome C with Pro-Caspase-9, ATP, and Apoptotic Protease Activating Factor-1. The effector Caspase-3 is activated when the Pro-Caspase is broken down by the Apoptosome into its active form, Caspase-9. The apoptosis process was then carried out by the active effector caspases digesting a variety of intracellular proteins. Additionally, microtubules typically work more efficiently in ATP-dependent ways in situations of high intracellular calcium, which results in ATP depletion and is a well-known sign of apoptosis. Additionally, the cytoskeleton is disrupted in the vacuoles that hold HA-NPs in the cytoplasm. In other words, it is believed that the presence of calcium content activates the Calpain, as Ca^{2+}-dependent protein kinases disrupt the cytoskeleton. This results in the disruption of the cytoskeleton around HA-NPs. Additionally, the high surface energy of HA-NPs due to the abundant Ca^{2+} ions can stimulate certain molecules and create free radicals. Actin filament damage caused by ROS can compromise the integrity of the cytoskeleton and cause cytoskeleton disruption [12]. Ca^{2+} can also activate NO synthases, transglutaminase, calcineurin, endonucleases, or phospholipases. These substances have been demonstrated to play a role in the different types of apoptotic cell death. The role of calcium-binding proteins including ALG-2 or calcium/calmodulin-dependent kinases such as the death-associated protein kinase and other enzymes known to be vital in apoptosis are only a few examples of other pathways that have been reported [13].

2. Materials and Methods

2.1. Materials

Altretamine (ALT) was received from Spectra Lab. Hyderabad, India, as a gift sample. HiMedia Lab Pvt. Ltd., Mumbai, India provided the calcium nitrate tetrahydrate $(Ca(NO_3)_2 \cdot 4H_2O)$, ammonium dihydrogen phosphate $(NH_4H_2PO_4)$, ammonia solution, methanol, and isopropyl alcohol that was needed. HPLC-grade water, methanol, and acetonitrile were purchased from Sigma-Aldrich, Bangalore, India. Internally prepared Milli-Q water was used during the trials. There were also analytical-grade reagents employed.

2.2. Synthesis ALT-Loaded HA-NPs (ALT-HA-NPs)

HA-NPs were prepared by using the wet chemical precipitation approach [14]. Firstly, separate aqueous solutions of 0.025 M $(Ca(NO_3)_2$ and 0.025 M of $(NH_4)_3PO_4$ were made using Milli-Q water. After that, the previously prepared $Ca(NO_3)_2$ solution in 500 mL of the three-necked round-bottom flask with a rosary-type condenser in the center neck was placed in a silicon oil thermal bath and kept at 90 °C under magnetic stirring conditions [15]. An aqueous $(NH_4)_3PO_4$ solution and NH_4OH solution were added dropwise via the left neck of the flask, and the pH was determined using a potentiometer mounted on the right neck of the flask. To produce HA particles, the solution was allowed to stir for 3 h until the required pH level was obtained [16]. Equation (1) depicts the chemical precipitation reaction for the production of HA. ALT was physically adsorbed onto the prepared HA-NPs.

$$6(NH_4)_2HPO_4 + 10Ca(NO_3)_2 \cdot 4H_2O + 8NH_4OH \rightarrow 20NH_4NO_3 + Ca_{10}(PO_4)_6(OH)_2 + 46H_2O \qquad (1)$$

2.3. Determination of the Encapsulation Efficiency % and Loading Capacity % of ALT-HA-NPs

The encapsulation efficiency % (EE %) of ALT in the prepared HA-NPs was determined by an indirect method where 2 mL of the prepared nanoparticle dispersion was centrifuged at 15,000 pm for 45 min. The supernatant was separated and analyzed spectrophotometrically at 226 nm after appropriate dilution to determine the free ALT [17]. The encapsulation efficiency was calculated using Equation (2):

$$(EE\%) = \frac{\text{Total amount of ALT} - \text{free ALT}}{\text{Total amount of ALT}} \times 100 \qquad (2)$$

Additionally, the drug loading capacity (DL%) was calculated [18] using Equation (3):

$$(DL\%) = \frac{\text{The amount of loaded ALT in nanoparticles (mg)}}{\text{weight of nanoparticles (mg)}} \times 100 \qquad (3)$$

2.4. Particle Size Analysis of ALT-HA-NPs

The particle size of the prepared ALT-HA-NPs was determined by dynamic light scattering technique using zetasizer (Malvern Instruments Ltd., Malvern, UK). The sample was diluted to the appropriate concentration, and the measurements were carried out at a temperature of 25 °C and an angle of 90° [19].

2.5. Determination of Surface Morphology of ALT-HA-NPs

2.5.1. Transmission Electron Microscopy (TEM)

The surface morphology was determined by TEM (JTEM model 1010, JEOL®, Tokyo, Japan). One drop of the prepared ALT-HA-NPs was added to the collodion-coated copper grid after being diluted with distilled water. The dried sample was stained with uranyl acetate solution and examined with TEM [20].

2.5.2. Scanning Electron Microscopy (SEM)

A small amount of the dry powder of the prepared ALT-HA-NPs was coated with approximately 15 nm gold (SPI-Module Sputter Coater). The coated sample was scanned by an analytical scanning electron microscope (JSEM-6360LA, JEOL®, Tokyo, Japan) under vacuum conditions at 15 kV acceleration voltage at room temperature [21].

2.6. In Vitro Release Studies

The drug release study was performed using the dialysis method. Where 2 mL (3 mg equivalent of ALT) of the prepared ALT-HA-NPs was transferred into a dialysis bag (cut-off 12kDa, Sigma). The dialysis bag was immersed in a beaker containing 100 mL of Phosphate Buffer Saline (PBS; pH 7.4) as a dissolution medium. The dissolution medium was stirred at 100 rpm and kept at 37 ± 1 °C. The samples were withdrawn at different time intervals up to 24 h and analyzed spectrophotometrically at 226 nm after appropriate dilution. The experiment was performed in comparison with the free ALT in triplicate and the mean ± SD was calculated [22,23].

2.7. Hemolytic Activity Determination

A previously reported procedure was used to evaluate the hemolytic activity of whole blood. Briefly, heparinized blood was obtained from dependable sources (Research Ethics Review Board (ERB) approval no. 2022/20137/MedAll/TRY; dated 11-02-2022). Before the experiment, human red blood cells were twice washed in PBS (pH 7.4). In 96-well microtiter plates, 100 µL of human RBC was plated with 0.4% (v/v) in PBS suspension and subsequently incubated for up to 24 h at 37 °C with an equal amount of ALT, ALT-HP-NPs, normal saline (0% hemolysis) aided as the negative control, and Milli-Q water (100% hemolysis) aided as the positive control. Equation (4) is the formula used to compute the % hemolysis in the experiment, which was done in triplicate [24]. In an ELISA reader, the lysed RBC absorbance was measured at 540 nm. PBS and 1% Triton-X 100 were used to determine 0% and 100% hemolysis.

$$\text{Hemolysis (\%)} = \frac{\text{Abs (sample)} - \text{Abs (negative control)}}{\text{Abs (positive control)} - \text{Abs (negative control)}} \times 100 \qquad (4)$$

2.8. In Vitro Cell Line Studies

Cytotoxicity Assessment

A previously described procedure was slightly modified to investigate the ALT, HA-NP, and ALT-HA-NP cytotoxicity. The MTT test on JURKAT cells was used to measure the percentage of cytotoxicity (E6-1; acute T cell leukemia cells). Briefly, the cells were seeded in a 96-well microtiter plate at a mass of 5×10^3 cells·well^{-1}, supplemented with fetal calf serum (2.5%), and then incubated at 37 °C for 24 h with a N_2 atmosphere of 90% with 5% of CO_2, and 5% O_2 for 24, 48, and 72 h, respectively. The cells were treated with two concentrations of the samples, i.e., 150 µg·mL^{-1}, and 300 µg·mL^{-1}. For this addition of 20 µL of MTT solution (5 mg·mL^{-1} in PBS at pH 7.4) to each well subsequently, the required amount of time had passed. Then, DMSO (100 µL) was used to dissolve the formazan crystals [25]. At 540 nm, the optical density (OD) was determined from an ELISA microplate reader after mixing with a mechanical plate mixer (Synergy HT, BioTek, Winooski, VT, USA). Three copies of each measurement were made. After 24 h, IC$_{50}$ values were collected for each sample, and the following equation (Equation (5)) was used to calculate the percentage of cytotoxicity:

$$\text{Toxicity (\%)} = \frac{\text{Abs (control)} - \text{Abs (sample)}}{\text{Abs (control)}} \times 100 \quad (5)$$

2.9. In Vivo Studies

2.9.1. Animals

The pharmacokinetic experiments were performed on male Wistar rats. The Institutional Animal Ethics Committee (IAEC), Anna University, Chennai, India approved the study protocol (Approval No. 1338). The animals were purchased from DORENCAMP, Bharathidasan University Animal House Capacity (IAEC/2021-2022; dated 28 August 2021). Utilizing Ehrlich's ascites model on Balb/c mice, tumor regression activity was assessed. The animals were kept in an animal house that was registered with CPCSEA (2276/RO/24/p/CPCSEA). IAEC authorized the protocol, which has the protocol number IN/TN/IAEC/2018/07. Animals were kept in normal laboratory cages made of polypropylene, two to a cage with unrestricted access to a normal laboratory diet and water (ambient temperatures of $25 \pm 2\,°C$ and $55 \pm 5\%$ relative humidity).

2.9.2. Pharmacokinetic Evaluation

Each of the two groups of animals contained six total individuals. One group received the ALT-HA-NPs (dispersed in PBS) for the studies, whereas the second group received the pure ALT (dispersed in PBS). Half a milliliter of the dispersions was administrated through the tail vein by intravenous administration. Each animal was given 0.2 mL diethyl ether anesthetic before the blood samples were taken after the retro-orbital plexus and immediately preserved within EDTA vacationers. The blood was withdrawn at the subsequent intervals: 0, 5, 15, 30, and 45 min, and 1, 2, 4, 6, 12, and 24 h. The blood-containing samples were then centrifuged at $4\,°C$ for 10 min using a 5000-rpm machine (Eppendorf). Before further estimation, in Eppendorf tubes, the supernatant was collected and kept at $-20\,°C$. The analysis method used by HPLC was modified from that used by Mohamed et al. [26]. The C_{max}, T_{max}, $AUC_{(0-t)}$, $t_{1/2}$, and the elimination rate constant was computed using the Microsoft Excel Addins-PK Solver and Pk1Pk2. To calculate relative bioavailability (Bio_{rel}), Equation (6) was used:

$$Bio_{rel} = \frac{AUC_{(test)} \times D_{(test)}}{AUC_{(Std)} \times D_{(Std)}} \quad (6)$$

where, AUC—Area under the Curve; D—dose.

2.9.3. Tumor Regression Evaluation

The Ehrlich's ascites (EAC) model in Balb/c mice was used to test the in vivo anti-cancer activity. Subcutaneously, the EAC cells (100 µL) were injected into the Balb/shaved dorsal surface. Seven days after the inoculum, measurable tumors formed ($0.08\,cm^3$). The mice were separated into four groups (n = 6) after the initial tumor development. PBS was injected into the first group as a control, ALT-HA-NPs was injected into the second group once every two days (1.5 mg/200 µL), free ALT was injected into the third group once in two days/mice (129 µg/200 µL), and HA-NPs were injected into the fourth group once every two days (1.5 mg/200 µL). Each group received intravenous care through a tail vein. Every other day, vernier calipers were used to measure the tumor length and width, and Equation (7) was used to compute the tumor volume [27].

$$\text{Tumor volume (TV)} = 0.5 \times \text{Length} \times \text{Width}^2 \quad (7)$$

The anti-tumor activity was then assessed in each case after measuring the tumor volume up to the 21st day.

2.10. Statistical Analysis

The mean and standard deviation of the data are the results of statistical analysis (mean ± SD). GraphPad (2018) Prism and Microsoft Excel (2019) were used to create bar graphs. ANOVA test was used to assess the significant differences among various experimental groups.

3. Results and Discussion

The most popular method for the preparation of HA-NPs was wet chemical precipitation from a solution, which has several benefits including a straightforward processing route, a high yield, being appropriate for industrial manufacturing, using cheap reagents, and the ability to create products with variable phase composition.

The prepared ALT-HA-NPs exhibited high EE% (96.27 ± 6.78%) and had drug loading of 8.2%. The particle size of the prepared ALT-HA-NPs was small in the nano range (156 ± 10.86 nm). The surface morphology of the prepared ALT-HA-NPs was examined by TEM and SEM. The prepared nanoparticle appeared spherical, as shown in Figure 1. Similar results were obtained by Ansari et al., who developed hydroxyapatite nanoparticles containing epirubicin for the treatment of cancer and examined the prepared nanoparticles with TEM [20]. Additionally, Soleimani et al. prepared Hydroxyapatite Nanoparticles for a human breast adenocarcinoma cell line and fibroblast examined the morphology with SEM and found that the prepared hydroxyapatite nanoparticles appeared spherical [28].

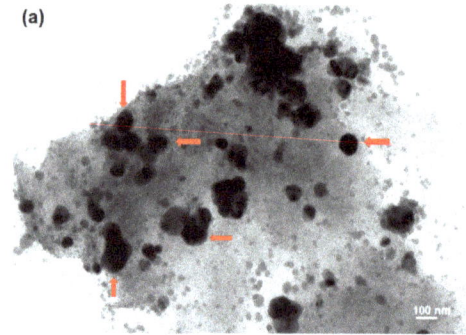
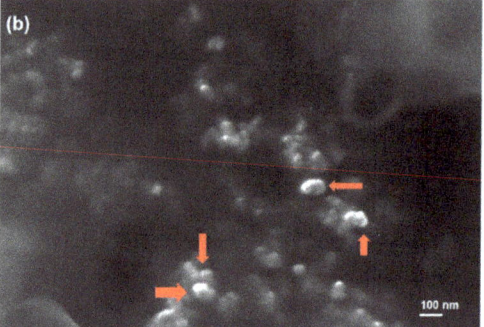

Figure 1. (**a**) TEM image of the ALT-HA-NPs and (**b**) SEM image of ALT-HA-NPs image, red arrows indicate NPs.

3.1. In Vitro Release Outcomes

The ALT in vitro release profile revealed a 24 h cumulative percentage of drug release up to 92.14 ± 4.45%. The ALT-HA-NPs, on the other hand, displayed a biphasic drug release profile, through an initial burst release up to 22.6 ± 1.2% in the initial 3 h, tailed by a continuous release (Figure 2). This first burst release of the ALT may be attributed to the drug molecules adhering to the nanoparticle surface [29]. The initial quick release may also be attributed to the nanoparticles' great surface-to-volume ratio [30]. The drug is confined inside the orifices of the porous nanoparticles, which results in the second phase of slower sustained release. In 24 h, as much as 71.2 ± 2.1% of the drug was released. An extended length of time will be favored by the therapeutic impact of gratitude to such a slow and steady drug release, which has been documented by Kumar et al. (2015) [31]. Similar results were obtained by Cai et al. who developed zoledronic acid-functionalized hydroxyapatite-loaded polymeric nanoparticles for the treatment of osteoporosis and observed that the drug release displayed a biphasic drug release profile [29].

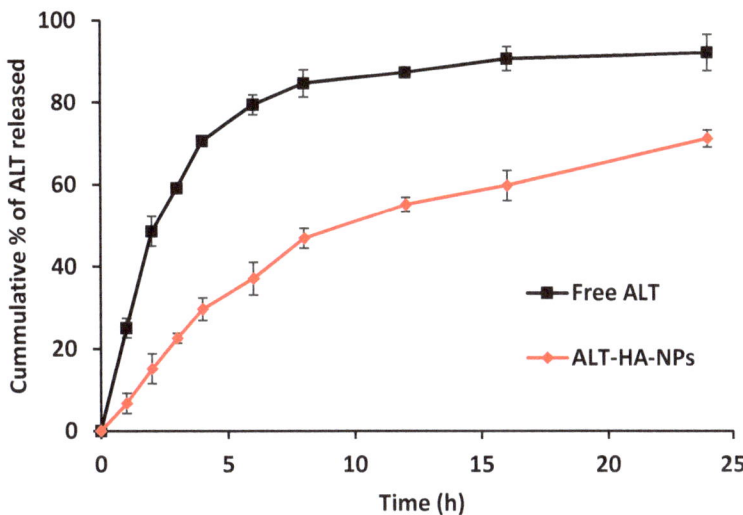

Figure 2. Cumulative percentage of ALT released from pure ALT and the ALT-HA-NPs (n = 3, mean ± SD).

3.2. Hemolysis Outcomes

To evaluate the NP biocompatibility and demonstrate their safety as a brand-new ALT carrier that satisfies preclinical requirements, a toxicity investigation was carried out. Wide-ranging hemolysis was seen in the case of Milli-Q water; however, isotonic saline was found to be minor. The ALT-HA-NPs had a hemolytic activity of 1.06 ± 0.05% and the unloaded HA-NPs had a hemolytic activity of 0.98 ± 0.04%, respectively (Figure 3). As a result, the NPs show no detectable hemolytic incompatibility ($p < 0.05$).

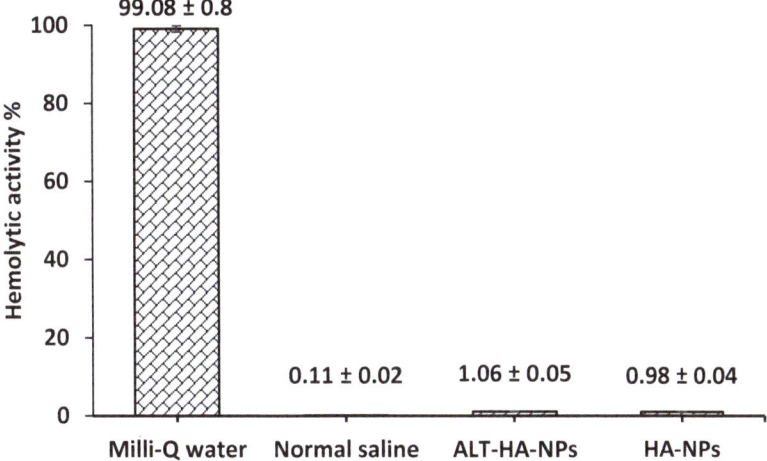

Figure 3. Hematolytic activity % for Milli-Q water, normal saline, ALT-HA-NPs, and HA-NPs (mean ± SD, n = 3, $p < 0.05$).

3.3. Cell Line Studies

MTT Assay

At three different time intervals, 24, 48, and 72 h, the cytotoxicity was assessed in a dose- and time-dependent method using dual doses, i.e., 300 and 150 µg·mL^{-1}. At a concentration of 300 (µg·mL^{-1}), the cytotoxicity percent of the free ALT, ALT-HA-NPs and HA-NPs were reported to be 96.7 ± 0.22%, 40.8 ± 1.99%, and 27.9 ± 4.01%, whereas at a concentration of 150 µg·mL^{-1}, the percentages were 94.1 ± 0.61%, 47.6 ± 2.03%, and 22.5 ± 2.08% after 24 h of treatment (Figure 4). At a high concentration of 300 µg·mL^{-1}, free ALT, ALT-HA-NPs, and HA-NPs, respectively, demonstrated 97.1 ± 0.33%, 80.4 ± 2.08%, and 43.6 ± 4.11% cytotoxicity after 48 h of treatment, although at a low concentration of 150 µg·mL^{-1}, 89.2 ± 0.41%, 77.8 ± 0.47%, and 29.9 ± 4.88% cytotoxicity was found. After 72 h of treatment, the percent cytotoxicity for the free ALT, ALT-HA-NPs, and HA-NPs, respectively, was observed to be 88.5 ± 2.11%, 96.2 ± 0.96%, and 58.36 ± 2.22%, respectively, whereas at 150 µg·mL^{-1}, the stated cytotoxicity percent values were 91.3 ± 0.53%, 89.66 ± 0.67%, and 50.2 ± 5.89%. The drug loading in HA-NPs is 8.2%. As a result, the ALT-HA-NPs can produce maximum drug concentrations of 20.7 µg·mL^{-1} and 10.4 µg·mL^{-1}, respectively, at concentrations of 300 and 150 µg·mL^{-1}. We found that the ALT-HA-NPs can produce a similar outcome as the free ALT at a concentration of 1/10th when compared to the concentrations of the free ALT tested (300 and 150 µg·mL^{-1}). The drug 24 h IC$_{50}$ was determined to be 32.44 µg·mL^{-1} for free ALT, 15.54 µg·mL^{-1} for ALT-HA-NPs, and 497.11 µg·mL^{-1} blank HA-NPs. However, ALT-HA-NPs showed that the cytotoxicity was markedly enhanced ($p < 0.01$) as compared to the free ALT (control).

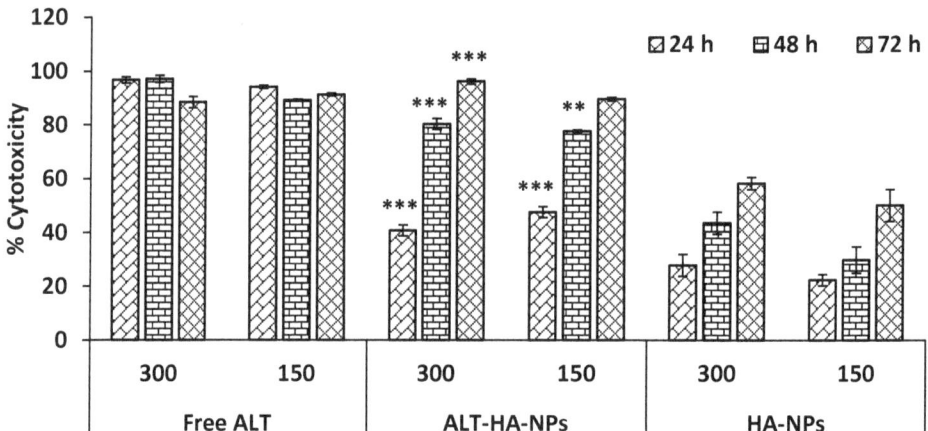

Figure 4. The outcome of ALT-HA-NPs, free ALT, and HA-NPs on the JURKAT cell line (n = 3, mean ± SD) is time- and dose-dependent. *** $p < 0.001$ and ** $p < 0.01$ denotes a significant difference between free ALT and ALT-HA-NPs.

The results of the hemolytic study, the cytotoxicity experiment (MTT assay), and a further identically high IC$_{50}$ value confirm the spherical-shaped HA-NPs exceptional biocompatibility and non-antigenicity, which were previously described in the literature [32,33]. When HA-NPs dissolve and release calcium ions into the cytoplasm after entering the cancer cell, it is believed that this disturbs intracellular calcium homeostasis. Calcium homeostasis is crucial because calcium plays a vital function as a secondary messenger, regulating crucial cellular processes including apoptosis and cell proliferation [34].

3.4. In Vivo Animal Model

3.4.1. Pharmacokinetic Parameters

Pharmacokinetic investigations were carried out, and many parameters were evaluated using a non-compartmental study to support our findings. Figure 5 shows the drug levels detected in blood for the mixture of lyophilized drug concentrate and ALT-HA-NPs. Calculations were made based on the data to determine T_{max}, C_{max}, $AUC_{(0-t)}$, drug half-life, elimination rate constant, and relative (Bio_{rel}) bioavailability.

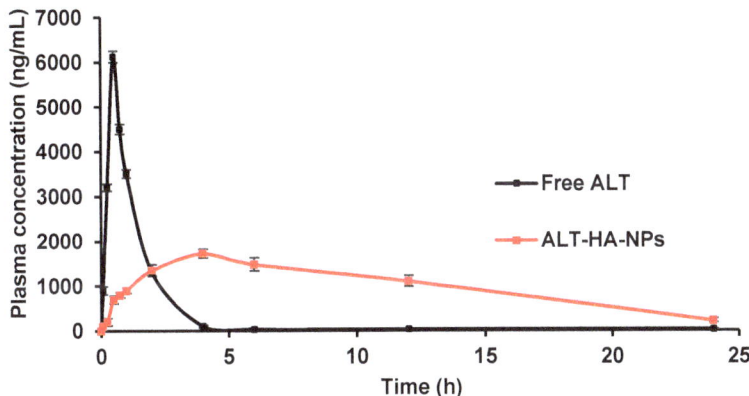

Figure 5. Plasma concentration–time curve after the intravenous injection of free ALT and ALT-HA-NPs in male Wistar rats ($p < 0.001$, mean ± SD, n = 3).

For the free ALT and the ALT-HA-NPs, the C_{max} was discovered to be 6124.4 ± 128.34 ng/mL and 1724.73 ± 98.46 ng/mL, respectively ($p < 0.001$). The T_{max} was determined to be 0.5 ± 0.24 h for the free ALT and 4 ± 0.31 h for the ALT-HA-NPs. The ALTs' AUC in solution was determined to be 8243.11 ± 6457.51 ng·h/mL, but when it was loaded into HA-NPs, it was much higher at 19,998.71 ± 8653.421 ng·h/mL ($p < 0.001$), increasing the ALTs' bioavailability by about 2.5 times. Drug-loaded HA-NPs were shown to have a significantly lower elimination rate constant (0.08756 ± 0.00279) than the free ALT (0.924567 ± 0.023456), and their half-life was found to be higher at 3.2 ± 0.29 h compared to the free ALTs of 0.87 ± 0.22 h.

ALT was thought to be rapidly eliminated from the body and to have a short half-life, which was well supported by Weber et al. (2015) [35]. As a result, it is clear from comparing the kinetic profiles of the two situations that the ALT was released from nanoparticles in a sustained manner and stays in the body for long time. The HA-NPs maintenance of constant plasma drug levels supports the increased $T_{1/2}$ values. Comparing the $AUC_{(0-t)}$ values with the extended T_{max} values made it clear that the body was exposed to the drug for a longer amount of time in the case of the drug-loaded HA-NPs. Enhancing bioavailability has advantages. Therefore, the HA nanoparticles of ALT are the best choice for safer therapy with increased drug bioavailability. To make it clinically feasible, further safety and efficacy studies are needed.

3.4.2. Tumor Regression Studies

Experiments on the 21-day tumor regression in Balb/c mice used as Ehrlich's ascites model were effective. As expected, the tumor volume was shown to significantly grow in the control group; after 21 days, an average tumor volume of 3221.45 mm^3 was documented. However, the tumor volume was significantly reduced in the other three groups (Figure 6). The ALT-HA-NPs produced the greatest reduction in tumor volume, with an average end volume of 506.25 mm^3 ($p < 0.001$). However, the average final tumor volume in the free ALT was reported to be 1151.05 mm^3 ($p < 0.01$). Furthermore, it was discovered that the blank HA-NPs significantly the reduced tumor size (1782.03 mm^3). Overall, the tumor decreased to 1/6th of its volume after being treated with ALT-HA-NPs, compared to 1/2 of its volume when treated with the free ALT and blank HA-NPs (Figure 6). The cellular uptake study thoroughly demonstrated that the nanoparticles can be readily internalized by the cells, and these findings further support the possibility of a synergistic interaction between the anticancer ALT activity, and the calcium ions released from the carrier, which would result in greater tumor volume reduction than with the anticancer drug alone or with blank HA-NPs [36]. Additionally, it was hypothesized that the drug-loaded NPs enhanced the permeation and retention mechanism, which causes them to collect and localize in the tumor area, where they reduce the tumor volume.

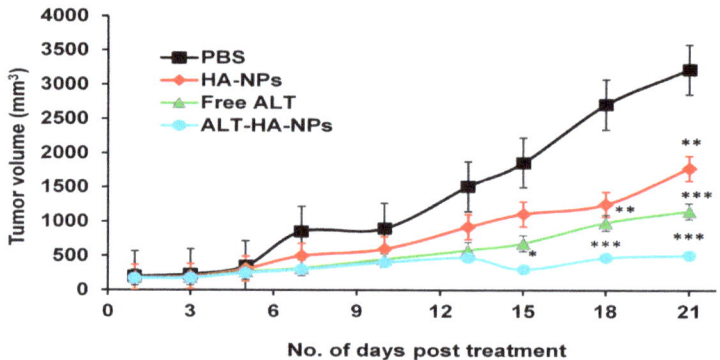

Figure 6. Anti-tumor activity of free ALT, ALT-HA-NPs, and blank HA-NPs (mean ± SD, n = 3). * significant compared to Control (PBS) group at $p < 0.05$, ** at p less than 0.01, *** at p less than 0.001.

4. Conclusions

According to our investigations, the ALT-HA-NPs exhibit superior combined anti-cancer effects compared to the free drug and blank HA-NPs. Due to its polar surface, HA with nanoscale dimensions is ideally adapted to interact with biomolecules in tissues and cells as well as with drugs. The cells may quickly ingest HA-NPs, and as they degrade, more Ca^{2+} eventually finds its way inside the cells. Altretamine anti-tumor action is then enhanced by calcium ion-induced proapoptotic pathways. It is necessary to conduct more research in this area to learn more about this synergism and its possible applications. Our investigation clearly shows that the formulation prepared can be used to treat CLL very successfully, minimizing the side effects such as diarrhea, weakness, nausea, and vomiting. For the research to advance, it is more important than ever to have a thorough understanding of the biomolecular effects of HA-NP-based systems on various cancer types. The experimental work undertaken for this purpose is quite complex, requiring the cooperation of biomolecular chemists, biomaterials scientists, oncologists, and biologists, in addition to the evaluation of full in vitro/in vivo toxicity profiles.

Author Contributions: Conceptualization, Y.A. and K.V.; Data curation, Y.A. and K.V.; Formal analysis, Y.A., K.V. and M.Q.; Funding acquisition, Y.A. and K.V.; Investigation, Y.A., K.V., K.P., M.E.-S., N.E. and M.Q.; Methodology, Y.A. and K.V.; Resources, Y.A., K.V., K.P., M.E.-S., N.E. and M.Q.; Software, Y.A., K.V., K.P., M.E.-S., N.E. and M.Q.; Validation, Y.A., K.V., K.P., M.E.-S., N.E. and M.Q.; Visualization, Y.A., K.V., K.P., M.E.-S., N.E. and M.Q.; Writing—original draft, Y.A. and K.V.; Writing—review and editing, Y.A., K.V., K.P., M.E.-S., N.E. and M.Q. All authors have read and agreed to the published version of the manuscript.

Funding: This research was funded by Deanship of Scientific Research at King Khalid University, grant number "RGP2/89/43".

Institutional Review Board Statement: The Institutional Animal Ethics Committee (IAEC), Anna University, Chennai, India approved the study protocol (Approval No. 1338).

Informed Consent Statement: Research Ethics Review Board (ERB) approval no. 2022/20137/MedAll/TRY; dated 11-02-2022.

Data Availability Statement: Data are available on request.

Acknowledgments: The authors are thankful to R. Vijaya, from Anna University (Chennai, India), for her full support to executing this study. The authors extend their sincere appreciation to the support by AlMaarefa Researchers Supporting program (MA-006), AlMaarefa University, Riyadh, Saudi Arabia.

Conflicts of Interest: The authors declare no conflict of interest.

References

1. Hassan, M.; Watari, H.; AbuAlmaaty, A.; Ohba, Y.; Sakuragi, N. Apoptosis and Molecular Targeting Therapy in Cancer. *BioMed Res. Int.* **2014**, *2014*, 150845. [CrossRef] [PubMed]
2. Kim, H.S.; Lim, J.M.; Kim, J.Y.; Kim, Y.; Park, S.; Sohn, J. Panaxydol, a Component of P Anax Ginseng, Induces Apoptosis in Cancer Cells through EGFR Activation and ER Stress and Inhibits Tumor Growth in Mouse Models. *Int. J. Cancer* **2016**, *138*, 1432–1441. [CrossRef]
3. Nagoor Meeran, M.F.; Javed, H.; Al Taee, H.; Azimullah, S.; Ojha, S.K. Pharmacological Properties and Molecular Mechanisms of Thymol: Prospects for Its Therapeutic Potential and Pharmaceutical Development. *Front. Pharmacol.* **2017**, *8*, 380. [CrossRef] [PubMed]
4. Levingstone, T.J.; Herbaj, S.; Dunne, N.J. Calcium Phosphate Nanoparticles for Therapeutic Applications in Bone Regeneration. *Nanomaterials* **2019**, *9*, 1570. [CrossRef]
5. Kargozar, S.; Mollazadeh, S.; Kermani, F.; Webster, T.J.; Nazarnezhad, S.; Hamzehlou, S.; Baino, F. Hydroxyapatite Nanoparticles for Improved Cancer Theranostics. *J. Funct. Biomater.* **2022**, *13*, 100. [CrossRef] [PubMed]
6. Ghate, P.; Prabhu, D.; Murugesan, G.; Goveas, L.C.; Varadavenkatesan, T.; Vinayagam, R.; Chi, N.T.L.; Pugazhendhi, A.; Selvaraj, R. Synthesis of Hydroxyapatite Nanoparticles Using Acacia Falcata Leaf Extract and Study of Their Anti-Cancerous Activity against Cancerous Mammalian Cell Lines. *Environ. Res.* **2022**, *214*, 113917. [CrossRef] [PubMed]
7. Zhang, K.; Zhou, Y.; Xiao, C.; Zhao, W.; Wu, H.; Tang, J.; Li, Z.; Yu, S.; Li, X.; Min, L. Application of Hydroxyapatite Nanoparticles in Tumor-Associated Bone Segmental Defect. *Sci. Adv.* **2019**, *5*, eaax6946. [CrossRef]
8. Tang, W.; Yuan, Y.; Liu, C.; Wu, Y.; Lu, X.; Qian, J. Differential Cytotoxicity and Particle Action of Hydroxyapatite Nanoparticles in Human Cancer Cells. *Nanomedicine* **2014**, *9*, 397–412. [CrossRef]
9. Singh, R.K.; Kumar, S.; Prasad, D.N.; Bhardwaj, T.R. Therapeutic Journery of Nitrogen Mustard as Alkylating Anticancer Agents: Historic to Future Perspectives. *Eur. J. Med. Chem.* **2018**, *151*, 401–433. [CrossRef]
10. Dabral, D.; Van den Bogaart, G. The Roles of Phospholipase A2 in Phagocytes. *Front. Cell Dev. Biol.* **2021**, *9*, 673502. [CrossRef]
11. Mohammadinejad, R.; Moosavi, M.A.; Tavakol, S.; Vardar, D.Ö.; Hosseini, A.; Rahmati, M.; Dini, L.; Hussain, S.; Mandegary, A.; Klionsky, D.J. Necrotic, Apoptotic and Autophagic Cell Fates Triggered by Nanoparticles. *Autophagy* **2019**, *15*, 4–33. [CrossRef]
12. Dmitry, B.; Juhaszova, M.; Sollot, S. Mitochondrial ROS-Induced ROS Release: An Update and Review. *Physiol. Rev.* **2014**, *94*, 909–950.
13. Swulius, M.T.; Waxham, M.N. Ca2+/Calmodulin-Dependent Protein Kinases. *Cell. Mol. Life Sci.* **2008**, *65*, 2637–2657. [CrossRef] [PubMed]
14. Ribeiro, T.P.; Monteiro, F.J.; Laranjeira, M.S. Duality of Iron (III) Doped Nano Hydroxyapatite in Triple Negative Breast Cancer Monitoring and as a Drug-Free Therapeutic Agent. *Ceram. Int.* **2020**, *46*, 16590–16597. [CrossRef]
15. Yelten-Yilmaz, A.; Yilmaz, S. Wet Chemical Precipitation Synthesis of Hydroxyapatite (HA) Powders. *Ceram. Int.* **2018**, *44*, 9703–9710. [CrossRef]
16. El-Bassyouni, G.T.; Eldera, S.S.; Kenawy, S.H.; Hamzawy, E.M. Hydroxyapatite Nanoparticles Derived from Mussel Shells for in Vitro Cytotoxicity Test and Cell Viability. *Heliyon* **2020**, *6*, e04085. [CrossRef] [PubMed]
17. Pandey, S.; Rai, N.; Mahtab, A.; Mittal, D.; Ahmad, F.J.; Sandal, N.; Neupane, Y.R.; Verma, A.K.; Talegaonkar, S. Hyaluronate-Functionalized Hydroxyapatite Nanoparticles Laden with Methotrexate and Teriflunomide for the Treatment of Rheumatoid Arthritis. *Int. J. Biol. Macromol.* **2021**, *171*, 502–513. [CrossRef] [PubMed]
18. AbouAitah, K.; Stefanek, A.; Higazy, I.M.; Janczewska, M.; Swiderska-Sroda, A.; Chodara, A.; Wojnarowicz, J.; Szałaj, U.; Shahein, S.A.; Aboul-Enein, A.M. Effective Targeting of Colon Cancer Cells with Piperine Natural Anticancer Prodrug Using Functionalized Clusters of Hydroxyapatite Nanoparticles. *Pharmaceutics* **2020**, *12*, 70. [CrossRef]
19. Sun, Y.; Devore, D.; Ma, X.; Yuan, Y.; Kohn, J.; Qian, J. Promotion of Dispersion and Anticancer Efficacy of Hydroxyapatite Nanoparticles by the Adsorption of Fetal Bovine Serum. *J. Nanoparticle Res.* **2019**, *21*, 1–12. [CrossRef]
20. Ansari, L.; Derakhshi, M.; Bagheri, E.; Shahtahmassebi, N.; Malaekeh-Nikouei, B. Folate Conjugation Improved Uptake and Targeting of Porous Hydroxyapatite Nanoparticles Containing Epirubicin to Cancer Cells. *Pharm. Dev. Technol.* **2020**, *25*, 601–609. [CrossRef] [PubMed]

21. Yedekci, Y.; Gedik, E.; Evis, Z.; Dogan, L.; Özyigit, G.; Gürkaynak, M. Radiosensitization Induced by Zinc-Doped Hydroxyapatite Nanoparticles in Breast Cancer Cells. *Int. J. Appl. Ceram. Technol.* **2021**, *18*, 563–572. [CrossRef]
22. Xu, Y.; Zhang, Z.; Wang, H.; Zhong, W.; Sun, C.; Sun, W.; Wu, H. Zoledronic Acid-Loaded Hybrid Hyaluronic Acid/Polyethylene Glycol/Nano-Hydroxyapatite Nanoparticle: Novel Fabrication and Safety Verification. *Front. Bioeng. Biotechnol.* **2021**, *9*, 629928. [CrossRef] [PubMed]
23. Dong, X.; Sun, Y.; Li, Y.; Ma, X.; Zhang, S.; Yuan, Y.; Kohn, J.; Liu, C.; Qian, J. Synergistic Combination of Bioactive Hydroxyapatite Nanoparticles and the Chemotherapeutic Doxorubicin to Overcome Tumor Multidrug Resistance. *Small* **2021**, *17*, 2007672. [CrossRef]
24. Yadav, K.; Yadav, D.; Kumar, S.; Narra, K.; El-Sherbiny, M.; Al-Serwi, R.H.; Othman, G.; Sendy, J.S.; Mohamed, J.M.M. Natural Biodegradable and Polymeric Nanoparticles for the Delivery of Noscapine for Cancer Treatment. *Biomass Convers. Biorefin.* **2022**, 1–13. [CrossRef]
25. Jamal Moideen, M.M.; Alqahtani, A.; Venkatesan, K.; Ahmad, F.; Krisharaju, K.; Gayasuddin, M.; Shaik, R.A.; Ibraheem, K.M.M.; Salama, M.E.M.; Abed, S.Y. Application of the Box–Behnken Design for the Production of Soluble Curcumin: Skimmed Milk Powder Inclusion Complex for Improving the Treatment of Colorectal Cancer. *Food Sci. Nutr.* **2020**, *8*, 6643–6659. [CrossRef] [PubMed]
26. Mohamed, J.M.; Alqahtani, A.; Ahmad, F.; Krishnaraju, V.; Kalpana, K. Pectin Co-Functionalized Dual Layered Solid Lipid Nanoparticle Made by Soluble Curcumin for the Targeted Potential Treatment of Colorectal Cancer. *Carbohydr. Polym.* **2021**, *252*, 117180. [CrossRef] [PubMed]
27. Mishra, S.; Tamta, A.K.; Sarikhani, M.; Desingu, P.A.; Kizkekra, S.M.; Pandit, A.S.; Kumar, S.; Khan, D.; Raghavan, S.C.; Sundaresan, N.R. Subcutaneous Ehrlich Ascites Carcinoma Mice Model for Studying Cancer-Induced Cardiomyopathy. *Sci. Rep.* **2018**, *8*, 5599. [CrossRef]
28. Soleimani, M.; Elmi, F.; Anijdan, S.H.M.; Elmi, M.M. Evaluating the Radiosensization Effect of Hydroxyapatite Nanoparticles on Human Breast Adenocarcinoma Cell Line and Fibroblast. *Iran. J. Med. Sci.* **2020**, *45*, 368.
29. Cai, Y.; Gao, T.; Fu, S.; Sun, P. Development of Zoledronic Acid Functionalized Hydroxyapatite Loaded Polymeric Nanoparticles for the Treatment of Osteoporosis. *Exp. Ther. Med.* **2018**, *16*, 704–710. [CrossRef]
30. Luo, H.; Zhang, Y.; Gan, D.; Yang, Z.; Ao, H.; Zhang, Q.; Yao, F.; Wan, Y. Incorporation of Hydroxyapatite into Nanofibrous PLGA Scaffold towards Improved Breast Cancer Cell Behavior. *Mater. Chem. Phys.* **2019**, *226*, 177–183. [CrossRef]
31. Kumar, P.; Ganure, A.L.; Subudhi, B.B.; Shukla, S. Design and Comparative Evaluation of In-Vitro Drug Release, Pharmacokinetics and Gamma Scintigraphic Analysis of Controlled Release Tablets Using Novel PH Sensitive Starch and Modified Starch-Acrylate Graft Copolymer Matrices. *Iran. J. Pharm. Res. IJPR* **2015**, *14*, 677. [PubMed]
32. Khan, S.; Ansari, A.A.; Rolfo, C.; Coelho, A.; Abdulla, M.; Al-Khayal, K.; Ahmad, R. Evaluation of in Vitro Cytotoxicity, Biocompatibility, and Changes in the Expression of Apoptosis Regulatory Proteins Induced by Cerium Oxide Nanocrystals. *Sci. Technol. Adv. Mater.* **2017**, *18*, 364–373. [CrossRef] [PubMed]
33. Yang, V.; Arumugam, S.R.; Pan, J.; Rajeshkumar, T.; Sun, Y.; Liu, X. Metal Oxide Nanoparticles as Biomedical Materials. *J. Colloid Interface Sci.* **2020**, *5*, 27.
34. Jones, C.A.; Hazlehurst, L.A. Role of Calcium Homeostasis in Modulating EMT in Cancer. *Biomedicines* **2021**, *9*, 1200. [CrossRef]
35. Weber, G.F. *Molecular Therapies of Cancer*; Springer: Berlin/Heidelberg, Germany, 2015.
36. Navarro-Ocón, A.; Blaya-Cánovas, J.L.; López-Tejada, A.; Blancas, I.; Sánchez-Martín, R.M.; Garrido, M.J.; Griñán-Lisón, C.; Calahorra, J.; Cara, F.E.; Ruiz-Cabello, F. Nanomedicine as a Promising Tool to Overcome Immune Escape in Breast Cancer. *Pharmaceutics* **2022**, *14*, 505. [CrossRef]

Disclaimer/Publisher's Note: The statements, opinions and data contained in all publications are solely those of the individual author(s) and contributor(s) and not of MDPI and/or the editor(s). MDPI and/or the editor(s) disclaim responsibility for any injury to people or property resulting from any ideas, methods, instructions or products referred to in the content.

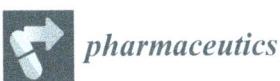

Article

Salbutamol Attenuates Diabetic Skeletal Muscle Atrophy by Reducing Oxidative Stress, Myostatin/GDF-8, and Pro-Inflammatory Cytokines in Rats

Anand Kumar [1], Priyanka Prajapati [1], Gurvinder Singh [2], Dinesh Kumar [2], Vikas Mishra [1], Seong-Cheol Kim [3], Chaitany Jayprakash Raorane [3,*], Vinit Raj [3,*] and Sapana Kushwaha [4,*]

[1] Department of Pharmaceutical Sciences, School of Pharmaceutical Sciences, Babasaheb Bhimrao Ambedkar University, Vidya Vihar, Raebareli Road, Lucknow 226025, India; anandkumarpharm@gmail.com (A.K.); priyankaprajapati243@gmail.com (P.P.); vikasmishra12@gmail.com (V.M.)

[2] Centre of Biomedical Research, SGPGIMS Campus, Lucknow 226014, India; gourav1752@gmail.com (G.S.); dineshcbmr@gmail.com (D.K.)

[3] School of Chemical Engineering, Yeungnam University, Gyeongsan 38541, Republic of Korea; sckim07@ynu.ac.kr

[4] National Institute of Pharmaceutical Education and Research (NIPER), Raebareli, New Transit Campus, Bijnor-Sisendi Road, Lucknow 226002, India

* Correspondence: chaitanyaraorane22@ynu.ac.kr (C.J.R.); drvinitraj@ynu.ac.kr (V.R.); sapana.kushwaha@niperrbl.ac.in (S.K.)

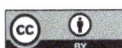

Abstract: Type 2 diabetes is a metabolic disorder that leads to accelerated skeletal muscle atrophy. In this study, we aimed to evaluate the effect of salbutamol (SLB) on skeletal muscle atrophy in high-fat diet (HFD)/streptozotocin (STZ)-induced diabetic rats. Male Sprague Dawley rats were divided into four groups (n = 6): control, SLB, HFD/STZ, and HFD/STZ + SLB (6 mg/kg orally for four weeks). After the last dose of SLB, rats were assessed for muscle grip strength and muscle coordination (wire-hanging, rotarod, footprint, and actophotometer tests). Body composition was analyzed in live rats. After that, animals were sacrificed, and serum and gastrocnemius (GN) muscles were collected. Endpoints include myofibrillar protein content, muscle oxidative stress and antioxidants, serum pro-inflammatory cytokines (interleukin-1β, interleukin-2, and interleukin-6), serum muscle markers (myostatin, creatine kinase, and testosterone), histopathology, and muscle ^{1}H NMR metabolomics. Findings showed that SLB treatment significantly improved muscle strength and muscle coordination, as well as increased lean muscle mass in diabetic rats. Increased pro-inflammatory cytokines and muscle markers (myostatin, creatine kinase) indicate muscle deterioration in diabetic rats, while SLB intervention restored the same. Also, Feret's diameter and cross-sectional area of GN muscle were increased by SLB treatment, indicating the amelioration in diabetic rat muscle. Results of muscle metabolomics exhibit that SLB treatment resulted in the restoration of perturbed metabolites, including histidine-to-tyrosine, phenylalanine-to-tyrosine, and glutamate-to-glutamine ratios and succinate, sarcosine, and 3-hydroxybutyrate (3HB) in diabetic rats. These metabolites showed a pertinent role in muscle inflammation and oxidative stress in diabetic rats. In conclusion, findings showed that salbutamol could be explored as an intervention in diabetic-associated skeletal muscle atrophy.

Keywords: diabetes; salbutamol; skeletal muscle atrophy; sarcosine; metabolomics

1. Introduction

Type 2 diabetes mellitus (T2DM) is a metabolic disorder that causes elevated blood glucose levels due to compromised insulin function and/or release [1]. Diabetes poses a significant global health challenge, with far-reaching implications that can impact patients' lives and well-being [2]. The interventions and management of microvascular (retinopathy, nephropathy, and neuropathy) and macro-vascular (cardiomyopathy) problems associated with diabetes are key goals of care for diabetic patients [3,4]. Diabetes is associated with diabetic myopathy, resulting in reduced skeletal and muscular strength [1,5,6]. However, this common condition lacks adequate research attention. It poses a significant clinical challenge, leading to a poorer quality of life for affected individuals. Skeletal muscle, constituting over 40% of total body mass in men and around 30% in women, is the predominant component in the human body [7]. Skeletal muscle is involved in a broad spectrum of physiological activities, such as metabolism, thermogenesis, and protein synthesis. These functions enable it to establish connections with other tissues, support an upright posture, and facilitate movement throughout the body [8]. Being the largest organ, skeletal muscle plays a crucial role in regulating glucose levels in the body. During the postprandial stage, it serves as a primary site for insulin-stimulated glucose absorption, facilitated by the translocation of glucose transporter type 4 (GLUT4) [9]. Oxidative stress and mild persistent inflammation are essential underlying causes of diabetic muscle dysfunction [1,10,11]. During oxidative stress and chronic inflammation, a multitude of intracellular signaling pathways undergo activation or inactivation [11]. This process results in detrimental effects such as apoptosis, impaired muscle progenitor cells (muscle satellite cells), and compromised myogenic capacity. Additionally, extracellular matrix (ECM) remodeling plays a pivotal role in the primary pathology, contributing to substantial muscle mass loss [1]. Findings suggest that oxidative stress and increased levels of transforming growth factor-β and tumor necrosis factor-α enhance ubiquitin proteolytic activity via specific E3 ubiquitin-ligase genes, including F-box-only protein 32 (FBXO32) and muscle-specific RING finger protein 1 (MuRF-1). This process leads to reduced protein synthesis and increased degradation of proteins in various skeletal muscles, including those affected by diabetic myopathy [12–14].

Salbutamol, known as albuterol, is a short-acting synthetic medication that is selective to β2-adrenoceptors (βAR). It is primarily used as a bronchodilator to manage bronchial asthma and chronic obstructive pulmonary disease (COPD). In previous research, it was observed that β2-adrenoceptors (βAR) and cyclic adenosine monophosphate (cAMP) mediated through the ubiquitin-proteasome system (UPS) [15]. Additionally, the selective β2-agonist clenbuterol, which belongs to the same drug category as salbutamoldemonstrated an anti-proteolytic effect during food deprivation. This effect is mediated through a cAMP/Akt-dependent pathway, leading to Foxo3a phosphorylation, suppression of atrogin-1, and inhibition of ubiquitination [16,17]. The study showed that short-term use of salbutamol increased voluntary muscle strength in humans [18]. However, the effect varied among different muscle groups. These findings suggest the therapeutic potential of β2-adrenoceptor agonists in modulating skeletal muscle function in humans. Both salbutamol and clenbuterol were administered to rats of different ages for three weeks, resulting in increased weight and protein content of hind-limb muscles in young and old rats. Additionally, both drugs increased the protein content of the whole body (carcass) and promoted muscle protein recovery in senescent rats [19]. Salbutamol has been found to enhance protein turnover rates in skeletal muscle after exercise in human subjects [20]. This effect involves the activation of cAMP/PKA and Akt2 signaling pathways and modulation of mRNA expression of growth-regulating proteins. These findings exhibit that salbutamol has the potential to enhance muscle protein synthesis and promote muscle growth in response to exercise [20]. Interestingly, a two-week course of salbutamol administration improved abilities in performing repeated sprints, physical performance, and muscle strength in athletic individuals [20]. Furthermore, salbutamol stimulates the transformation of muscle fiber isoforms, specifically myosin-heavy-chain (MHC)-I to MHC IIa, and enhances the hypertrophy of MHC IIa fibers after weight exercise [21]. A recent clinical trial demonstrates that albuterol (salbutamol) improved muscle function in Pompe disease and showed potential benefit as an adjunctive treatment along with enzyme replacement therapy [22].

Taken together, these promising findings suggest that salbutamol could be repurposed for the treatment of muscle atrophy. Based on these findings, we hypothesized that salbutamol might provide protection against skeletal muscle atrophy in diabetic rats induced by a high-fat diet (HFD)/streptozotocin (STZ). Furthermore, studies suggest that specific metabolites identified through plasma and skeletal muscle metabolomics profiles of well-phenotype diabetes patients may play a role in the pathophysiological pathway leading to the development of type 2 diabetes [23,24]. ^{1}H nuclear magnetic resonance (NMR) is a new technique used to detect these metabolites in the muscle tissue of diabetic patients [25] and enables researchers to provide insights into the metabolic disruptions in diabetic skeletal muscle. We further investigated how salbutamol modulates these altered metabolites in the skeletal muscle of diabetic rats.

2. Materials and Methods

2.1. Chemicals and Reagents

Salbutamol was received as a gift sample from Cipla Ltd., Mumbai, India. All the chemicals used in the present study were purchased from Sigma, St. Louis, MO, USA, and MP Biomedicals, Santa Ana, CA, USA, unless specified. The ELISA kits, IL-6 (Cat#550319) was purchased from BD Biosciences, San Jose, CA, USA. IL-2 ELISA kit (Cat# RAB0288) kit was purchased from Sigma, St. Louis, MO, USA. IL-1β (Cat #E-EL-R0012) kit was purchased from Elab Biosciences, Houston, TX, USA. Creatine kinase (Cat #3100709) and testosterone (Cat #3110023) ELISA kits were purchased from Real Gene Labs, Los Angeles, CA, USA GDF-8 ELISA kit (Cat #DGDF80) was purchased from the R&D System, Minneapolis, MN, USA. LiquiMax HDL Direct, LDL Cholesterol Direct, LiquiMax Cholesterol, Triglycerides kits were purchased from Avecon Health Care Pvt. Ltd., Haryana, India. High-fat diet was purchased by Bharat Ansh Scientific Industries, Lucknow, India. All the solvents used in the present study were of analytical grade.

2.2. Experimental Design

The animal experiments were performed according to the Committee for Control and Supervision of Experiments on Animals (CCSEA) guidelines approved by the Institutional Animal Ethical Committee (IAEC) of Babu Banarasi Das Northern India Institute of Technology (BBDNIIT) Lucknow, India (IAEC approval no. BBDNIIT/IAEC/2019/19). Twenty-four male Sprague Dawley (SD) rats aged 8–10 weeks and weighing 200 ± 30 g were purchased from the Central Drug Research Institute (CDRI), Lucknow, India. Standard laboratory conditions were maintained (22 ± 4 °C), and the animals were kept under an ambient environment (12 h light/dark cycles), humidity (50–60%), and water ad libitum. Animals were housed in polypropylene cages, and one week before starting the experiment, the rats were acclimatized to workable conditions. Twenty-four rats were allocated and randomized into four groups (n = 6): group I (control) received citrate buffer as a vehicle; group II (salbutamol, per se) was the control group treated with 6 mg/kg salbutamol (SLB) orally for four weeks once daily; group III (HFD/STZ) had a high-fat diet ad libitum for two weeks and injected as a single low dose of 35 mg/kg of streptozotocin (STZ) intraperitoneally (i.p.) (hereafter named as HFD/STZ group); and group IV served as HFD/STZ + salbutamol. SLB was prepared in distilled water at administered 6 mg/kg per oral for four weeks once daily. Blood samples were collected from the retro-orbital plexus under light anesthesia, and serum was separated and stored at −20 °C for further endpoints. Rats were sacrificed humanely by cervical dislocation, and the gastrocnemius muscle (GN) was isolated and preserved in 10% formalin for histology and kept at −80 °C for other endpoint parameters. The gastrocnemius (GN) muscle is chosen for its unique composition of both type 1 and type 2 muscle fibers. Additionally, it has been extensively studied in previous research [26,27].

2.2.1. Induction of Type 2 Diabetes

The Srivansan et al. model was used for the induction of type 2 diabetes [28]. In brief, SD male rats were given ad libitum access to a high-fat diet (HFD), having fat (58%), protein (25%), and carbohydrate (17%) for two weeks. After the initial two weeks of HFD diet, a single intraperitoneal injection of a low dose of STZ (35 mg/kg) was administered, and the animals were then continued on the HFD feeding for an additional two weeks. At the end of the four weeks, fasting plasma glucose, insulin, and lipid profile (triglyceride and cholesterol) were measured to confirm the induction of type-2 diabetes. Rats with fasting plasma glucose levels of $\geq$250 mg/dL or higher were considered diabetic and were used in the present experiments. The STZ was prepared in a citrate buffer (pH of 4.5, while the respective control rats were given a vehicle (citrate buffer) in volume of 1 mL/kg, intraperitoneally. Blood glucose levels were recorded with a glucometer (Dr Morepen GlucoOne, model-BG3).

2.2.2. Rationale of Selection of Salbutamol Dose

Based on an extensive literature review, it was observed that salbutamol is commonly administered in microgram doses, primarily in studies focusing on asthma. Furthermore, two findings were identified that repurposed salbutamol for different research purposes, specifically sepsis [29] and in the central nervous system [30]. In these studies, rats were administered salbutamol at doses of 4 mg/kg and 10 mg/kg for specific research objectives. Based on these findings, we carefully selected a dose within the range of these two studies. Therefore, in the present study, we chose a dose of 6 mg/kg of salbutamol.

2.3. Estimation of Body Weight, Gastrocnemius (GN) Muscle Weight, and Blood Glucose Levels

The body weight and gastrocnemius muscle weight of the rats were weighed using an analytical balance at the beginning and end of the experiment. Next, blood glucose levels were assessed using a glucometer at the start and end of the four-weeks experiment.

2.4. Estimation of Body Composition

The body composition of rats, specifically lean mass and fat mass, was assessed using the EchoMRI-500 body composition analyzer (EchoMRI Corporation Pvt. Ltd., Singapore). All the animals were gently placed in a specially designed, clear plastic holder without the need for anesthesia. The holder was then inserted into a designated tubular space on the side of the EchoMRI™ machine. By pressing a key on the keyboard, we initiated the scanning process and recorded the values for fat mass (in grams), lean body mass (in grams), free water (in grams), total water (in grams), and body weight (in grams) of each rat. The body weight, fat mass, and lean body mass were extracted from the collected data. These parameters were utilized to calculate the percentage change in lean mass and fat mass. These calculations were carried out to analyze the body composition, with a specific focus on the distribution of lean and fat mass. The data were expressed in percentages [31,32].

2.5. Behavioral Parameters

2.5.1. Assessment of Forelimb Grip Strength by Grip Strength Meter

Rats were raised by their tails and forced to grab a hard bar connected to a mechanical force sensor of grip strength meter (LEGSM-01; Milton Enterprises, Nashik, India). Each rat was gently dragged backward by the tail, and grip strength was determined by tension reading on the digital force gauge shortly before the rat let go of the bar [33,34].

2.5.2. Assessment of Locomotor Activity by Actophotometer Test

Random locomotor activity was measured using an actophotometer. Each animal was monitored for 5 min in a $14 \times 14 \times 14$ cm^2 closed-field arena with six photocells on the outside wall. A six-digit counter was used to track the photocell light interruptions (locomotor activity). The actophotometer was turned on, and each rat was placed in the cage independently for 5 min to measure locomotor activity [35].

2.5.3. Assessment of Muscle Strength by Wire-Hanging Test

The hanging wire analysis was performed to determine the coordination and muscle strength of the rats. It involves suspending the rat from a one-meter height at a stainless-steel wire of approximately 2.5 cm width over a soft fall area for three minutes. The number of falls of each animal was recorded using a digital camera with a cut-off of 10 falls [36].

2.5.4. Assessment of Muscle Coordination by Rotarod Test

The rotarod instrument assessed motor coordination and balance in the forelimbs and hind limbs. The latency to fall was determined after each rat was placed on the rotarod for 5 min at a constant speed of 5 rpm during the trial phase. Each experiment included three runs. Each rat was placed on the rotarod for a maximum of 5 min at a speed that increased from 4–40 rpm during the test, and the latency to fall was recorded [35].

2.5.5. Assessment of Gait Speed by Footprint Test

At the end of the experiment, the gait cycle of the respective groups (control, salbutamol, HFD/STZ, and HFD/STZ + salbutamol) animals was assessed using the footprint test. The forefeet and hind feet of the different groups rats (control, salbutamol, HFD/STZ, and HFD/STZ + salbutamol) were painted with different non-toxic colors to obtain footprints. Subsequently, the rats were allowed to walk on white paper. The average distance moved forward between the steps was used to compute the stride length. The average distance between the left and right hind footprints was used to calculate the width of the hind and front bases. To assess step alternation homogeneity, the distance between the left-to-left and right-to-right front footprint/hind footprint overlap was measured. For the assessment, a set of six steps was chosen, eliminating impressions created at the start and end of the run [37].

2.6. Estimation of Total and Myofibrillar Protein Concentration

Total and myofibrillar proteins from rats GN skeletal muscles have been estimated as per previous protocol [38]. In brief, 50 mg of GN muscles were homogenized on ice-cold buffer, pH 6.8, containing sucrose (8.5%), EDTA (5 mM), KCl (50 mM), and $MgCl_2$ (100 mM). This homogenate was used to measure the concentration of total protein. Further, GN homogenate was centrifuged at $2500\times g$ for 15 min at 4 °C. The supernatant was then discarded, and the remaining pellet was re-suspended in a solution (pH-6.8, 100 mM KCl, 5 mM $MgCl_2$, 5 mM EDTA, and 0.1% Triton X-100. This process was repeated twice. Further, the remaining pellet was washed in buffer (pH-6.8, 5 mM EDTA, and 100 mM KCl) and then centrifuged at $2500\times g$ for 10 min. This washing step was repeated once more. The obtained myofibrillar pellet was then re-suspended in a buffer solution (5 mM tris-hydroxymethyl aminomethane and 150 mM KCl, pH-7.4). The supernatant was used to calculate the amount of myofibrillar protein. The concentrations of both total protein and myofibrillar protein were assessed using a Lowry assay [39]. Bovine serum albumin (BSA) was used as the standard.

2.7. Assessment of Oxidative Stress Markers and Antioxidative Status

To conduct the oxidative stress and antioxidant assay, 100 mg of the gastrocnemius (GN) muscle was homogenized in 1 mL of cold phosphate-buffered saline (pH 7.4). The homogenate was subsequently used for all biochemical estimations.

2.7.1. Estimation of Lipid Peroxidation by Malondialdehyde

The measurement of malondialdehyde (MDA) content by thiobarbituric acid (TBA) directly determines the non-enzymatic oxidative state for lipid peroxidation [40]. In brief, 500 µL of 30% trichloroacetic acid (TCA), 500 µL of 0.8% TBA, and 1 mL of homogenized GN muscles in phosphate-buffered saline were mixed and incubated for 10 min at room temperature. The resulting reaction mixture was then heated at 80 °C for 30 min. After the mixture was cooled, it was centrifuged at $5000\times g$ for 15 min, and the absorbance of the resulting supernatant was measured at 540 nm. The results are expressed in nM/mg protein.

2.7.2. Estimation of Protein Carbonyl Content

The protein carbonyl content (PC) is determined based on the reaction of 2,4-Dinitrophenylhydrazine (DNPH) and serves as an indicator of oxidative stress [41]. Briefly, 500 µL of 10% TCA and 150 µL of GN muscle homogenate were mixed and incubated at room temperature for ten minutes. After centrifuging the reaction mixture at 13,000× g for 2 min, the supernatant was discarded, and the pellet was collected. Next, the pellet was suspended in 250 µL of 0.2% DNPH and incubated for 30 min. After incubation, 50 µL of 100% TCA was added to the mixture and centrifuged at 13,000× g for 5 min. The supernatant was then discarded, and the remaining cell pellets were 500 µL of washed with 1:1 v/v ethanol: ethyl acetate solution. The pellets were further dissolved in 6 M guanidine HCl and vortexed. Subsequently, the absorbance of the supernatant was measured at 360 nm. The results are expressed in µM/mg protein.

2.7.3. Estimation of Catalase Activity by H_2O_2 Decomposition

Catalase activity was directly estimated by monitoring the rate of H_2O_2 breakdown. In brief, 50 µL of GN muscle homogenates were mixed with 250 µL of 19 mM of H_2O_2. Next, immediately after the reaction, we measured the absorbance at 240 nm for 3 min. Catalase activity was calculated using an extinction value of 0.0719 $mM^{-1}cm^{-1}$. The results are expressed as the number of moles of H_2O_2 that were broken down/min/mg of protein in the sample.

2.7.4. Estimation of Reduced Glutathione Activity by Ellman's Reagent

The amount of glutathione (GSH) was determined by reducing 5,5'-dithiobis-(2-nitrobenzoic acid) (also known as DTNB or Ellman's reagent) by the thiol group of GSH, which resulted in a yellow-colored GS-TNB complex [42]. In brief, 250 µL of 50% TCA and 120 µL GN muscles homogenate was incubated for 10 min at room temperature. After centrifugation at 5000× g for 10 min, the precipitate was removed. In a reaction mixture comprising 3 µL of 0.6 mM DTNB and 130 µL of 0.2 M sodium phosphate-buffered (pH 8), free -SH groups in the supernatant were measured (pH 8.0). The absorbance was determined at 405 nm, and the results were expressed in nanomoles/mg of protein.

2.7.5. Estimation of Superoxide Dismutase Activity by Pyrogallol Activity

Superoxide dismutase (SOD) activity was determined by inhibiting the reduction in pyrogallol activity by SOD present in the sample [43]. In brief, 2.9 mL of 0.5 M tris buffer (pH 8.0) having tris HCl (50 mM), EDTA (1 mM) was mixed with 100 µL of GN muscles homogenate. After that, incubation for 5 min was carried out at room temperature. A total of 25 µL of 2.6 mM pyrogallol was then added to stop the reaction. The change in absorbance after the addition of pyrogallol for 3 min was measured at 420 nm. SOD activity was evaluated in millimoles of reduced pyrogallol/min/mg of protein.

2.8. Estimation of Cellular Toxicity by Histological Analysis

The gastrocnemius (GN) muscles were preserved by fixing them in 10% formalin. Next, the muscles were subjected to a series of treatments involving graded alcohol and xylene, followed by embedding in paraffin wax. The sections were cut with a thickness of 5 µm using a Thermo HM325 rotary microtome and were taken on pre-coated slides. Then, the sections were dewaxed in xylene for 2–5 min and processed according to the previous protocol [44]. The muscle sections were stained with Hematoxylin and Eosin (H&E) and subsequently processed and mounted with DPX. Furthermore, the slides were observed at 20× magnification by using an Olympus Microscope (BX53, Hamburg, Germany). The cross-sectional area (CSA) and Feret's diameter of the muscle fibers were analyzed by

ImageJ software (NIH, Bethesda, MD, USA) [44]. A total of 15–20 tissue sections were utilized for analysis, with 3 slides per group.

2.9. Estimation of Serum Testosterone, GDF-8, Inflammatory Markers, and Lipid Markers

Serum levels of testosterone, GDF-8, IL-2, IL-6, IL-1β, creatine kinase, total cholesterol (TC), low-density lipoprotein (LDL), high-density lipoprotein (HDL), and triglycerides (TG) were measured using the procedure provided by the manufacturer. The very-low-density lipoprotein (VLDL) lipid level was determined using Friedewald's formula as follows:

$$\text{VLDL (mg/dL)} = \text{TC} - \text{HDL} - \text{LD}$$

2.10. ^{1}H NMR-Based GN Muscle Metabolomics Profiling

2.10.1. Sample Preparation

In total, 50 mg GN muscle was homogenized in 500 µL of ice-cold normal saline. Homogenates were vortexed and sonicated for 30 s. After that, GN muscle homogenates were centrifuged at 16,278× g for 5 min at 4 °C. After homogenization, the supernatant was collected, and from this, 250 µL of supernatant was mixed with 250 µL of 100% deuterium oxide (D_2O). Following this step, 450 µL of this mixture was put in 5 mm NMR tubes (Wilmad Glass, Vineland, NJ, USA). A sealed capillary tube containing sodium salt of 3-trimethylsilyl-(2,2,3,3-d4)-propionic acid (1.0 mM) (TSP) dissolved in D_2O as a co-solvent was used as an internal standard reference and inserted in the NMR tubes [45].

2.10.2. NMR Measurements

A Bruker 800 MHz NMR spectrometer (AVANCE-III, equipped with a cryoprobe) was used for NMR experiments at 298 K. The metabolic profiles of the muscles were determined using one-dimensional (1D) ^{1}H CPMG (Carr–Purcell–Meiboom–Gill) pulse sequence NMR. The tests were performed on all muscle samples with pre-saturation of the water signal during a recycle delay (RD) of 5 s using the Bruker standard library pulse program "cpmgpr1d". The other acquisition parameters were as follows: the width of the ^{1}H spectral sweep was 12 ppm, the number of transients was 128, and the T2 filtering time (to suppress the broad signals of higher molecular weight macromolecules, including proteins) was obtained with an echo time of 200 s repeated 300 times, which resulted in a total effective echo time of 60 ms. All NMR spectra were processed using the Bruker NMR data processing program Topspin (v2.1), employing a typical Fourier transformation (FT) technique, as well as manual phase and baseline correction. Before the FFT was performed, each FID was zero-filled to a total of 65,536 data points and then multiplied by an exponential line-broadening function operating at 0.3 Hz.

2.10.3. Spectral Assignment and Concentration Profiling

Using the Chenomx NMR suite's 800 MHz compound spectral database library with pH set at 7.2 for all samples (Chenomx Inc., Edmonton, AB, Canada), various peaks in the ^{1}D ^{1}H CPMG NMR spectra were identified and annotated for different muscle tissue metabolites. This was performed in conjunction with 2D homonuclear ^{1}H-^{1}H TOCSY and heteronuclear ^{1}H-^{13}C HSQC NMR [46]. The metabolic assignments were further confirmed using publicly accessible databases (such as HMBD: http://www.hmdb.ca (accessed on 21 October 2022) and BMRB: www.bmrb.wisc.edu/metabolomics (accessed on 15 September 2022) and and the NMR assignments of metabolites published in several previous metabolomics studies [47–50]. All CPMG pulse NMR spectra that were collected were visually inspected to determine whether they were acceptable. Additional analyses were performed using the NMR suite of the commercial software CHENOMX (Chenomx Inc., Edmonton, AB, Canada). First, all of the NMR spectra were baseline corrected and calibrated internally to ^{1}H NMR peak of formate (at δ = 8.43 ppm and with the concentration set to 0.01 mM). Next, concentration profiling of the 40 muscle tissue metabolites was carried out following the procedure described in the previous section [51]. Then, 3-hydroxy-butyrate

(3HB), acetone, alanine, betaine, acetate, choline, citrate, dimethyl sulfone (DMS), creatine, dimethylamine (DMA), glutamine, glucose, glutamate, glycine, glycerol, isoleucine, isobutyrate (IsoB), leucine, lactate, phenylalanine, methanol, pyruvate, succinate, proline, serine, threonine, valine, tyrosine, histidine, and myoinositol. Following this, the metabolic profiles were utilized to estimate five key metabolic ratios, including the phenylalanine-to-tyrosine ratio (PTR), histidine-to-tyrosine ratio (HTR), and glutamate-to-glutamine ratio (EQR), as discussed in the preceding section [52,53].

2.10.4. Multivariate Data Analysis

The resultant metabolic concentrations and ratio values were then transferred to the MS Office Excel program and transformed into a comma-separated values (CSV) text format file, which was then utilized for multivariate data analysis in MetaboAnalyst 4.0., which is an open-access web-based metabolomics data processing tool [54,55]. Principal component analysis, often known as PCA, was applied to locate data outliers and offer a concise picture of the trending grouping of the data set. Subsequently, supervised Partial Least Squares Discriminant Analysis (PLS-DA) was applied to discover group separations and locate the discriminating metabolites that accounted for group separations. A 10-fold cross-validation approach was used to prevent overfitting of the PLS-DA model. For GN muscle metabolic profiling, NMR spectra acquired from the muscle tissue were processed using the PROFILER-Module of CHENOMX. Following this, the quantities of the selected metabolites were determined for each of the three sets of muscle tissue samples. PLS-DA analysis was used to evaluate the quantitative muscle metabolic profiles of the control, salbutamol, HFD/STZ, and HFD/STZ + salbutamol groups. Permutation analysis was performed to cross-validate the PLS-DA models a hundred times, and the resultant goodness-of-fit parameter R^2 and goodness-of-prediction parameter Q2 were utilized to evaluate the characteristics of the PLS-DA models. The VIP score, also known as the variable significance on projection score, must have a value larger than 1.0 to be employed in the PLS-DA model's process of identifying the metabolites responsible for discrimination. The metabolite concentration profile data matrix was then exposed to a random forest (RF) classification model (a supervised machine learning method), and discriminatory metabolic profiles were cross-validated using a Mean Decrease Accuracy (MDA) score plot [56,57]. In summary, MDA reflects how much accuracy the model loses when each variable is removed from the RF classification model when comparing the study groups. The greater the loss of accuracy, the more critical the variable is for effective categorization. The statistical analysis module of MetaboAnalyst (https://www.metaboanalyst.ca (accessed on 21 October 2022)) was used to analyze the RF classification model. Analysis of variance (ANOVA) with multiple group comparisons was used to assess the statistical significance of the discriminating factors. The benchmark for statistical significance was a significance level of 0.05 or a p-value of 0.05. Chenomx NMR Suite v8.1 was used to quantitatively estimate the key metabolites.

2.11. Statistical Analysis

The data were analyzed using GraphPad Prism software (version 8.01). All the values were expressed as the mean ± standard deviation (SD). Statistical analysis was performed on the data from the four groups using a one-way analysis of variance (ANOVA), followed by Tukey's multiple comparisons *post hoc* test. The differences were considered statistically significant at $p < 0.05$.

3. Results

3.1. Effect of Salbutamol on Blood Glucose Levels, Body Weight, and GN Muscle Weight in HFD/STZ-Induced Diabetic Rats

There was no change in blood glucose levels between the HFD/STZ and HFD/STZ + salbutamol groups (Table 1). These results suggest that salbutamol treatment did not have a significant effect on blood glucose levels. Similarly, the fasting insulin levels were

399.75 ± 9.35 pg/mL in diabetic rats when compared to control (860.58 ± 11.58 pg/mL). SLB treatment for 4 weeks led to a significant increase in body weight as compared to the HFD/STZ group ($p < 0.001$). These results indicate that SLB treatment leads to a decrease in body weight in the HFD/STZ group. The finding also showed that SLB treatment significantly increased the GN weight as compared to the HFD/STZ group ($p < 0.001$) (Table 1). Findings indicate that SLB treatment increased the weight of the GN muscle in HFD/STZ rats. These results led us to further investigate body composition, specifically the measurements of lean mass and fat mass.

Table 1. Effect of salbutamol on blood glucose level (mg/dL), body weight (g), and GN muscle (mg) weight in HFD/STZ-induced diabetic rats. Data were represented as mean ± SD ($n = 6$). Statistical significance was determined using one-way ANOVA with Tukey's multiple comparisons post hoc test. Table depict *** $p < 0.001$ vs. control and ### $p < 0.001$ vs. HFD/STZ and ns: non significant.

Parameters	Time Points	Control	Salbutamol	HFD/STZ	HFD/STZ + Salbutamol
Blood Glucose level (mg/dL)	0 week	124.83 ± 1.47	124.33 ± 1.21	124.66 ± 3.26	124.66 ± 2.94
	4 weeks	124.83 ± 1.94	125.16 ± 1.72	371.16 ± 14.90 ***	370.83 ± 15.43 ns
Body weight (g)	0 week	185.16 ± 2.31	194.50 ± 3.08	184.50 ± 2.07	175.00 ± 3.03
	4 weeks	206.66 ± 2.80	226.66 ± 1.96	306.33 ± 3.01 ***	203.50 ± 1.51 ###
GN muscle weight (mg)	4 weeks	783.50 ± 2.88	804.66 ± 2.73	338.66 ± 2.50 ***	776.16 ± 6.76 ###

3.2. Effect of Salbutamol on Body Composition in HFD/STZ-Induced Diabetic Rats

The results demonstrated that SLB treatment significantly increased the percentage of lean mass compared to the HFD/STZ group ($p < 0.001$) (Figure 1A). This suggests that SLB treatment led to an increase in lean tissue or muscle mass in HFD-induced diabetic rats. The SLB treatment group exhibited a reduced percentage of fat mass compared to the HFD/STZ group ($p < 0.001$) (Figure 1B). This indicates that SLB treatment was associated with a decrease in fat tissue in HFD/STZ-induced diabetic rats. These findings suggest that SLB may have a positive effect on body composition by promoting an increase in lean mass and reduced fat mass in HFD/STZ-induced diabetic rats. The reduced percentage of fat mass and the greater percentage of lean mass in the SLB treatment group imply that SLB could potentially ameliorate muscle atrophy associated with the HFD/STZ-induced diabetic condition. These results further evaluate muscle strength and coordination in HFD/STZ-induced diabetic rats.

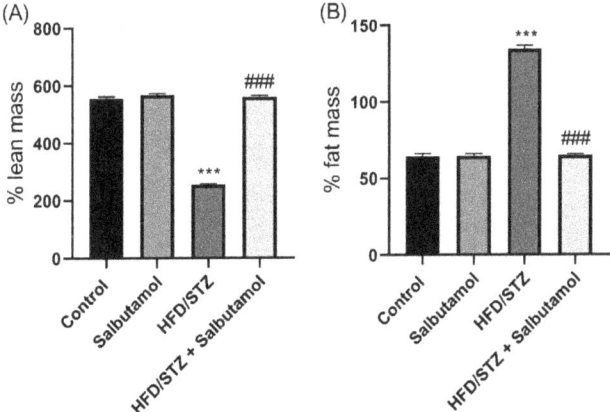

Figure 1. Effect of salbutamol on the lean muscle mass in HFD/STZ -induced diabetic rats. (**A**) Lean mass (%) and (**B**) fat mass (%). Data were represented as mean ± SD ($n = 6$). Statistical significance

was determined using one-way ANOVA with Tukey's multiple comparisons post hoc test. Bar graphs depict *** $p < 0.001$ vs. control and ### $p < 0.001$ vs. HFD/STZ.

3.3. Effect of Salbutamol on Muscle Strength and Motor Coordination in HFD/STZ-Induced Diabetic Rats

Next, diabetic rats exhibited a significant decrease in grip strength and wire-hanging ability, indicating compromised muscle strength compared to the control group. However, the SLB treatment improved grip strength and wire-hanging performance compared to the control group ($p < 0.001$) (Figure 2A,B). SLB treatment significantly increased muscle coordination and balance. This was demonstrated by increased latency to fall ($p < 0.001$) (Figure 2C) and longer stride lengths (right-to-right and left-to-left) ($p < 0.001$) (Figure 2D,E) in diabetic rats. SLB treatment also resulted in increased locomotion time in diabetic rats ($p < 0.001$) (Figure 2F). This suggests an improvement in motor coordination and balance due to SLB intervention. Overall, the results indicate that SLB treatment effectively improved muscle strength, coordination, function, and balance in HFD/STZ-induced diabetic rats. The improvements observed in grip strength, wire-hanging ability, latency time, stride lengths, and locomotion time suggest that SLB can improve muscle strength and enhance motor coordination.

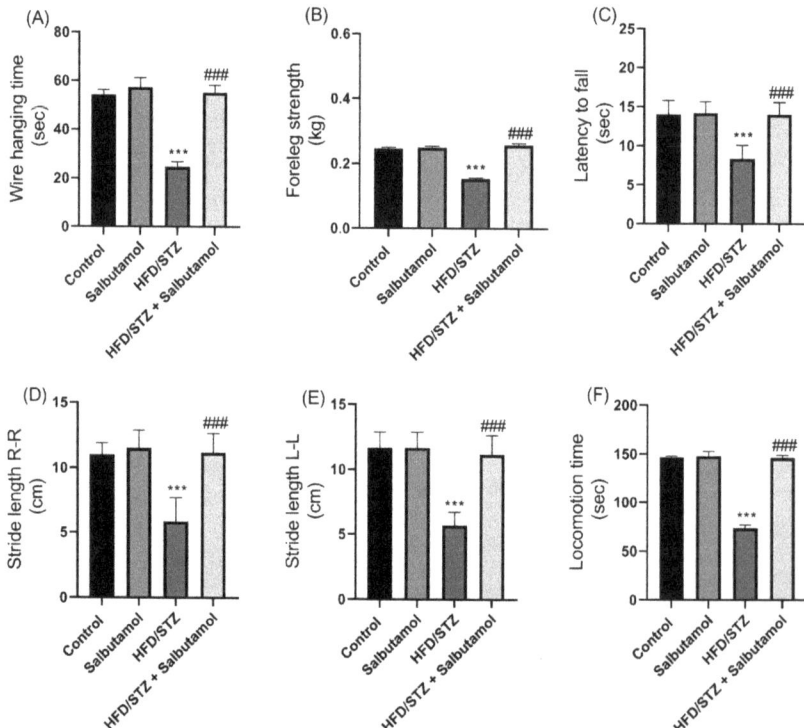

Figure 2. Effect of salbutamol on muscle strength, function and coordination in HFD/STZ-induced diabetic rats. (**A**) Hanging time (s), (**B**) Foreleg grip strength (kg), (**C**) Latency to fall (s), (**D**) Stride length (cm) R-R, (**E**) Stride length (cm) L-L, and (**F**) Locomotion time (s). Data were represented as mean ± SD ($n = 6$). Statistical significance was determined using one-way ANOVA with Tukey's multiple comparisons post hoc test. Bar graphs depict *** $p < 0.001$ vs. control and ### $p < 0.001$ vs HFD/STZ.

3.4. Effect of Salbutamol on Total and Myofibrillar Protein Concentration in HFD/STZ-Induced Diabetic Rats

Next, the total protein content in the GN muscles was significantly decreased in the HFD/STZ group compared to the control group ($p < 0.001$). SLB treatment was able to restore the total protein content compared to the HFD/STZ group (Figure 3B). Similarly, the myofibrillar protein content was found to be significantly decreased in the HFD/STZ group compared to the control group ($p < 0.001$). However, SLB treatment restored the myofibrillar protein content (Figure 3A). These results suggest that the HFD/STZ-induced diabetic condition led to a reduction in both total protein contents and myofibrillar protein in the GN muscles. However, SLB treatment significantly increased the protein contents, indicating its potential to counteract the negative effects of the HFD/STZ-induced diabetic condition on skeletal muscle protein.

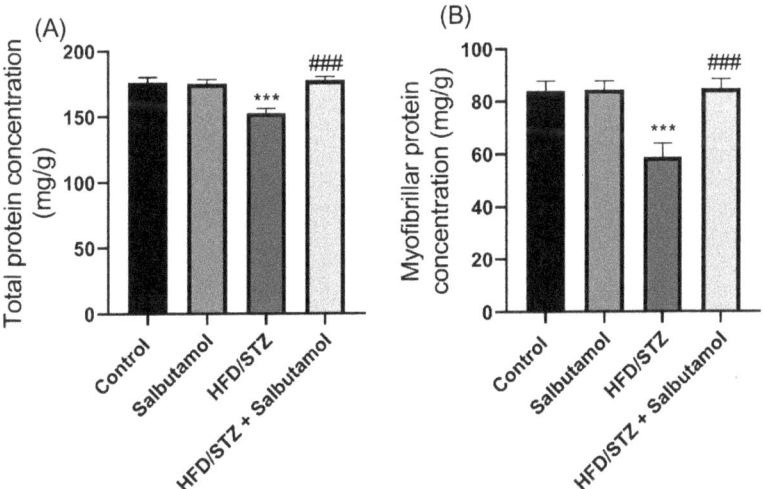

Figure 3. Effect of salbutamol on the protein concentration of GN muscle in HFD/STZ-induced diabetic rats. (**A**) Total protein concentration (mg/g) and (**B**) myofibrillar protein concentration (mg/g). Data were represented as mean ± SD ($n = 6$). Statistical significance was determined using one-way ANOVA with Tukey's multiple comparisons *post hoc* test. Bar graphs depict *** $p < 0.001$ vs. control and ### $p < 0.001$ vs. HFD/STZ.

3.5. Effect of Salbutamol on Oxidative Stress and Antioxidant Status in HFD/STZ-Induced Diabetic Rats

Next, the levels of superoxide dismutase (SOD), catalase, and reduced glutathione (GSH) antioxidant enzymes were found to be significantly decreased in the HFD/STZ group compared to the control group ($p < 0.001$). However, SLB treatment restored the antioxidant status by increasing the levels of SOD, catalase, and GSH, similar to the control group (Figure 4A–C). The levels of malondialdehyde (MDA), which is a marker of lipid peroxidation, and protein carbonyl (PC), which is a marker of protein peroxidation, were significantly increased in the HFD/STZ group compared to the control group ($p < 0.001$). However, SLB treatment resulted in decreased levels of oxidative stress, as evidenced by reduced levels of MDA and PC (Figure 4D,E). These results indicate that the diabetic condition resulted in increased oxidative stress and decreased antioxidant status in the GN muscles. Furthermore, the treatment with SLB significantly increased the antioxidant status and reduced oxidative stress in the diabetic muscle.

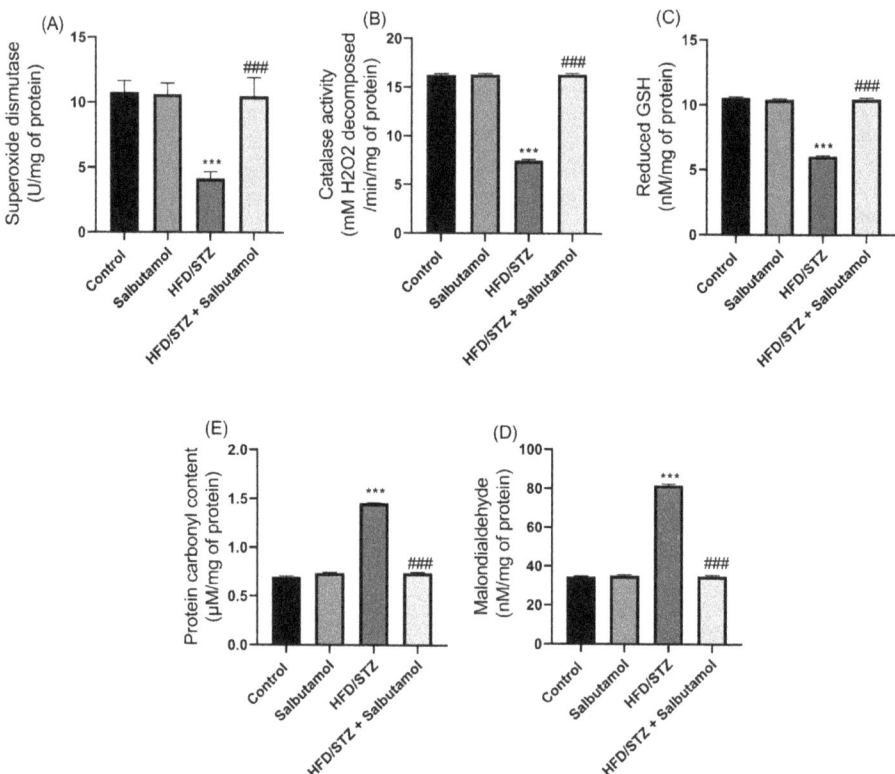

Figure 4. Effect of salbutamol on antioxidant status and oxidative stress markers of GN muscle in HFD/STZ-induced diabetic rats. (**A**) Superoxide dismutase (U/mg of protein), (**B**) catalase activity (U/mg), (**C**) reduced GSH (nM/mg of protein), (**D**) MDA (nM/mg of protein), and (**E**) protein carbonyl content (μmoles/mg of protein). Data were represented as mean ± SD ($n = 6$). Statistical significance was determined using one-way ANOVA with Tukey's multiple comparisons post hoc test. Bar graphs depict *** $p < 0.001$ vs. control and ### $p < 0.001$ vs. HFD/STZ.

3.6. Effect of Salbutamol on the Cellular Architecture of GN Muscle in HFD/STZ-Induced Diabetic Rats

The GN muscles in the control group showed a regular and organized structure, indicating normal muscle morphology (Figure 5A). In diabetic rats, the GN muscles exhibited shrinkage and varying myofiber sizes with significant gaps when compared to the control group. This suggests muscle damage and disorganization associated with the HFD/STZ-induced diabetic condition (Figure 5A). SLB treatment restored the muscle architecture in the HFD/STZ group, indicating a reversal of the structural abnormalities induced by diabetes (Figure 5A). In addition, quantitative measurements of the cross-sectional area (CSA) and Feret's diameter of myofibers were decreased in the HFD/STZ group compared to the control group and were performed using ImageJ software 1.44 (NIH, USA). The results demonstrated that salbutamol treatment significantly increased the CSA and Feret's diameter of myofibers in diabetic rats compared to the control group ($p < 0.001$). This indicates an improvement in myofiber size and morphology following salbutamol intervention (Figure 5B,C). These findings suggest that the intervention of salbutamol effectively improved the cellular changes and structural abnormalities in the GN muscle associated with HFD/STZ-induced diabetes. The restoration of muscle architecture, as evidenced by the increased cross-sectional area (CSA) and Feret's diameter of myofibers, indicates the potential of salbutamol in ameliorating muscle cellular architecture in diabetic conditions.

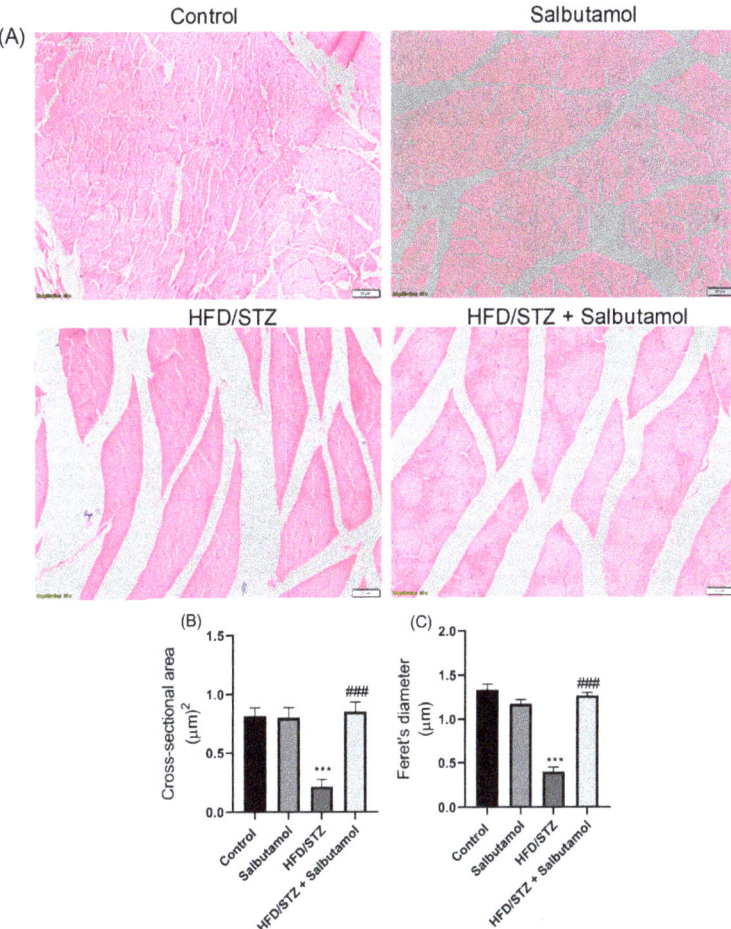

Figure 5. Effect of salbutamol on muscle architecture in HFD/STZ-induced diabetic rats (**A**) H&E-stained images of GN muscle, (**B**) cross-sectional area (μm)^2, and (**C**) Feret's diameter (μm). Data were represented as mean ± SD (n = 6). Statistical significance was determined using one-way ANOVA with Tukey's multiple comparisons post hoc tests. Bar graphs depict *** $p < 0.001$ vs. control and ### $p < 0.001$ vs. HFD/STZ.

3.7. Effect of Salbutamol on Serum Level of Creatine Kinase, GDF-8, Testosterone, and Pro-Inflammatory Markers in HFD/STZ-Induced Diabetic Rats

Next, the serum creatine kinase (CK) and growth differentiation factor 8 (GDF-8) muscle damage markers were found to be significantly elevated in HFD/STZ group compared to the control group ($p < 0.001$). However, SLB treatment significantly decreased serum CK and GDF-8 levels in the diabetic group (Figure 6A,B). These results suggest that the decreased levels or inhibition of myostatin and CK, in combination with SLB treatment, may enhance skeletal muscle mass. The serum testosterone level was increased in the SLB treatment group compared to the HFD/STZ group ($p < 0.001$). This increase in testosterone level was positively correlated with muscle mass, suggesting a potential role of testosterone in the modulation of muscle mass (Figure 6C). Also, the serum pro-inflammatory markers IL-1β, IL-2, and IL-6 were found to be significantly increased in the HFD/STZ group compared to the control group ($p < 0.001$). However, SLB intervention resulted in reduced levels of these pro-inflammatory cytokines (IL-1β, IL-2, and IL-6) (Figure 7A–C). This indicates that lowered pro-inflammatory cytokine levels may attenuate muscle atrophy. These results suggest that HFD/STZ-induced diabetic conditions lead to alterations in circulating markers associated with muscle mass, inflammation, and testosterone levels. SLB treatment appears to have a beneficial effect by restoring the levels of CK and GDF-8, positively influencing testosterone levels, and reducing pro-inflammatory cytokine levels. These findings highlight the potential of SLB in reducing muscle inflammation in diabetic rats.

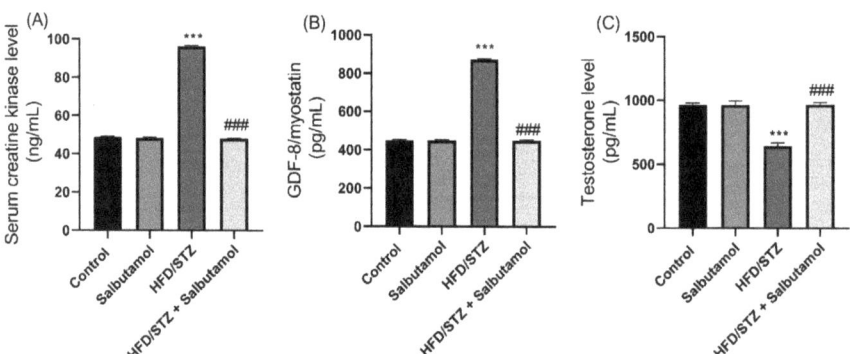

Figure 6. Effect of salbutamol on muscle damage markers in HFD/STZ-induced diabetic rats. (**A**) Serum creatine kinase (ng/mL), (**B**) GDF-8 level (pg/mL), and (**C**) Testosterone level (pg/mL). Data were represented as mean ± SD ($n = 6$). Statistical significance was determined using one-way ANOVA with Tukey's multiple comparisons post hoc test. Bar graphs depict *** $p < 0.001$ vs. control and ### $p < 0.001$ vs. HFD/STZ.

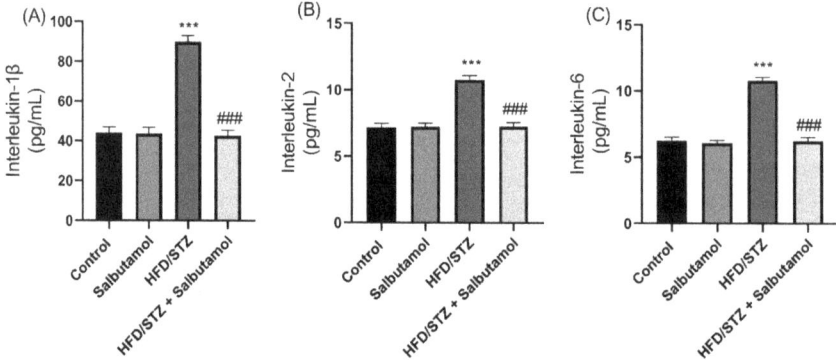

Figure 7. Effect of salbutamol on serum inflammatory markers in HFD/STZ-induced diabetic rats. (**A**) IL-1β (pg/mL), (**B**) IL-2 (pg/mL), and (**C**) IL-6 (pg/mL). Data were represented as mean ± SD ($n = 6$). Statistical significance was determined using one-way ANOVA with Tukey's multiple comparisons post hoc test. Bar graphs depict *** $p < 0.001$ vs. control and ### $p < 0.001$ vs. HFD/STZ.

3.8. Effect of Salbutamol on Serum Lipid Profile in HFD/STZ-Induced Diabetic Rats

The HFD/STZ group exhibited significantly higher levels of total cholesterol (TC), triglyceride (TG), low-density lipoprotein (LDL), and very-low-density lipoprotein (VLDL) compared to the control group ($p < 0.001$) (Figure 8A–D). These findings indicate an elevation in circulating lipid levels associated with the diabetic condition. The HDL levels in the HFD/STZ group were significantly lower than those in the control group ($p < 0.001$) (Figure 8E). This indicates a reduction in the levels of protective HDL cholesterol in diabetic rats. SLB intervention significantly restored the serum lipid profiles, indicating a reversal of the lipid abnormalities induced by diabetes (Figure 8A–E). These results suggest that the diabetic condition leads to dysregulation of serum lipid profiles, characterized by elevated levels of TC, LDL, VLDL, and TG, as well as reduced levels of HDL. The administration of SLB appears to ameliorate these lipid abnormalities by restoring the lipid profile to levels compared to the control group. These findings suggest that excessive lipid levels may contribute to muscle damage, and the intervention with SLB helps in mitigating this effect.

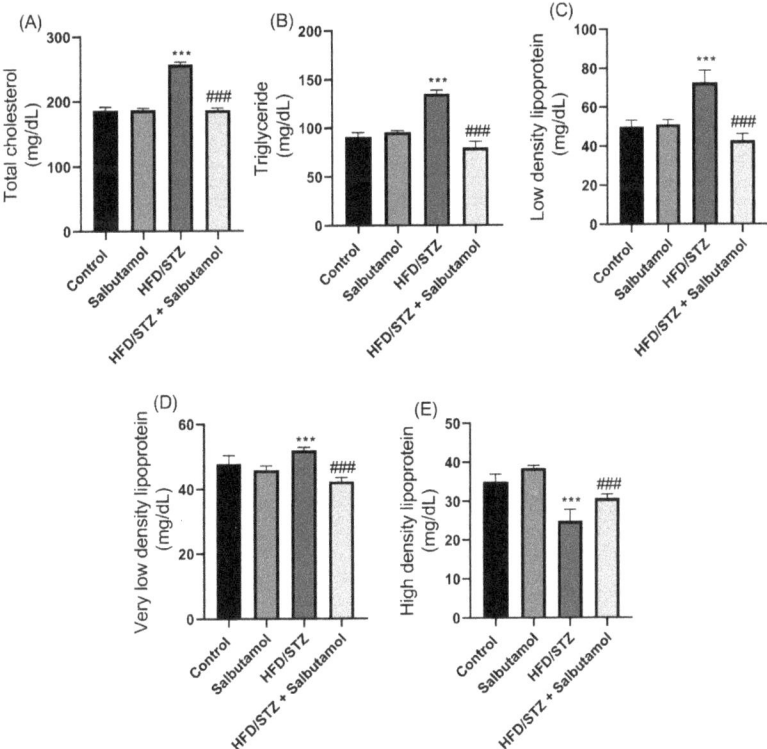

Figure 8. Effect of salbutamol on serum lipidemic profile in HFD/STZ-induced diabetic rats. (**A**) Total cholesterol (mg/dL), (**B**) Triglyceride (mg/dL), (**C**) HDL (mg/dL), (**D**) LDL (mg/dL), and (**E**) VLDL (mg/dL). Data were represented as mean ± SD (n = 6). Statistical significance was determined using one-way ANOVA with Tukey's multiple comparisons post hoc test. *** $p < 0.001$ vs. control and ### $p < 0.001$ vs. HFD/STZ.

3.9. Effect of Salbutamol on GN Muscle Metabolomics Using ^{1}H NMR-Based Technique in HFD/STZ-Induced Diabetic Rats

Figure S1 shows the typical 1D and ^{1}H NMR spectra of rat GN muscle samples acquired from the control, salbutamol, HFD/STZ, and HFD/STZ + salbutamol groups. NMR peaks of the different metabolites were annotated. They mainly show the signals of metabolites, such as (a) amino acids, viz. alanine, glycine, glutamate, glutamine, π-methylhistidine, leucine, isoleucine, phenylalanine, methionine, sarcosine, proline, threonine, serine, valine, and tyrosine; (b) energy metabolites, viz. acetate, creatine, fumarate, formate, glycerol, lactate, pyruvate, and succinate; (c) lipoproteins (VLDL and LDL); (d) ketone body content, viz. acetone, betaine, 3-hydroxybutyrate; and (e) additional metabolites were also estimated in the subsequent combinations or ratios, viz. phenylalanine-to-tyrosine ratio (PTR), histidine-to-tyrosine ratio (HTR), and glutamate-to-glutamine ratio (EQR). Next, to investigate the effect of salbutamol on metabolites in diabetic rats, the GN muscle metabolic profile was obtained using 1D ^{1}H NMR spectroscopy. This profile was then subjected to multivariate statistical analysis to determine the metabolic patterns that were altered. This was carried out with the help of MetaboAnalyst (v4.0, a free web-based software [58]. The 3D score plot obtained from PLS-DA analysis showed a distinct separation among the four groups, demonstrating a substantial metabolic difference between the HFD/STZ and HFD/STZ + salbutamol groups as opposed to the control group and the salbutamol group by itself. (Figure S2A). In addition, compared with the standard HFD/STZ group, there was a discernible tendency toward clustering treatment groups (HFD/STZ + salbutamol) and shifting toward the control group (Figure S2A). The PLS-DA model validation parameters ($R2 > 0.57$ and $Q2 > 0.38$) and predictive capability (Q2) were significantly high, suggesting a significant metabolic variation between the study groups (Figure S2B). The metabolic features of discriminatory relevance were first identified using the PLS-DA model based on variable importance in projection (VIP) score values > 1.0 (Figure S2C). Statistical significance was evaluated using ANOVA. We also performed machine learning random forest (RF) classification analysis (RFA) to confirm the discriminatory potential of metabolic profiles for classifying the data. The variables are presented from descending importance in the mean decrease accuracy (MDA) score plot derived from the RF clustering approach. Integrative analysis (based on VIP and MDA score plots and ANOVA statistics) identified several metabolic entities with discriminatory potential. It could predict the therapeutic response to salbutamol, as shown in Figures S2C,D. Compared to control rats, GN muscle levels of 3-hydroxybutyrate, sarcosine, succinate, HTR, PTR, and EQR were elevated, and creatine and glycine levels were decreased in the HFD/STZ group (Figure S2B,D). Quantitative variations in these discriminatory features are shown through box-cum-whisker plots (Figure 9). As evident from the results, several GN muscle metabolites showed a metabolic reprogramming trend (Figure 9), suggesting that salbutamol could potentially alleviate metabolic alterations in diabetic rat muscle.

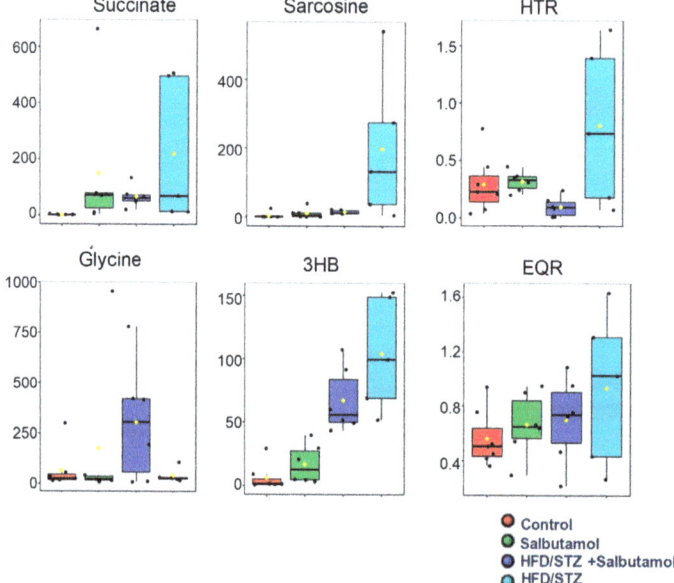

Figure 9. Representative box-cum-whisker plots showing quantitative variations of concentration pertinent GN muscle metabolites. The black round dots along the Y axis in the box plots denote the

concentrations of metabolites, while the yellow rhombus denotes mean concentrations of the group. In the box plots, the boxes denote interquartile ranges, horizontal lines inside the box denote the median, and the bottom and top boundaries of boxes are 25th and 75th percentiles, respectively. Lower and upper whiskers are 5th and 95th percentiles, respectively. Key acronyms are HTR: histidine-to-tyrosine ratio 3-HB: 3-hydroxybutyrate; EQR: glutamate-to-glutamine ratio.

3.10. Disturbed Interlinking Metabolic Pathways in Diabetes-Induced Skeletal Muscle Atrophy

After analyzing significant muscle metabolites (sarcosine, PTR, EQR, HTR, succinate, and 3-hydroxybutyrate) in HFD/STZ and HFD/STZ + salbutamol groups, we investigated how those metabolites are involved and utilized in glycolysis, TCA cycle, and other metabolic pathways. These pathways included the tricarboxylic acid (TCA) cycle (succinate), ketogenesis (3-hydroxybutyrate), histidine metabolism (histidine), glycine metabolism (sarcosine), and other metabolic pathways (PTR, HTR, and EQR) in Figure 10 and are detailed in the Section 4.

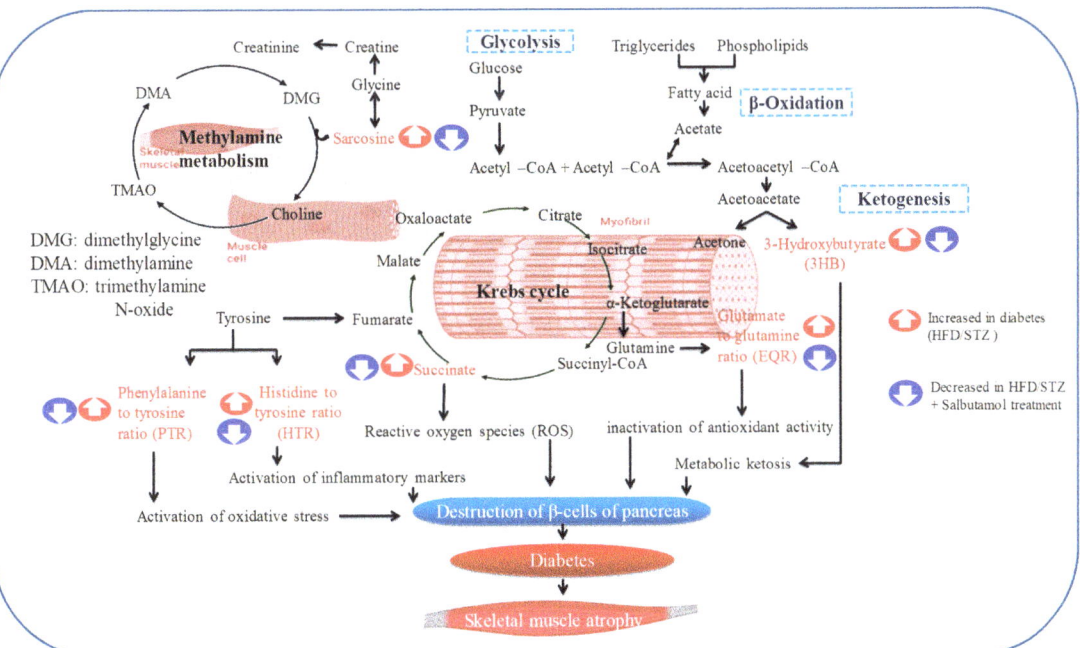

Figure 10. The figure illustrates the involvement of specific enzymes and their impact on interconnected pathways, offering valuable insights into understanding the intricacies of muscle metabolism. The representative altered key metabolites in the figure depict interlinked pathways, including glycolysis, the tricarboxylic acid (TCA) cycle, and methylamine metabolism. The blue color signifies the restored metabolites due to salbutamol intervention, demonstrating the ameliorating effect of salbutamol on diabetic skeletal muscle. In contrast, the dark red color indicates the altered status of metabolites in the diabetic condition, indicating significant increases and imbalances within different pathways of skeletal muscle.

4. Discussion

In the present study, salbutamol significantly improved muscle mass, grip strength, antioxidant levels, and muscle architecture in HFD/STZ-induced diabetic rats. Furthermore, muscle metabolomics analysis showed that salbutamol significantly restored the altered metabolites such as sarcosine, HTR, PTR, EQR, succinate, and 3-hydroxybutyrate in diabetic rats. Taken together, these findings showed that salbutamol attenuated skeletal muscle atrophy in HFD/STZ-induced diabetic rats. The results showed that salbutamol significantly increased body weight and gastrocnemius (GN) muscle weight but did not alter blood glucose levels in HFD/STZ-induced diabetic rats. Emery et al. showed that 16 days of treatment with β2 agonists, viz. clenbuterol and fenoterol, increased the body weight and GN muscle mass as compared to the control rat [59]. A low dose of clenbuterol improved glucose homeostasis in insulin-resistant rats. This was most likely mediated by increasing glucose absorption in skeletal muscle, which increased insulin sensitivity. A finding showed that salbutamol increased the GN muscle weight and protein content in both young and senescent rats [19]. Clinical studies in human subjects demonstrate that salbutamol treatment increased lean body mass, muscle strength, and endurance [20]. Our findings also showed that salbutamol significantly increased the lean mass and grip strength in diabetic rats. These findings indicate that salbutamol has the potential to increase muscle mass. Furthermore, protein accretion is linked to skeletal muscle growth, and muscle protein pools primarily contain myofibril, mitochondrial, and sarcoplasmic proteins [20]. Our results showed that salbutamol had a higher myofibrillar protein content in GN muscle as compared to diabetic rats. Recent findings have demonstrated that the β2-agonist salbutamol promotes the transition of the muscle fiber isoform from MHC-I to MHCIIa [21]. Moreover, salbutamol intervention in resistance exercise increased the myofibrillar protein fractionation rate and turnover in young men [20]. Next, we checked the levels of testosterone and muscle damage markers, viz. creatine kinase and myostatin. Intriguingly, treatment with salbutamol increased testosterone levels in diabetic rats, which is consistent with the finding that salbutamol considerably increased plasma testosterone levels in athletic men following submaximal exercise [60]. Myostatin (also known as GDF-8) is a negative regulator that affects skeletal muscle growth [61]. Our results showed that salbutamol significantly decreased myostatin levels in diabetic rats. The results were also in line with findings where type 2 diabetic subjects showed increased mRNA expression of muscle myostatin linked to metabolism and systemic inflammation [62]. Contrary to the results presented here, salbutamol was shown to increase myostatin mRNA levels; however, this effect could be neutralized by the concomitant downregulation of activinRIIB, which is associated with resistance training [20]. Our results showed that salbutamol significantly decreased serum creatine kinase (CK) levels in diabetic rats. Because muscle has a large phosphocreatine reserve, changes in CK levels are associated with muscle injury and inflammation. Increased activity in the muscle implies muscular damage and CK leakage from the muscles. Earlier findings showed that creatine kinase levels were elevated in diabetic rats [63]. Thus, elevated serum CK levels observed in exercise-induced muscle damage can lead to the activation of pro-inflammatory markers. This activation can occur due to the destabilization of the cell and membrane, resulting in the infiltration of leukocytes during the process of repair. Next, we assessed the levels of serum inflammatory markers, including IL-2, IL-6, and IL-1β, and observed a significant increase in these markers in diabetic rats. However, our findings indicated that salbutamol treatment significantly restored these levels, suggesting that salbutamol possesses anti-inflammatory properties. Further, our results demonstrated that salbutamol significantly restored the levels of superoxide dismutase, catalase, and glutathione in the GN muscle of diabetic rats. These enzymes and molecules act as antioxidants, and their restoration by salbutamol suggests its potential role in mitigating oxidative stress in diabetic conditions.

Furthermore, GN muscle oxidative stress (MDA and protein carbonyl content) levels were significantly decreased by salbutamol treatment in diabetic rats. Previous studies have shown that salbutamol exerts significant antioxidative effects in rat models [64]. Moreover, our results showed that salbutamol treatment significantly increased the muscle fiber size and cross-sectional area in diabetic muscle. These findings demonstrate that salbutamol can attenuate muscle cellular architecture, highlighting its potential anti-atrophy properties in diabetic-induced skeletal muscle wasting.

Previous findings have demonstrated that the β-2 agonist formoterol significantly increases muscle fiber size, area, and contractile performance in skeletal muscles [17]. Taken together, our findings support the notion that beta-2 agonists could be effective interventions against muscle wasting disorders.

Next, we carried the ^{1}H NMR muscle metabolomics to investigate the effects of salbutamol on diabetes-induced alterations in muscle metabolites. Findings showed that amino acids metabolites (e.g., glycine, histidine, tyrosine, and sarcosine), energy metabolites (e.g., choline, acetate, creatine, lactate, and succinate), and ketone bodies (e.g., betaine, 3-hydroxybutyrate, and isobutyrate) were significantly altered in diabetic skeletal muscles. Furthermore, metabolites levels of succinate, 3-hydroxybutyrate (3-HB), and the ratios of histidine-to-tyrosine (HTR), phenylalanine-to-tyrosine (PTR), and glutamate-to-glutamine ratio (EQR), were elevated in the HFD/STZ-induced diabetic group, and salbutamol treatment restored these levels (Figure 10). Succinate is primarily recognized as a metabolite that serves as an intermediate in the tricarboxylic acid (TCA) cycle and plays a vital role in mitochondrial metabolism and ATP generation. However, recent studies have revealed that succinate has broader implications beyond being a substrate for succinate dehydrogenase and the respiratory chain [65]. Our findings indicated a significant increase in succinate levels in diabetic muscle while salbutamol treatment restored the same. Changes in the altered levels of succinate (an intermediate of the TCA cycle) may affect energy balance and muscle insulin sensitivity [66]. Moreover, recent in vitro and in vivo studies have demonstrated that succinate supplementation can disrupt skeletal muscle homeostasis and impair muscle regeneration [65]. These findings suggest that defects in the TCA cycle are commonly observed in wasting skeletal muscle, and diabetic muscle is not an exception. Furthermore, previous metabolomics and transcriptomic studies have shown that the loss of succinate dehydrogenase (SDH) results in an excessive accumulation of succinate [67], which is consistent with the findings of our study. These studies have also revealed that SDH deficiency leads to the inappropriate activation of the mTORC1 pathway in β-cells, subsequently leading to mitochondrial dysfunction [67]. Overall, succinate appears to have multifaceted roles beyond its traditional function in the TCA cycle. Its dysregulation may contribute to skeletal muscle dysfunction and impaired regeneration observed in various pathological conditions, including diabetes [65]. Furthermore, intervention with salbutamol resulted in the restoration of the altered skeletal muscle metabolites. Our findings demonstrated a significant increase in 3-HB levels in the skeletal muscle of diabetic rats compared to the control group. Further, increased production of ketone bodies, such as β-hydroxybutyrate and acetoacetate, results in ketonemia. Moreover, the findings revealed that α-hydroxybutyrate, an organic acid derived from α-ketobutyrate, is a potential biomarker of insulin sensitivity in individuals with normal glucose tolerance. These findings suggest that impaired glucose metabolism and disrupted insulin regulation in diabetes indicate disturbances in fatty acid oxidation [68,69]. An elevated level of circulatory PTR (for oxidative markers) and HTR (for inflammatory markers) indicates that disease-induced oxidative stress and inflammation, and hyper-activation of the immune system led to predicated disease [53,70]. PTR and HTR assess the body's capacity to convert phenylalanine to tyrosine and the histidine-to-tyrosine ratio. The conversion enzyme requires cofactors, such as tetrahydrobiopterin (BH4), niacin (B3), and iron. Increasing the muscle PTR ratio may aid in diagnosing inflammatory disease and a person's catabolic stage [71]. To preserve physiological homeostasis and fulfill the energy demands of muscle cells, it is necessary to increase their dependence on additional energy sources [72]. As a direct result, several gluconeogenic amino acids, including glutamine and glutamate, were present at lower concentrations in the diabetic group. The consumption of glutamine is directly associated with the suppression of inflammatory reactions in skeletal muscle [73]. In addition, extracellular glutamine concentration can control the production of the adaptor protein GRB10 and has a direct impact on the muscle's inflammatory response [73]. Next, sarcosine, chemically known as N-methyl glycine, is an intermediate in glycine biosynthesis and degradation and a glycine transporter inhibitor. However, sarcosine levels are governed by sarcosine dehydrogenase, an enzyme that converts sarcosine to glycine, and dimethylglycine dehydrogenase, which produces sarcosine from dimethylglycine. Owing to their capacity to regulate sarcosine levels in myonuclei cells, these enzymes may be essential for controlling sarcomere protein degradation [74]. Our ^{1}H-NMR metabolomics analysis identified an intriguing and less-studied metabolite called sarcosine. It revealed a significant increase in sarcosine levels in diabetic muscle compared to the control group. Only one study has shown elevated sarcosine levels in rats exposed to a high-fructose and high-fat diet, utilizing LC/TOF-MS urine metabolomics analysis [75]. Interestingly, sarcosine has drawn attention as a potential biomarker for aggressive and metastatic prostate cancer, as elevated levels have been observed in tumors associated with this condition [76]. Sarcosine has been shown to activate autophagy in cultured cells and boosts autophagic flux in vivo, suggesting that it may play a role in the induction of autophagy caused by dietary constraints [77]. Additionally, a recent study published in the 'Lancet' found higher sarcosine levels in individuals who exhibited resistance to dietary changes following exercise training. This study involved muscle metabolomics combined with MS/MS analysis of plasma amino acids [78]. Taken together, these findings suggest that sarcosine may play a role in metabolic diseases and provide new evidence highlighting its significance in diabetic skeletal muscles. However, further research is necessary to fully elucidate the role of sarcosine in these conditions and explore its potential as a diagnostic or therapeutic target.

5. Conclusions

In conclusion, the findings of this study suggest that salbutamol has the potential to improve skeletal muscle atrophy in diabetic rats. Our results demonstrated that salbutamol significantly increased grip strength and lean muscle mass in diabetic rats. Also, salbutamol treatment results in increased levels of antioxidants in the muscles and reduced muscle atrophy and inflammatory markers, and restored muscle damage biomarkers that indicate its potential to reduce muscle inflammation and oxidative stress. Furthermore, the GN muscle metabolomics markers identified in this study could serve as valuable prognostic markers for diabetic skeletal muscle atrophy. Overall, these findings highlight the potential of salbutamol as a therapeutic intervention for managing skeletal muscle atrophy associated with diabetes.

6. Limitation of the Study

In the present study, our focus was solely on investigating the effects of salbutamol on lean mass, oxidative stress, inflammatory markers, and muscle metabolomics of gastrocnemius muscles in HFD/STZ-induced type 2 diabetic rats. The main limitation of this study is that we did not assess the protein expressions of muscle damage markers or investigate the specific mechanism by which salbutamol balances protein synthesis and degradation. Further, more preclinical studies and detailed molecular mechanisms will provide a comprehensive understanding of how salbutamol reduces muscle atrophy in diabetic skeletal muscle.

Supplementary Materials: The following supporting information can be downloaded at https://www.mdpi.com/article/10.3390/pharmaceutics15082101/s1. Figure S1: Stack plot of representative 800 MHz one-dimensional ^{1}H CPMG NMR spectra of rat GN muscle of rat samples of four study groups; Figure S2: Multivariate statistical analysis.

Author Contributions: Conceptualization, A.K. and S.K.; methodology, A.K.; software, P.P. and G.S.; validation, A.K., D.K. and V.M.; formal analysis, A.K.; investigation, A.K.; resources, S.-C.K.; data curation, A.K., P.P., D.K. and V.M.; writing—original draft preparation, A.K. and S.K.; writing—review and editing, A.K., S.-C.K., C.J.R., V.R. and S.K.; visualization, A.K. and G.S.; supervision, C.J.R., V.R. and S.K.; project administration, C.J.R., V.R. and S.K.; funding acquisition, A.K., S.-C.K., C.J.R., V.R. and S.K. All authors have read and agreed to the published version of the manuscript.

Funding: This work was supported by a University Grants Commission (UGC) startup grant (F. 30-460/2019) (BSR) to Sapana Kushwaha and Indian Council of Medical Research-Senior Research Fellowship (ICMR-SRF) (File no-3/1/3/8/Dis & Rehab/2022-NCD-II) to Anand Kumar. This research was also supported by the Basic Science Research Program through the National Research Foundation of Korea (NRF), funded by the Ministry of Education (2020R1I1A3052258) and by the Technology Development Program (S3060516) funded by the Ministry of SMEs and Startups (MSS, Republic of Korea) 2021.

Institutional Review Board Statement: The animal study procedure was approved by the Institutional Review Board (Institutional Animal Care and Use Committee) of BBDNIT, Lucknow (IAEC no. BBDNIIT/IAEC/2019/10; dated 27 March 2019).

Informed Consent Statement: Not applicable.

Data Availability Statement: The data supporting the findings of this study are available upon request from the corresponding author.

Acknowledgments: The authors are grateful to Babasaheb Bhimrao Ambedkar University, Lucknow, India, for providing the infrastructure required for this study. We thank the Centre of Biomedical Research (CBMR), Lucknow, India, for providing the NMR facility. Anand Kumar acknowledges the Indian Council of Medical Research (ICMR) in New Delhi, India, for a research fellowship under the ICMR-SRF scheme. We express our gratitude to N Chattopadhyay, Chief Scientist at the Central Drug Research Institute, Lucknow, India, for generously granting us access to their Echo MRI facility to assess body mass composition.

Conflicts of Interest: The authors declare no conflict of interest.

References

1. D'Souza, D.M.; Al-Sajee, D.; Hawke, T.J. Diabetic myopathy: Impact of diabetes mellitus on skeletal muscle progenitor cells. *Front. Physiol.* **2013**, *4*, 379. [CrossRef] [PubMed]
2. Cho, N.H.; Shaw, J.E.; Karuranga, S.; Huang, Y.; da Rocha Fernandes, J.D.; Ohlrogge, A.W.; Malanda, B. IDF Diabetes Atlas: Global estimates of diabetes prevalence for 2017 and projections for 2045. *Diabetes Res. Clin. Pract.* **2018**, *138*, 271–281. [CrossRef]
3. Chawla, A.; Chawla, R.; Jaggi, S. Microvasular and macrovascular complications in diabetes mellitus: Distinct or continuum? *Indian J. Endocrinol. Metab.* **2016**, *20*, 546–551. [CrossRef]
4. Viigimaa, M.; Sachinidis, A.; Toumpourleka, M.; Koutsampasopoulos, K.; Alliksoo, S.; Titma, T. Macrovascular Complications of Type 2 Diabetes Mellitus. *Curr. Vasc. Pharmacol.* **2020**, *18*, 110–116. [CrossRef] [PubMed]
5. Hernández-Ochoa, E.O.; Llanos, P.; Lanner, J.T. The Underlying Mechanisms of Diabetic Myopathy. *J. Diabetes Res.* **2017**, *2017*, 7485738. [CrossRef] [PubMed]
6. Rusbana, T.B.; Agista, A.Z.; Saputra, W.D.; Ohsaki, Y.; Watanabe, K.; Ardiansyah, A.; Budijanto, S.; Koseki, T.; Aso, H.; Komai, M.; et al. Supplementation with Fermented Rice Bran Attenuates Muscle Atrophy in a Diabetic Rat Model. *Nutrients* **2020**, *12*, 2409. [CrossRef] [PubMed]
7. Csapo, R.; Gumpenberger, M.; Wessner, B. Skeletal Muscle Extracellular Matrix—What Do We Know about Its Composition, Regulation, and Physiological Roles? A Narrative Review. *Front. Physiol.* **2020**, *11*, 253. [CrossRef] [PubMed]
8. Pedersen, B.K.; Febbraio, M.A. Muscles, exercise and obesity: Skeletal muscle as a secretory organ. *Nat. Rev. Endocrinol.* **2012**, *8*, 457–465. [CrossRef]
9. Yang, J. Enhanced skeletal muscle for effective glucose homeostasis. *Prog. Mol. Biol. Transl. Sci.* **2014**, *121*, 133–163.
10. Yaribeygi, H.; Sathyapalan, T.; Atkin, S.L.; Sahebkar, A. Molecular Mechanisms Linking Oxidative Stress and Diabetes Mellitus. *Oxid. Med. Cell Longev.* **2020**, *2020*, 8609213. [CrossRef]
11. Aragno, M.; Mastrocola, R.; Catalano, M.G.; Brignardello, E.; Danni, O.; Boccuzzi, G. Oxidative stress impairs skeletal muscle repair in diabetic rats. *Diabetes* **2004**, *53*, 1082–1088. [CrossRef] [PubMed]
12. Okun, J.G.; Rusu, P.M.; Chan, A.Y.; Wu, Y.; Yap, Y.W.; Sharkie, T.; Schumacher, J.; Schmidt, K.V.; Roberts-Thomson, K.M.; Russell, R.D.; et al. Liver alanine catabolism promotes skeletal muscle atrophy and hyperglycaemia in type 2 diabetes. *Nat. Metab.* **2021**, *3*, 394–409. [CrossRef]
13. Webster, J.M.; Kempen, L.; Hardy, R.S.; Langen, R.C.J. Inflammation and Skeletal Muscle Wasting During Cachexia. *Front. Physiol.* **2020**, *11*, 597675. [CrossRef] [PubMed]
14. Price, S.R.; Bailey, J.L.; Wang, X.; Jurkovitz, C.; England, B.K.; Ding, X.; Phillips, L.S.; Mitch, W.E. Muscle wasting in insulinopenic rats results from activation of the ATP-dependent, ubiquitin-proteasome proteolytic pathway by a mechanism including gene transcription. *J. Clin. Investig.* **1996**, *98*, 1703–1708. [CrossRef]
15. Gonçalves, D.A.P.; Lira, E.C.; Baviera, A.M.; Cao, P.; Zanon, N.M.; Arany, Z.; Bedard, N.; Tanksale, P.; Wing, S.S.; Lecker, S.H.; et al. Mechanisms Involved in 3′,5′-Cyclic Adenosine Monophosphate-Mediated Inhibition of the Ubiquitin-Proteasome System in Skeletal Muscle. *Endocrinology* **2009**, *150*, 5395–5404.

16. Gonçalves, D.A.; Silveira, W.A.; Lira, E.C.; Graca, F.A.; Paula-Gomes, S.; Zanon, N.M.; Kettelhut, I.C.; Navegantes, L.C.C. Clenbuterol suppresses proteasomal and lysosomal proteolysis and atrophy-related genes in denervated rat soleus muscles independently of Akt. *Am. J. Physiol. Endocrinol. Metab.* **2012**, *302*, 123–133. [CrossRef]
17. Gonçalves, D.A.; Silveira, W.A.; Manfredi, L.H.; Graca, F.A.; Amrani, A.; Bertaggia, E.; Neill, B.T.O.; Lautherbach, N.; Machado, J.; Nogara, J.; et al. Insulin/IGF1 signalling mediates the effects of β(2)-adrenergic agonist on muscle proteostasis and growth. *J. Cachexia Sarcopenia Muscle* **2019**, *10*, 455–475. [CrossRef]
18. Hostrup, M.; Kalsen, A.; Auchenberg, M.; Bangsbo, J.; Backer, V. Effects of acute and 2-week administration of oral salbutamol on exercise performance and muscle strength in athletes. *Scand J. Med. Sci. Sports* **2016**, *26*, 8–16. [CrossRef] [PubMed]
19. Carter, W.J.; Lynch, M.E. Comparison of the effects of salbutamol and clenbuterol on skeletal muscle mass and carcass composition in senescent rats. *Metabolism* **1994**, *43*, 1119–1125. [CrossRef] [PubMed]
20. Hostrup, M.; Reitelseder, S.; Jessen, S.; Kalsen, A.; Nyberg, M.; Egelund, J.; Kreiberg, M.; Kristensen, C.M.; Thomassen, M.; Pilegaard, H.; et al. Beta$_2$-adrenoceptor agonist salbutamol increases protein turnover rates and alters signalling in skeletal muscle after resistance exercise in young men. *J. Physiol.* **2018**, *596*, 4121–4139. [CrossRef] [PubMed]
21. Jessen, S.; Reitelseder, S.; Kalsen, A.; Kreiberg, M.; Onslev, J.; Gad, A.; Ørtenblad, N.; Backer, V.; Holm, L.; Bangsbo, J.; et al. β$_2$-Adrenergic agonist salbutamol augments hypertrophy in MHCIIa fibers and sprint mean power output but not muscle force during 11 weeks of resistance training in young men. *J. Appl. Physiol.* **2021**, *130*, 617–626. [CrossRef] [PubMed]
22. Koeberl, D.D.; Case, L.E.; Desai, A.; Smith, E.C.; Walters, C.; Han, S.-O.; Thurberg, B.L.; Young, S.P.; Bali, D.; Kishnani, P.S. Improved muscle function in a phase I/II clinical trial of albuterol in Pompe disease. *Mol. Genet. Metab.* **2020**, *129*, 67–72. [CrossRef] [PubMed]
23. Menni, C.; Fauman, E.; Erte, I.; Perry, J.R.; Kastenmüller, G.; Shin, S.Y.; Petersen, A.K.; Hyde, C.; Psatha, M.; Ward, K.J.; et al. Biomarkers for type 2 diabetes and impaired fasting glucose using a nontargeted metabolomics approach. *Diabetes* **2013**, *62*, 4270–4276. [CrossRef] [PubMed]
24. Mora-Ortiz, M.; Nuñez Ramos, P.; Oregioni, A.; Claus, S.P. NMR metabolomics identifies over 60 biomarkers associated with Type II Diabetes impairment in db/db mice. *Metabolomics* **2019**, *15*, 89. [CrossRef]
25. Del Coco, L.; Vergara, D.; De Matteis, S.; Mensà, E.; Sabbatinelli, J.; Prattichizzo, F.; Bonfigli, A.R.; Storci, G.; Bravaccini, S.; Pirini, F.; et al. NMR-Based Metabolomic Approach Tracks Potential Serum Biomarkers of Disease Progression in Patients with Type 2 Diabetes Mellitus. *J. Clin. Med.* **2019**, *8*, 720. [CrossRef] [PubMed]
26. Andreassen, C.S.; Jensen, J.M.; Jakobsen, J.; Ulhøj, B.P.; Andersen, H. Striated muscle fiber size, composition, and capillary density in diabetes in relation to neuropathy and muscle strength. *J. Diabetes* **2014**, *6*, 462–471. [CrossRef]
27. Ato, S.; Kido, K.; Sato, K.; Fujita, S. Type 2 diabetes causes skeletal muscle atrophy but does not impair resistance training-mediated myonuclear accretion and muscle mass gain in rats. *Exp. Physiol.* **2019**, *104*, 1518–1531. [CrossRef] [PubMed]
28. Srinivasan, K.; Viswanad, B.; Asrat, L.; Kaul, C.; Ramarao, P. Combination of high-fat diet-fed and low-dose streptozotocin-treated rat: A model for type 2 diabetes and pharmacological screening. *Pharmacol. Res.* **2005**, *52*, 313–320. [CrossRef] [PubMed]
29. Ozogul, B.; Halici, Z.; Cadirci, E.; Karagoz, E.; Bayraktutan, Z.; Yayla, M.; Akpinar, E.; Atamanalp, S.S.; Unal, D.; Karamese, M. Comparative study on effects of nebulized and oral salbutamol on a cecal ligation and puncture-induced sepsis model in rats. *Drug Res.* **2015**, *65*, 192–198. [CrossRef] [PubMed]
30. Caccia, S.; Fong, M.H. Kinetics and distribution of the β-adrenergic agonist salbutamol in rat brain. *J. Pharm. Pharmacol.* **1984**, *36*, 200–202. [CrossRef]
31. Nixon, J.P.; Zhang, M.; Wang, C.; Kuskowski, M.A.; Novak, C.M.; Levine, J.A.; Billington, C.J.; Kotz, C.M. Evaluation of a quantitative magnetic resonance imaging system for whole body composition analysis in rodents. *Obesity* **2010**, *18*, 1652–1659. [CrossRef] [PubMed]
32. China, S.P.; Pal, S.; Chattopadhyay, S.; Porwal, K.; Kushwaha, S.; Bhattacharyya, S.; Mittal, M.; Gurjar, A.A.; Barbhuyan, T.; Singh, A.K.; et al. Globular adiponectin reverses osteo-sarcopenia and altered body composition in ovariectomized rats. *Bone* **2017**, *105*, 75–86. [CrossRef] [PubMed]
33. Meyer, O.A.; Tilson, H.A.; Byrd, W.C.; Riley, M.T. A method for the routine assessment of fore- and hindlimb grip strength of rats and mice. *Neurobehav. Toxicol.* **1979**, *1*, 233–236.
34. Cabe, P.A.; Tilson, H.A.; Mitchell, C.L.; Dennis, R. A simple recording grip strength device. *Pharmacol. Biochem. Behav.* **1978**, *8*, 101–102. [CrossRef] [PubMed]
35. Sachan, N.; Saraswat, N.; Chandra, P.; Khalid, M.; Kabra, A. Isolation of Thymol from Trachyspermum ammi Fruits for Treatment of Diabetes and Diabetic Neuropathy in STZ-Induced Rats. *Biomed. Res. Int.* **2022**, *2022*, 8263999. [CrossRef]
36. Mu, S.; OuYang, L.; Liu, B.; Zhu, Y.; Li, K.; Zhan, M.; Liu, Z.; Jia, Y.; Lei, W.; Reiner, A. Preferential interneuron survival in the transition zone of 3-NP-induced striatal injury in rats. *J. Neurosci. Res.* **2011**, *89*, 744–754. [CrossRef] [PubMed]
37. Mendes, C.S.; Bartos, I.; Márka, Z.; Akay, T.; Márka, S.; Mann, R.S. Quantification of gait parameters in freely walking rodents. *BMC Biol.* **2015**, *13*, 50. [CrossRef] [PubMed]
38. Koopman, R.; Gehrig, S.M.; Léger, B.; Trieu, J.; Walrand, S.; Murphy, K.T.; Lynch, G.S. Cellular mechanisms underlying temporal changes in skeletal muscle protein synthesis and breakdown during chronic β-adrenoceptor stimulation in mice. *J. Physiol.* **2010**, *588*, 4811–4823. [CrossRef] [PubMed]
39. Hornberger, T.A., Jr.; Farrar, R.P. Physiological hypertrophy of the FHL muscle following 8 weeks of progressive resistance exercise in the rat. *Can. J. Appl. Physiol.* **2004**, *29*, 16–31. [CrossRef] [PubMed]

40. Ohkawa, H.; Ohishi, N.; Yagi, K. Assay for lipid peroxides in animal tissues by thiobarbituric acid reaction. *Anal. Biochem.* **1979**, *95*, 351–358. [CrossRef]
41. Wehr, N.B.; Levine, R.L. Quantification of protein carbonylation. *Methods Mol. Biol.* **2013**, *965*, 265–281. [PubMed]
42. Rahman, I.; Kode, A.; Biswas, S.K. Assay for quantitative determination of glutathione and glutathione disulfide levels using enzymatic recycling method. *Nat. Protoc.* **2006**, *1*, 3159–3165. [CrossRef] [PubMed]
43. Weydert, C.J.; Cullen, J.J. Measurement of superoxide dismutase, catalase and glutathione peroxidase in cultured cells and tissue. *Nat. Protoc.* **2010**, *5*, 51–66. [CrossRef] [PubMed]
44. Takada, S.; Kinugawa, S.; Hirabayashi, K.; Suga, T.; Yokota, T.; Takahashi, M.; Fukushima, A.; Homma, T.; Ono, T.; Sobirin, M.A.; et al. Angiotensin II receptor blocker improves the lowered exercise capacity and impaired mitochondrial function of the skeletal muscle in type 2 diabetic mice. *J. Appl. Physiol.* **2013**, *114*, 844–857. [CrossRef] [PubMed]
45. Beckonert, O.; Keun, H.C.; Ebbels, T.M.; Bundy, J.; Holmes, E.; Lindon, J.C.; Nicholson, J.K. Metabolic profiling, metabolomic and metabonomic procedures for NMR spectroscopy of urine, plasma, serum and tissue extracts. *Nat. Protoc.* **2007**, *2*, 2692–2703. [CrossRef] [PubMed]
46. Guleria, A.; Misra, D.P.; Rawat, A.; Dubey, D.; Khetrapal, C.L.; Bacon, P.; Misra, R.; Kumar, D. NMR-Based Serum Metabolomics Discriminates Takayasu Arteritis from Healthy Individuals: A Proof-of-Principle Study. *J. Proteome Res.* **2015**, *14*, 3372–3381. [CrossRef] [PubMed]
47. Wishart, D.S.; Jewison, T.; Guo, A.C.; Wilson, M.; Knox, C.; Liu, Y.; Djoumbou, Y.; Mandal, R.; Aziat, F.; Dong, E.; et al. HMDB 3.0--The Human Metabolome Database in 2013. *Nucleic Acids Res.* **2013**, *41*, D801–D807. [CrossRef] [PubMed]
48. Guleria, A.; Bajpai, N.K.; Rawat, A.; Khetrapal, C.L.; Prasad, N.; Kumar, D. Metabolite characterisation in peritoneal dialysis effluent using high-resolution (1) H and (1) H-(13) C NMR spectroscopy. *Magn. Reson. Chem.* **2014**, *52*, 475–479. [CrossRef] [PubMed]
49. Guleria, A.; Pratap, A.; Dubey, D.; Rawat, A.; Chaurasia, S.; Sukesh, E.; Phatak, S.; Ajmani, S.; Kumar, U.; Khetrapal, C.L.; et al. NMR based serum metabolomics reveals a distinctive signature in patients with Lupus Nephritis. *Sci. Rep.* **2016**, *6*, 35309. [CrossRef] [PubMed]
50. Walejko, J.M.; Chelliah, A.; Keller-Wood, M.; Gregg, A.; Edison, A.S. Global Metabolomics of the Placenta Reveals Distinct Metabolic Profiles between Maternal and Fetal Placental Tissues Following Delivery in Non-Labored Women. *Metabolites* **2018**, *8*, 10. [CrossRef] [PubMed]
51. Singh, A.; Prakash, V.; Gupta, N.; Kumar, A.; Kant, R.; Kumar, D. Serum Metabolic Disturbances in Lung Cancer Investigated through an Elaborative NMR-Based Serum Metabolomics Approach. *ACS Omega* **2022**, *7*, 5510–5520. [CrossRef] [PubMed]
52. Kumar, U.; Kumar, A.; Singh, S.; Arya, P.; Singh, S.K.; Chaurasia, R.N.; Singh, A.; Kumar, D. An elaborative NMR based plasma metabolomics study revealed metabolic derangements in patients with mild cognitive impairment: A study on north Indian population. *Metab. Brain Dis.* **2021**, *36*, 957–968. [CrossRef] [PubMed]
53. Kumar, U.; Sharma, S.; Durgappa, M.; Gupta, N.; Raj, R.; Kumar, A.; Sharma, P.N.; Krishna, V.P.; Kumar, R.V.; Guleria, A.; et al. Serum Metabolic Disturbances Associated with Acute-on-chronic Liver Failure in Patients with Underlying Alcoholic Liver Diseases: An Elaborative NMR-based Metabolomics Study. *J. Pharm. Bioallied Sci.* **2021**, *13*, 276–282. [PubMed]
54. Cassiède, M.; Nair, S.; Dueck, M.; Mino, J.; McKay, R.; Mercier, P.; Quémerais, B.; Lacy, P. Assessment of (1)H NMR-based metabolomics analysis for normalization of urinary metals against creatinine. *Clin. Chim. Acta* **2017**, *464*, 37–43. [CrossRef] [PubMed]
55. Bassit, R.A.; Sawada, L.A.; Bacurau, R.F.; Navarro, F.; Costa Rosa, L.F. The effect of BCAA supplementation upon the immune response of triathletes. *Med. Sci. Sports Exerc.* **2000**, *32*, 1214–1219. [CrossRef] [PubMed]
56. Shah, M.; Mamyrova, G.; Targoff, I.N.; Huber, A.M.; Malley, J.D.; Rice, M.M.; Miller, F.W.; Rider, L.G. The clinical phenotypes of the juvenile idiopathic inflammatory myopathies. *Medicine* **2013**, *92*, 25–41. [CrossRef] [PubMed]
57. Chen, T.; Cao, Y.; Zhang, Y.; Liu, J.; Bao, Y.; Wang, C.; Jia, W.; Zhao, A. Random forest in clinical metabolomics for phenotypic discrimination and biomarker selection. *Evid. Based Complement. Altern. Med.* **2013**, *2013*, 298183. [CrossRef]
58. Xia, J.; Wishart, D.S. Using MetaboAnalyst 3.0 for Comprehensive Metabolomics Data Analysis. *Curr. Protoc. Bioinform.* **2016**, *55*, 14.10.11–14.10.91. [CrossRef] [PubMed]
59. Emery, P.W.; Rothwell, N.J.; Stock, M.J.; Winter, P.D. Chronic effects of beta 2-adrenergic agonists on body composition and protein synthesis in the rat. *Biosci. Rep.* **1984**, *4*, 83–91. [CrossRef] [PubMed]
60. Collomp, K.; Candau, R.; Lasne, F.; Labsy, Z.; Préfaut, C.; De Ceaurriz, J. Effects of short-term oral salbutamol administration on exercise endurance and metabolism. *J. Appl. Physiol.* **2000**, *89*, 430–436. [CrossRef] [PubMed]
61. McPherron, A.C.; Lawler, A.M.; Lee, S.J. Regulation of skeletal muscle mass in mice by a new TGF-beta superfamily member. *Nature* **1997**, *387*, 83–90. [CrossRef] [PubMed]
62. Brandt, C.; Nielsen, A.R.; Fischer, C.P.; Hansen, J.; Pedersen, B.K.; Plomgaard, P. Plasma and muscle myostatin in relation to type 2 diabetes. *PLoS ONE* **2012**, *7*, e37236. [CrossRef] [PubMed]
63. Yadav, A.; Singh, A.; Phogat, J.; Dahuja, A.; Dabur, R. Magnoflorine prevent the skeletal muscle atrophy via Akt/mTOR/FoxO signal pathway and increase slow-MyHC production in streptozotocin-induced diabetic rats. *J. Ethnopharmacol.* **2021**, *267*, 113510. [CrossRef] [PubMed]

64. Uzkeser, H.; Cadirci, E.; Halici, Z.; Odabasoglu, F.; Polat, B.; Yuksel, T.N.; Ozaltin, S.; Atalay, F. Anti-inflammatory and antinociceptive effects of salbutamol on acute and chronic models of inflammation in rats: Involvement of an antioxidant mechanism. *Mediat. Inflamm.* **2012**, *2012*, 438912. [CrossRef]
65. Arneson-Wissink, P.C.; Hogan, K.A.; Ducharme, A.M.; Samani, A.; Jatoi, A.; Doles, J.D. The wasting-associated metabolite succinate disrupts myogenesis and impairs skeletal muscle regeneration. *JCSM Rapid Commun.* **2020**, *3*, 56–69. [CrossRef]
66. Jessen, S.; Baasch-Skytte, T.; Onslev, J.; Eibye, K.; Backer, V.; Bangsbo, J.; Hostrup, M. Muscle hypertrophic effect of inhaled beta$_2$-agonist is associated with augmented insulin-stimulated whole-body glucose disposal in young men. *J. Physiol.* **2022**, *600*, 2345–2357. [CrossRef]
67. Lee, S.; Xu, H.; Van Vleck, A.; Mawla, A.M.; Li, A.M.; Ye, J.; Huising, M.O.; Annes, J.P. β-Cell Succinate Dehydrogenase Deficiency Triggers Metabolic Dysfunction and Insulinopenic Diabetes. *Diabetes* **2022**, *71*, 1439–1453. [CrossRef] [PubMed]
68. Mahendran, Y.; Vangipurapu, J.; Cederberg, H.; Stancáková, A.; Pihlajamäki, J.; Soininen, P.; Kangas, A.J.; Paananen, J.; Civelek, M.; Saleem, N.K.; et al. Association of ketone body levels with hyperglycemia and type 2 diabetes in 9,398 Finnish men. *Diabetes* **2013**, *62*, 3618–3626. [CrossRef] [PubMed]
69. Gall, W.E.; Beebe, K.; Lawton, K.A.; Adam, K.P.; Mitchell, M.W.; Nakhle, P.J.; Ryals, J.A.; Milburn, M.V.; Nannipieri, M.; Camastra, S.; et al. alpha-hydroxybutyrate is an early biomarker of insulin resistance and glucose intolerance in a nondiabetic population. *PLoS ONE* **2010**, *5*, e10883. [CrossRef] [PubMed]
70. Muhammed, H.; Kumar, D.; Dubey, D.; Kumar, S.; Chaurasia, S.; Guleria, A.; Majumder, S.; Singh, R.; Agarwal, V.; Misra, R. Metabolomics analysis revealed significantly higher synovial Phe/Tyr ratio in reactive arthritis and undifferentiated spondyloarthropathy. *Rheumatology* **2020**, *59*, 1587–1590. [CrossRef] [PubMed]
71. Wannemacher, R.W., Jr.; Klainer, A.S.; Dinterman, R.E.; Beisel, W.R. The significance and mechanism of an increased serum phenylalanine-tyrosine ratio during infection. *Am. J. Clin. Nutr.* **1976**, *29*, 997–1006. [CrossRef]
72. Armstrong, R.B.; Ianuzzo, C.D. Decay of succinate dehydrogenase activity in rat skeletal muscle following streptozotocin injection. *Horm. Metab. Res.* **1976**, *8*, 392–394. [CrossRef] [PubMed]
73. Dollet, L.; Kuefner, M.; Caria, E.; Rizo-Roca, D.; Pendergrast, L.; Abdelmoez, A.M.; Karlsson, H.K.R.; Björnholm, M.; Dalbram, E.; Treebak, J.T.; et al. Glutamine Regulates Skeletal Muscle Immunometabolism in Type 2 Diabetes. *Diabetes* **2022**, *71*, 624–636. [CrossRef] [PubMed]
74. Benarrosh, A.; Garnotel, R.; Henry, A.; Arndt, C.; Gillery, P.; Motte, J.; Bakchine, S. A young adult with sarcosinemia. No benefit from long duration treatment with memantine. *JIMD Rep.* **2013**, *9*, 93–96. [PubMed]
75. Huang, C.F.; Chen, A.; Lin, S.Y.; Cheng, M.L.; Shiao, M.S.; Mao, T.Y. A metabolomics approach to investigate the proceedings of mitochondrial dysfunction in rats from prediabetes to diabetes. *Saudi J. Biol. Sci.* **2021**, *28*, 4762–4769. [CrossRef] [PubMed]
76. Cavaliere, B.; Macchione, B.; Monteleone, M.; Naccarato, A.; Sindona, G.; Tagarelli, A. Sarcosine as a marker in prostate cancer progression: A rapid and simple method for its quantification in human urine by solid-phase microextraction-gas chromatography-triple quadrupole mass spectrometry. *Anal. Bioanal. Chem.* **2011**, *400*, 2903–2912. [CrossRef] [PubMed]
77. Walters, R.O.; Arias, E.; Diaz, A.; Burgos, E.S.; Guan, F.; Tiano, S.; Mao, K.; Green, C.L.; Qiu, Y.; Shah, H.; et al. Sarcosine Is Uniquely Modulated by Aging and Dietary Restriction in Rodents and Humans. *Cell Rep.* **2018**, *25*, 663–676.e666. [CrossRef]
78. Pileggi, C.A.; Blondin, D.P.; Hooks, B.G.; Parmar, G.; Alecu, I.; Patten, D.A.; Cuillerier, A.; O'Dwyer, C.; Thrush, A.B.; Fullerton, M.D.; et al. Exercise training enhances muscle mitochondrial metabolism in diet-resistant obesity. *eBioMedicine* **2022**, *83*, 104192. [CrossRef]

Disclaimer/Publisher's Note: The statements, opinions and data contained in all publications are solely those of the individual author(s) and contributor(s) and not of MDPI and/or the editor(s). MDPI and/or the editor(s) disclaim responsibility for any injury to people or property resulting from any ideas, methods, instructions or products referred to in the content.

/ pharmaceutics

Article

Development and Evaluation of Solid Lipid Nanoparticles for the Clearance of Aβ in Alzheimer's Disease

Meghana Goravinahalli Shivananjegowda [1], Umme Hani [2], Riyaz Ali M. Osmani [1], Ali H. Alamri [2], Mohammed Ghazwani [2], Yahya Alhamhoom [2], Mohamed Rahamathulla [2], Sathishbabu Paranthaman [3], Devegowda Vishakante Gowda [4,*] and Ayesha Siddiqua [5]

[1] Department of Pharmaceutics, JSS College of Pharmacy, JSS Academy of Higher Education and Research, Mysuru 570015, India
[2] Department of Pharmaceutics, College of Pharmacy, King Khalid University, Abha 61421, Saudi Arabia
[3] Department of Cell Biology and Molecular Genetics, Sri Devaraj Urs Medical College, Sri Devaraj Urs Academy of Higher Education and Research, Kolar 563101, India
[4] Department of Pharmaceutics, Cauvery College of Pharmacy, Mysuru 570028, India
[5] Department of Clinical Pharmacy, College of Pharmacy, King Khalid University, Abha 62529, Saudi Arabia
* Correspondence: dvgccp3@gmail.com

Abstract: Aggregation of Amyloid-β (Aβ) leads to the formation and deposition of neurofibrillary tangles and plaques which is the main pathological hallmark of Alzheimer's disease (AD). The bioavailability of the drugs and their capability to cross the BBB plays a crucial role in the therapeutics of AD. The present study evaluates the Memantine Hydrochloride (MeHCl) and Tramiprosate (TMPS) loaded solid lipid nanoparticles (SLNs) for the clearance of Aβ on SHSY5Y cells in rat hippocampus. Molecular docking and in vitro Aβ fibrillation were used to ensure the binding of drugs to Aβ. The in vitro cell viability study showed that the M + T SLNs showed enhanced neuroprotection against SHSY5Y cells than the pure drugs (M + T PD) in presence of Aβ (80.35μM ± 0.455 μM) at a 3:1 molar ratio. The Box–Behnken Design (BBD) was employed to optimize the SLNs and the optimized M + T SLNs were further characterized by %drug entrapment efficiency (99.24 ± 3.24 of MeHCl and 89.99 ± 0.95 of TMPS), particle size (159.9 ± 0.569 nm), PDI (0.149 ± 0.08), Zeta potential (−6.4 ± 0.948 mV), Transmission Electron Microscopy (TEM), Atomic Force Microscopy (AFM) and in vitro drug release. The TEM & AFM analysis showed irregularly spherical morphology. In vitro release of SLNs was noted up to 48 h; whereas the pure drugs released completely within 3 h. M + T SLNs revealed an improved pharmacokinetic profile and a 4-fold increase in drug concentration in the brain when compared to the pure drug. Behavioral tests showed enhanced spatial memory and histological studies confirmed reduced Aβ plaques in rat hippocampus. Furthermore, the levels of Aβ decreased in AlCl$_3$-induced AD. Thus, all these noted results established that the M + T SLNs provide enhanced neuroprotective effects when compared to pure and individual drugs and can be a promising therapeutic strategy for the management of AD.

Keywords: drug delivery; nanotechnology; alzheimer's disease; Amyloid-β; solid lipid nanoparticles; SHSY5Y cells

1. Introduction

Alzheimer's disease (AD) is a progressive neurodegenerative disorder whose pathology is mainly driven by the presence of plaques and neurofibrillary tangles containing Amyloid-β (Aβ) and hyper-phosphorylated tau protein [1]. According to recent WHO reports, AD is the seventh leading cause of death and more than 55 million people live with dementia worldwide. The number is expected to rise to 78 million in 2030 and 139 million in 2050 [2]. Aβ is a protein that is produced in normal physiology, and is involved in reducing the excitatory activity of potassium channels and reducing neuronal apoptosis [3]. Impaired Aβ clearance and mutations in the human APP gene cause the development of

Aβ plaques and AD-like brain pathology [4]. Until June 2021 there was no particular drug targeting Aβ except a few symptomatic treatments such as acetylcholinesterase inhibitors & NMDA antagonists [5]. An Aβ antibody Aducanumab was recently approved by FDA which targets Aβ plaques the main hallmark [6]. The attributes that play a crucial role in delivering drugs to achieve a desired therapeutic outcome for treating AD are the blood brain barrier (BBB) penetration and bioavailability [7]. Nanotechnology-based delivery systems emerge as a ray of hope to overcome these drawbacks [8]. The lipid-based nanodelivery systems are promising tools for delivering drugs across BBB in comparison with conventional forms [9–11].

Solid lipid nanoparticles (SLN), among other nanoparticulate formulations, have lately received new consideration as a possible drug delivery system for brain targeting [12–14]. In order to treat neurodegenerative disorders in a nontoxic, safe, and efficient manner by crossing the BBB, solid lipid nanoparticles (SLNs) are one of the safest and least expensive drug carriers [12,13]. SLNs' functionality and effectiveness depend on their constituents, size, shape, physico-chemical properties, and the synthetic processes by which they are formed [14–16]. Here we make use of the SLNs in encapsulating memantine Hydrochloride (MeHCl) and Tramiprosate (TMPS). MeHCl is an NMDA antagonist and is known to slow down the neurotoxicity and reduce Aβ levels involved in AD [17]. Tramiprosate is an orally administered compound that binds to various amino acid residues of $Aβ_{1-42}$ [18] which results in the stabilization of Aβ monomers thereby preventing the formation of oligomers and fibrils.

This inhibition leads to neuroprotection by preventing subsequent deposition of Aβ. In order to improve its efficacy and reduce the adverse effects lipid-based nanoparticulate delivery would be feasible. The current study aims at targeting amyloid-β fibrillation [19] using lipid-based nanoparticles [20,21] carrying Aβ inhibitors (TMPS) [22] along with anti-glutaminergic drugs (MeHCl) which are proposed to be a very vital target in the management of Alzheimer's disease.

2. Materials and Methods

2.1. Materials

Memantine Hydrochloride (MeHCl) was a generous gift sample from Strides Pharmasciences ltd., Bangalore, Tramiprosate (TMPS), Thioflavin-T, MTT, and Aluminium chloride was procured from Sigma Aldrich. Labrafil, labrasol and gelucire 43/04 was a gift sample from Gattefosse, Germany. $Aβ_{1-42}$ was procured from Tocris Bioscience, UK. Fetal Bovine Serum, Penicillin-Streptomycin, and GlutaMAX TM were procured from Thermo Fisher Scientific, Pittsburgh, PA, USA. DMEM Hams F12 media, MEM Media, and Dialysis membrane with a molecular weight cut off of 12 kD were procured from Himedia Laboratories Pvt, Ltd., Mumbai.

2.2. Methods

2.2.1. Molecular Docking Studies of TMPS and MeHCl

The docking is carried out using a CDOCKER algorithm from Discovery studio that is based on simulated annealing which is simulated using a CHARMm force field. The 3D structure of $Aβ_{1-42}$ (2BEG) was downloaded from a protein data bank before docking and processed to remove side chains, loops, and conformers. Simultaneously the preparation of ligands was carried out to remove the duplicates and fix valences after which the protein and ligands were subjected to docking. The binding site of the protein was identified through a receptor cavity tool using a site search and flood-filling algorithm. The compounds memantine hydrochloride and tramiprosate were docked with the defined sphere site using random conformations with 1000 steps of dynamics to choose the best possible result for interaction analysis [22].

2.2.2. In Vitro Aβ Fibrillation Studies

The Aβ fibrillation study was conducted using a thioflavin-T assay which uses $A\beta_{1\text{-}42}$ human peptide at a concentration of 10 μM combined with or without various concentrations of Memantine Hydrochloride (500, 250, 125, 63, and 31.5 μM) and Tramiprosate (300, 150, 75, 37.5 and 18.75 μM). The $A\beta_{1\text{-}42}$ solution was incubated with the drug solution for 48 h and then 20 μM Thioflavin-T was added. The fluorescence was measured at 450 nm for excitation and 485 nm for emission. Curcumin was used as a positive control and 0.1% DMSO was diluent for all compounds [23].

2.2.3. Neuroprotective Effects of MeHCl & TMPS

Neuronal Cell Line Procurement and Maintenance

Human Neuronal cells SHSY5Y (ATCC® No. CRL-2266) were obtained from American Type Culture Collection (ATCC, Rockville, MD, USA). The cells were maintained using the complete media of DMEM Hams F12: MEM media (1:1 ratio), 10% v/v FBS, 1% v/v Penicillin-Streptomycin, and glutaMAX TM solution at 37 ± 0.5 °C, with 5% CO_2 in a sterile condition.

Cell Viability of $A\beta_{1\text{-}42}$

In order to establish a model of Aβ-induced toxicity, SH-SY5Y cells were treated with different concentrations of $A\beta_{1\text{-}42}$ (200, 100, 50, 25, 12.5, 6.25 & 3.125 μM) for 24 h. We examined the cell viability using MTT assay and ThT assay, respectively.

In-Vitro Cytotoxicity Studies

The main aim of this study was to identify the better active compound which is having maximum inhibition of Aβ aggregation with less drug concentration against SHSY5Y cells. The SHSY5Y cells (10×10^3 cells/well) were dispersed in 96 well plates (100 μL/well) of complete MEM media for 36 h to attain 80% confluence. The cells were treated with $A\beta_{1\text{-}42}$ and with various concentrations of MeHCl and TMPS as mentioned below. Cisplatin (100 μM) was used as a positive control (PC) and blank SLNs were used as vehicle control (VC). The plates were incubated with 5% CO_2 at 37 ± 0.5 °C for 24 h and then MTT solution was added and was incubated for 1hr. The formed formazone crystals were dissolved using DMSO after discarding the media and the optical density (OD) was measured using a microplate reader at 570nm [24,25]. The mean OD of each set of wells was calculated and the % of cell viability was calculated using Equation (1).

% Cell viability = Mean OD (test − blank)/mean OD (control − blank) × 100   (1)

Simultaneous Combination Assay

Based on the individual Neuroprotective assay of drugs, we determined the combinational neuroprotective effects of MeHCl & TMPS against SHSY5Y cells by using simultaneous combination assay. SHSY5Y cells were seeded at a density of 10×10^3 cells per well on 96-well plates, and after 36 h of incubation, the cells were treated simultaneously with $A\beta_{1\text{-}42}$, MeHCl & TMPS for 24 h.

At constant ratios (MeHCl 3: TMPS 1 molar ratio), different drug doses were combined using the IC_{50} values calculated from the previous cytotoxicity studies. The SHSY5Y cells were treated with different doses of MeHCl (30, 15, 7.5, 3.75, 1.87, 0.93 & 0.46 μM) and TMPS (10, 5, 2.5, 1.25, 0.625, 0.312 & 0.156 μM) for simultaneous estimation [26].

Memantine Hydrochloride (MeHCl)

The primary stock solution of pure MeHCl (100 mM) was prepared using DMSO. Then, SHSY5Y cells were treated with various concentrations of pure MeHCl (3.9, 7.81, 15.62, 31.25, 62.5, 125, 250 μM).

Tramiprosate (TMPS)

The primary stock solution of pure TMPS, (100 mM) was prepared using DMSO. Then, SHSY5Y cells were treated with various concentrations of pure TMPS (7.81, 15.62, 31.25, 62.5, 125, 250, and 500 µM).

2.2.4. Formulation of Solid Lipid Nanoparticles

SLNs were prepared by the homogenization-ultrasonication method [27]. The drug was dispersed in the lipid phase of labrasol and gelucire 43/04 (2:1) and heated to a temperature higher than the melting point of the lipid. A Smix of tween 80 and labrafil (3:1) finalized in the DoE was dissolved in the aqueous phase and heated to the same temperature as that of the lipid mixture. The aqueous phase was added into the lipid phase dropwise to form a primary emulsion. The formed primary emulsion was homogenized and probe sonicated for a specific time. The mixture was left to cool down to form solid lipid nanoparticles. Further, the formed nanoparticles were characterized for morphology and particle size.

2.2.5. Experimental Design

In order to demonstrate the response of the surface model by attaining different combinations of values JMP pro software was employed. Without using the 3-level factorial design, we used the Box Behnken design to form a quadratic. A 3-factor, 3-level Box Behnken design was used to optimize the procedure for the formulation of SLNs. The selected independent variables are Smix, homogenization time, and homogenization speed, while the selected dependent variables were particle size and polydispersity index. This leads to the optimization of SLNs with a small experimental design (17 runs).

2.3. Evaluation of Drug Loaded SLNs

2.3.1. %Drug Entrapment Efficiency (%DEE)

The entrapment efficiency of MeHCl and TMPS loaded and was determined by centrifuging a fixed amount of desired SLNs for 1 h at 10,000 RPM to obtain the supernatant. This supernatant was diluted further and the %DEE of both MeHCl and TMPS was determined using HPLC. The %DEE was calculated using Equation (2).

$$\text{Entrapment Efficiency} = \left(\text{Wd} - \frac{\text{Ws}}{\text{Wd}}\right) \times 100 \qquad (2)$$

2.3.2. In Vitro Drug Release Studies

Release studies of pure drug memantine hydrochloride and tramiprosate pure drug (M + T PD) and memantine hydrochloride and tramiprosate loaded solid lipid nanoparticles (M + T SLNs) were performed by using a dialysis membrane to which a solution equivalent to 1mg/mL concentration of pure drug and drug loaded SLNs were loaded. The loaded dialysis bags were placed in 7.4 pH PBS at 37 ± 0.5 °C with 100 RPM stirring in an orbital shaker incubator. 1ml Aliquots were withdrawn and replaced at various time points (0.15, 0.5, 1, 1.5, 2, 2.5, 3, 4, 8, 12, 24, and 48 h). The concentration of MeHCl and TMPS in the sample aliquots was determined using the HPLC method.

2.3.3. Transmission Electron Microscopy (TEM)

TEM was employed for morphological analysis and particle size confirmation. An arrangement of bright field imaging at collective magnification and diffraction approach was employed to disclose the form and size of the SLNs. The sample was prepared by diluting the optimized M + T SLNs in distilled water (1:100), and a sample was loaded on a copper grid and blemished with uranyl acetate for 30 s. The stained grid was dried, positioned on a glass slide and a coverslip, and observed under the microscope [28].

2.3.4. Atomic Force Microscopy (AFM)

Atomic force microscopy (5600 LS, Agilent, Santa Clara, CA, USA) was used to perceive the surface morphology of M + T SLNs. The samples were dehydrated by placing them on silicon wafers at room temperature. The morphology of M + T SLNs was examined using contact scanning probe microscopy.

2.4. Animals

All experimental animals were acclimated to the laboratory environment for a week prior to the start of the experiment for in vivo pharmacokinetic, bio-distribution, and pharmacodynamics measurements. The Institutional Animal Ethics Committee (IAEC) granted approval for the submitted study procedure. The studies were carried out in accordance with the guidelines established by the institutional ethical committee of the JSS Academy of Higher Education and Research's central animal facility.

2.5. Pharmacokinetics and Bio-Distribution

The 37 rats were divided into 2 groups, i.e., group I (M + T PD) and group II (M + T SLNs). Albino Wister Rats were injected intraperitoneally (i.p.) with 10 mg/kg of TMPS and 20 mg/kg of MeHCl in both pure drug and SLNs form. Following was the administration of both M + T.

PD and M + T SLNs the blood was withdrawn from the retro-orbital sinus at 0.15, 0.30, 1, 6, 12, 24, and 48 h. The obtained blood samples were centrifuged at 4000 RPM for the separation of plasma and stored at -80 °C until the analysis of MeHCl and TMPS content. All of the animals were anesthetized using ketamine before sacrificing. Brain tissues and other major organs, such as livers, kidneys, and spleens were excised, rinsed, and store at -80 °C to assess the bio-distribution of MeHCl and TMPS. The organs were homogenized individually using a tissue homogenizer and centrifuged at 12,000 RPM to separate the supernatant. The obtained supernatant was analyzed for the MeHCl and TMPS content using HPLC [29,30].

2.6. Pharmacodynamics

The animals were alienated into eight groups I–VIII. Group I was used as a control, whereas group II–VIII animals were administered with 100 mg/kg of $AlCl_3$ orally for 4 weeks to provoke AD along with 0.9% of NaCl (5 mL/kg), $AlCl_3$ + 10 mg/kg of MeHCl PD, $AlCl_3$ + 20 mg/kg of TMPS PD, $AlCl_3$ + 30 mg/kg of M + T PD, $AlCl_3$ + 10 mg/kg of MeHCl SLN, $AlCl_3$ + 20 mg/kg of TMPS SLN and M + T SLN single dose every day for 4 weeks respectively [31]. After the treatment period, the learning and memory of the animals were examined by the Morris Water Maze test. The brain tissues were excised, rinsed, and stored in neutral buffered formalin (NBF) which will further be used for histopathology studies. ELISA will be used for the quantification of $A\beta_{1-42}$ in both control and treated groups using the commercial assay kits as per the protocols suggested by the manufacturer.

2.6.1. Morris Water Maze Test

The strength of the learned spatial search bias was assessed during a probe trial on the 6th day without the platform. The MWM test was conducted as per the standard method by [32], with a minor modification to determine the impact of $AlCl_3$-induced AD on spatial memory in Wistar rats. A circular drum (diameter: 125 cm; height: 36 cm) filled with water was split equally into four quadrants. Skimmed milk was used to make the water turbid. The platform was placed in the NW quadrant, 1 cm underneath the water. The rats were exposed to the acquisition trial (exercise to find the hidden platform) twice a day for five days. A probe test was carried out on the 6th day; the platform was removed to test the retention memory of the rats. The rats were allowed to swim in the drum for a period of 60 s, the assessment was video recorded and ANY-maze software was used to determine the escape latency, distance travelled, and the number of entries in the target quadrant and track plot of the mice.

2.6.2. Histopathology

A 10% neutral buffered formalin (NBF) was used as a fixing solution for rat brains. Brain tissues were embedded in paraffin and coronal sections (3–5 μm) of the hippocampus region were cut using a microtome. Sections were mounted on a slide, washed and dehydrated with 95% ethanol, and stained with congo red dye for histopathological examination [33].

2.6.3. ELISA

The Aβ content was measured using ELISA Kit following the kit's protocol (Cloud Clone Corp., Katy, TX, USA).

3. Results

3.1. Docking Analysis

The hydrophobic interactions and the salt bridge between Asp23/Glu22 and Lys28 residue in $A\beta_{1-42}$ is mainly responsible for the formation of insoluble aggregates and changes in β-sheet conformation. In order to demonstrate the binding modes of MeHCl and TMPS with $A\beta_{1-42}$ we used the CDOCKER application where figures were generated through visualization. A 2BEG was a form Aβ which was chosen for the docking study of Aβ with MeHCl and TMPS. All docked conformations are ranked based on docking scores.

As shown in Figure 1, TMPS was mainly stabilized by conventional hydrogen bonding with Glu22 and Ala21. Furthermore, van der Waals interaction was seen with the Leu34, Val36, Ala21, and Glu22 and Carbon hydrogen bond interaction with Asp23, Glu22, and Leu34. However, there was a presence of an unfavorable bump in the interaction of MeHCl with $A\beta_{1-42}$, thus proving that there is no role of memantine in the deaggregation of $A\beta_{1-42}$, but is made use of in the study due to its effect as an NMDA antagonist in the treatment of AD.

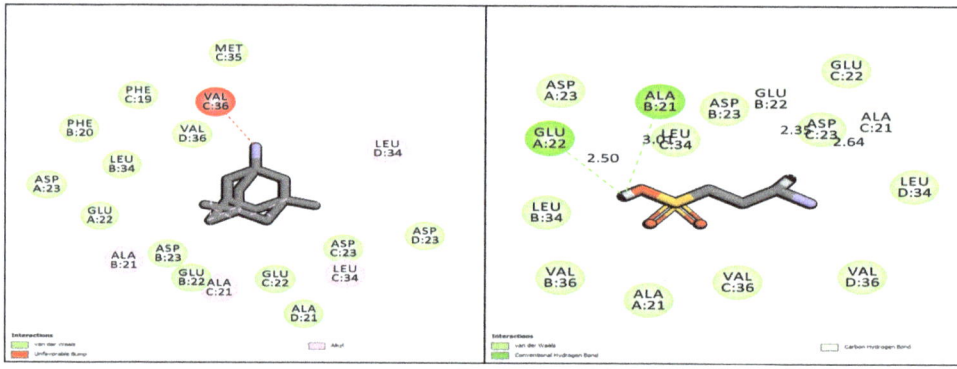

Figure 1. 2D molecular docking simulations of MeHCl and TMPS.

3.2. In Vitro Aβ Fibrillation Studies

Thioflavin-T is a dye that particularly binds to Aβ protein and helps in monitoring Aβ fibrillation. This study was used to evaluate the anti-amyloidogenic activity of MeHCl and TMPS. Both the drugs studied exhibited bioactivity. Tramiprosate showed higher bioactivity by inhibiting 16.56% of Aβ while Memantine Hydrochloride showed 3.22% inhibition of aggregation (Figure 2).

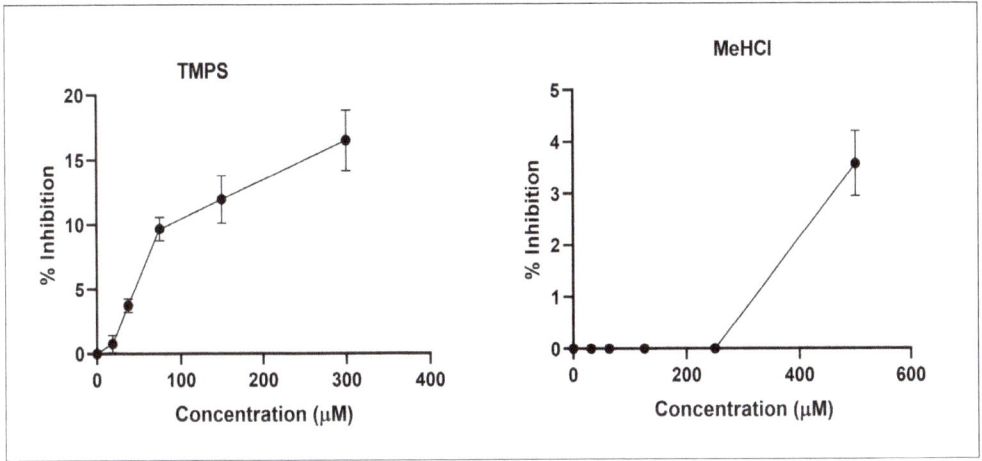

Figure 2. Amyloid-β anti-aggregation assay (data points represented as mean ± SD, where $n = 3$ and $p < 0.05$).

3.3. Neuroprotective Effects of MeHCl & TMPS
3.3.1. Aβ$_{1-42}$

The morphological changes and dose dependent responses of SHSY5Y on the treatment of Aβ$_{1-42}$ are represented in Figure 3. As the dose increased (200, 100, 50, 25, 12.5, 6.25 & 3.125 μM) the aggregation around the cells also increased which was assessed using MTT & ThT assay. These results indicated that the cells were sensitive to Aβ$_{1-42}$ exposure. The obtained IC 50 value for SHSY5Y cells with Aβ$_{1-42}$ was 80.35 μM ± 0.455 μM.

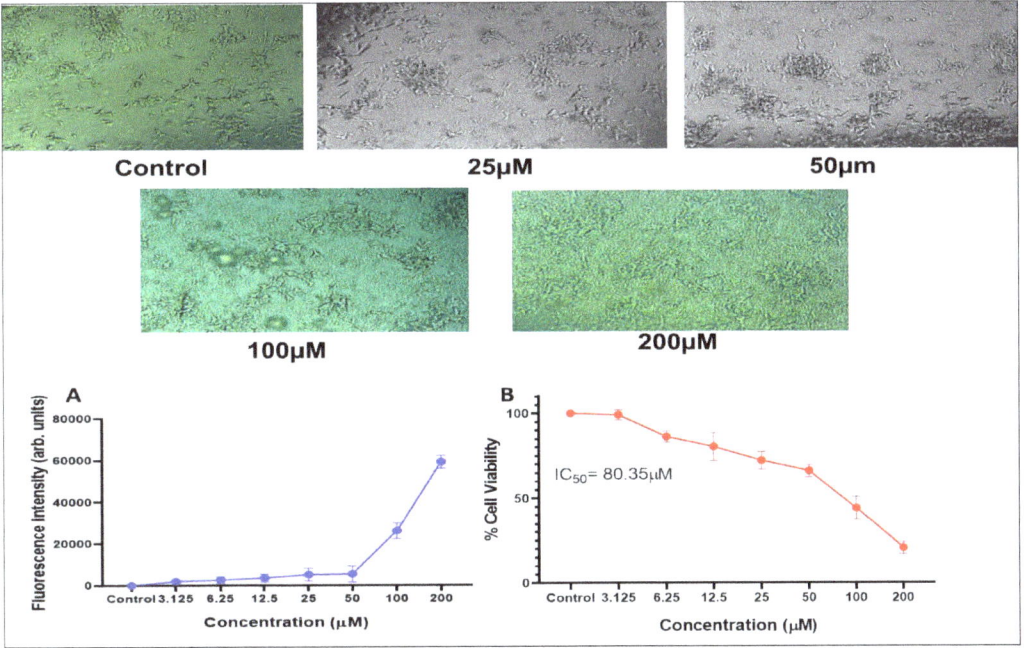

Figure 3. Effect of different Aβ$_{1-42}$ concentrations on the viability of SHSY5Y cells (**A**) ThT assay (**B**) MTT assay (data points mean ± SD, $n = 3$).

3.3.2. MeHCl

The morphological changes and dose dependent responses of SHSY5Y on the treatment of MeHCl was represented in Figure 4A. With the increase in the dose (3.9, 7.81, 15.62, 31.25, 62.5, 125, 250 µM) the aggregation around the cells also decreased. The obtained IC 50 value for SHSY5Y cells with MeHCl PD, MeHCl SLN, MeHCl PD + Aβ & MeHCl SLN + Aβ was 582.6 ± 2.098, 485.9 ± 4.196, 30.28 ± 4.196 & 10.67 ± 4.268 respectively (Figure 4).

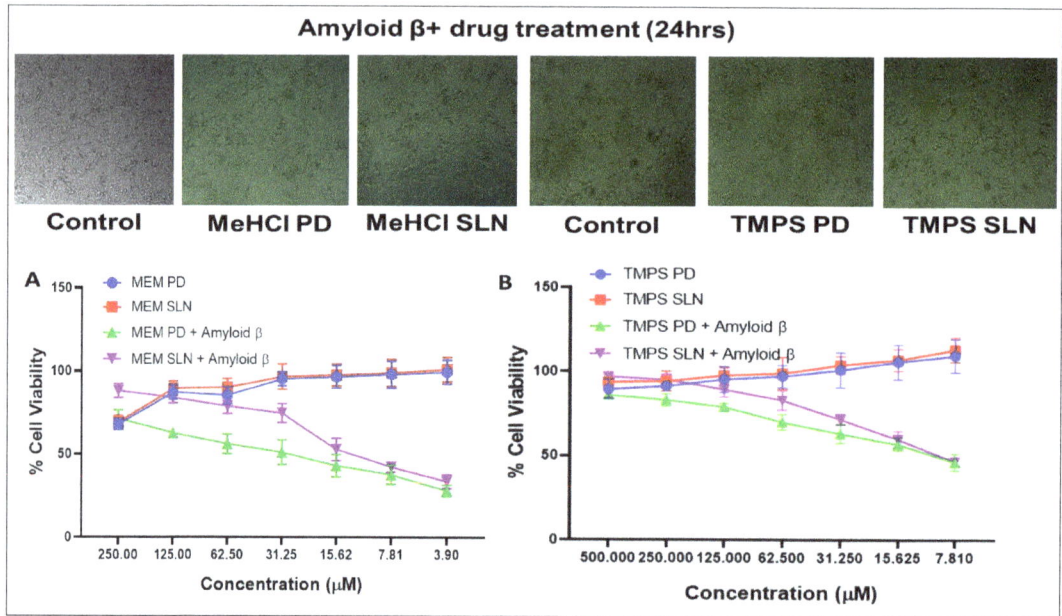

Figure 4. The % of Cell viability assay. (**A**) The dose dependent response of SHSY5Y cells on the treatment of MeHCl (**B**) The dose dependent response of SHSY5Y cells on the treatment of TMPS. Data is represented in mean ± SD (n = 3).

3.3.3. TMPS

The morphological changes and dose dependent responses of SHSY5Y in the treatment of TMPS are represented in Figure 4B. With the increase in the dose (7.81, 15.62, 31.25, 62.5, 125, 250, and 500 µM) the aggregation around the cells also decreased. The obtained IC 50 value for SHSY5Y cells with TMPS PD + Aβ & TMPS SLN + Aβ was 9.892 ± 1.56 & 9.535 ± 1.651 respectively (Figure 4).

3.3.4. Simultaneous Estimation

Then, we examined the combinational neuroprotective effects of the MeHCl & TMPS combination against the SHSY5Y cell line (Figure 5). The cell viability effects of different drug combinations were assessed. As anticipated, the MeHCl & TMPS treatment exhibited the highest neuro-protective effect against SHSY5Y cells when used in combination. Ten µM of TMPS + 20 µM of MeHCl showed a cell viability of 89.159 ± 1.916 which is much higher than the individual cell viability. The IC50 of M + T PD and M + T SLN was found to be 5.235 ± 0.41 and 3.627 ± 0.56. This shows that the drugs used in combination show enhanced neuroprotection.

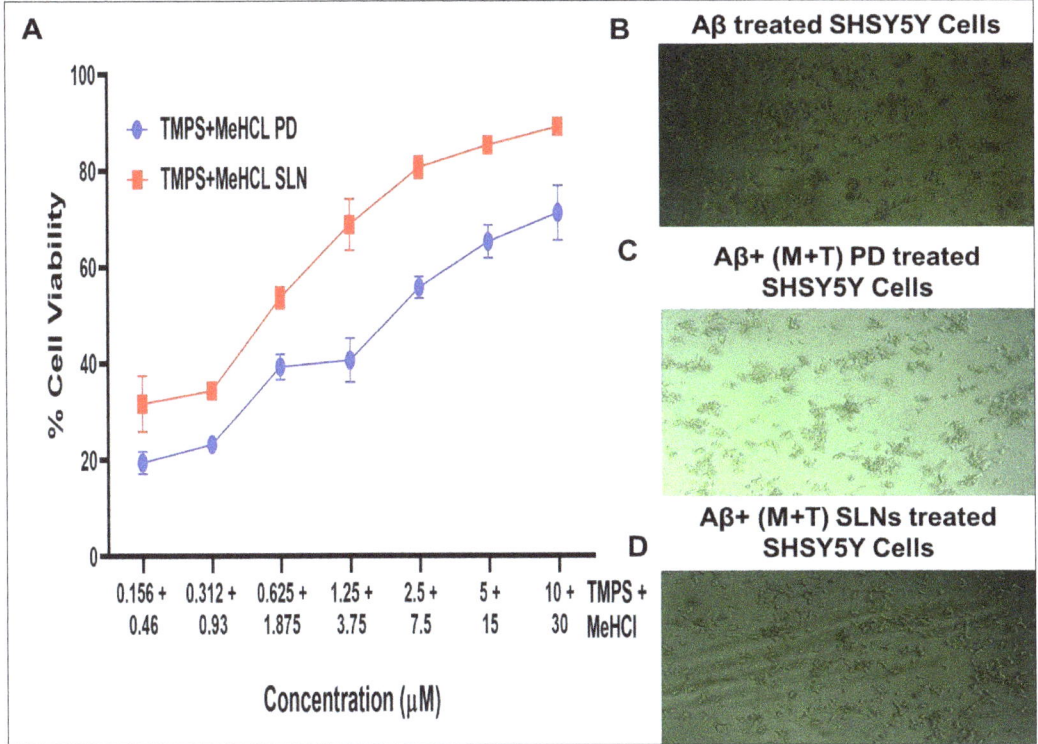

Figure 5. (**A**) The dose dependent activity of MeHCl & TMPS combination on SHSY5Y cells, (**B**) Aβ treated SHSY5Y cells, (**C**) Aβ+ (M+T) PD treated SHSY5Y cells and (**D**) Aβ+ (M+T) SLNs treated SHSY5Y cells. Data is represented in mean ± SD (n = 3).

3.4. Formulation of Solid Lipid Nanoparticles

3.4.1. Model Fitting

To fit the two target variables, statistical analysis and joint model fitting based on the actualized experimental design were carried out using JMP Pro®. The *p*-value was used to evaluate the significance of the overall effects and investigated interactions. After manual backward exclusion of the 95% confidence level, Table 1 displays the significant effects and interactions present in the model. From top to bottom, the associated *p*-values are decreasing. The impact of the associated effects or interactions on the responses increases with decreasing *p*-value. The "^" denotes the main effects with higher-level interactions (Table 1). Table 2 lists the results of an independent analysis of the data about the corresponding impact of each factor on each response.

3.4.2. Effect of Independent Variables on Responses

The mean PDI of the prepared SLNs was in the range of 0.12 ± 0.002 to 0.455 ± 0.025, and the mean diameter of the prepared SLNs was in the range of 65.04 ± 0.515 to 490 ± 1.63. Analysis of variance (ANOVA) based on Fisher's ratio (F-ratio) of 0.267 indicates that the model established for PDI and PS is statistically significant. The ratio of the model of sum squares to the overall sum of squares, or the value known as r-squared (r^2), was calculated and found to be 0.90 for PS and 0.96 for PDI. This shows that the regression model accounts for 90% and 96% of the variation in the response for PS and PDI respectively. Figure 6 shows the significant correlation between the determined values and those anticipated by the PS & PDI fitted model. The limited range of points along the red line and inside the 95% confidence interval for model significance corroborates this (Figure 6).

3.4.3. Verification of the Model

The formulation was replicated at the optimal conditions (15% Smix, 6 min of homogenization, and 15,000 RPM homogenization speed) predicted by the prediction profiler obtained from the box-Behnken design, thereby validating the desirability equations for response prediction (Figure 7). PS and PDI both had projected response values of 193.94 nm and 0.146, respectively. The experimental results of PS (159.90.081) and PDI (0.1540.0036) were in good agreement with the projected results. The experiment was performed in triplicate.

Table 1. Effect Summary of factors and observed responses for MeHCl + TMPS SLNs.

Source	Log Worth	p Value
Homogenization speed*Homogenization speed	3.612	0.00024
Homogenization time*Homogenization time	3.492	0.00032
Homogenization speed (10,20)	3.475	0.00033 ^
Smix*Homogenization time	2.669	0.00214
Homogenization time*homogenization speed	2.3922	0.00406
Homogenization time (4,8)	1.916	0.01212 ^
Smix*Smix	1.811	0.01545
Smix*Homogenization speed	1.401	0.03970
Smix (10,20)	1.158	0.06957 ^

(^ denotes effects with containing effects above them).

Table 2. Box Behnken design factors and observed responses for MeHCl and TMPS loaded SLNs (* Mean ± SD, n = 3).

Pattern	S_{mix}	Homogenization Time	Homogenization Speed	Particle Size * (Mean ± SD)	PDI * (Mean ± SD)
0	15	6	15	159.9 ± 0.569	0.154 ± 0.04
0	15	6	15	163 ± 0.070	0.192 ± 0.0007
+0−	20	6	10	252 ± 0.212	0.259 ± 0.0007
0−+	15	4	20	106.5 ± 0.424	0.399 ± 0.0007
−−0	10	4	15	576 ± 0.572	0.284 ± 0.0014
−0−	10	6	10	65.04 ± 0.282	0.397 ± 0.0007
0	15	6	15	333 ± 0.424	0.123 ± 0.0007
+0+	20	6	20	157 ± 0.282	0.149 ± 0.0007
+−0	20	4	15	282.1 ± 1.414	0.274 ± 0.0028
−0+	10	6	20	295.4 ± 0.353	0.196 ± 0.0014
0	15	6	15	158 ± 0.282	0.12 ± 0.0028
0	20	8	15	490 ± 0.353	0.211 ± 0.0028
−+0	10	8	15	174.1 ± 0.353	0.213 ± 0.0014
0+−	15	8	10	70.43 ± 0.296	0.455 ± 0.0028
0	15	6	15	155 ± 0.424	0.144 ± 0.0028
0++	15	8	20	280.4 ± 0.141	0.175 ± 0.0028

* n = 3.

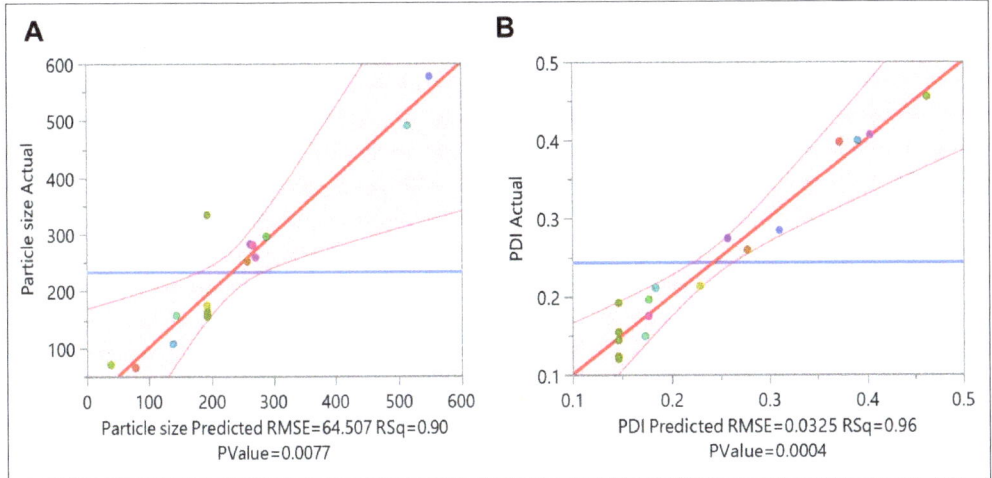

Figure 6. Statistical evaluation of prepared SLNs of (**A**) Predicted v/s actual plot for Particle size and (**B**) Predicted v/s actual plot for PDI.

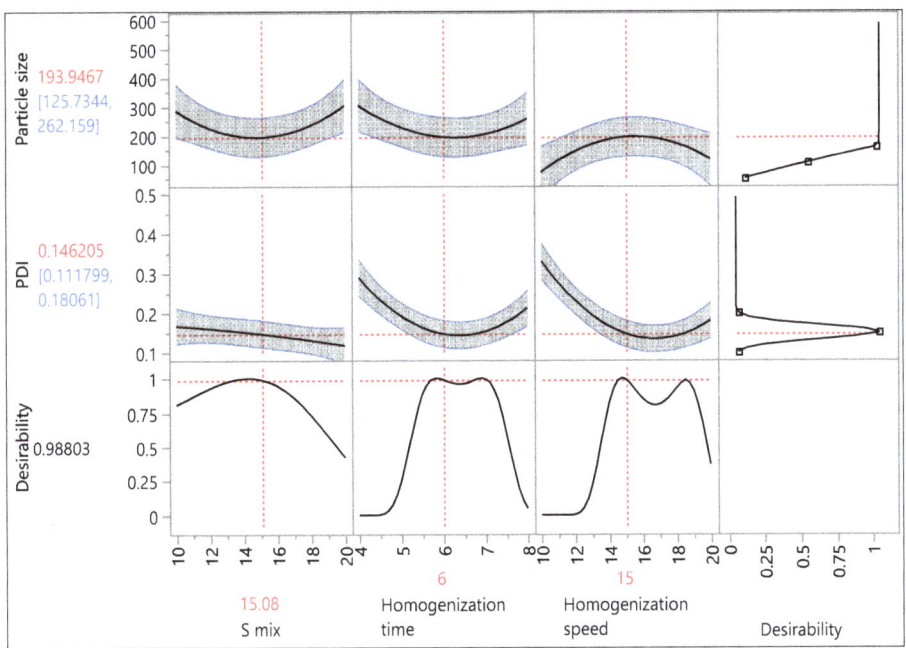

Figure 7. Prediction profile of prepared SLNs where the actual values are similar to that of the predicted values.

3.5. Evaluation of Drug Loaded SLNs

3.5.1. %Drug Entrapment Efficiency (%DEE)

%DEE of MeHCl & TMPS was found to be 99.24 ± 3.24 and 89.99 ± 0.95, respectively.

3.5.2. Determination of Particle Size (PS), Polydispersity Index (PDI), and Zeta Potential of Optimized Formulation

The particle size of the developed MeHCl + TMPS SLNs and Placebo formulations were found to be 159.9 ± 0.569 nm and 157 ± 0.623 nm with a PDI value of 0.149 ± 0.08 and 0.161 ± 0.04. The Zeta potential of the MeHCl + TMPS SLNs and Placebo formulations were found to be −6.4 ± 0.948 mV and −6.15 ± 0.854 mV.

3.5.3. Transmission Electron Microscopy (TEM)

The morphological analysis of optimized M + T SLNs was examined using TEM micrographs. The particles were spherical with sizes varying in 0.5μm scale. The obtained data were in good agreement with the particle size analysis of the M + T SLNs formulation (Figure 8C).

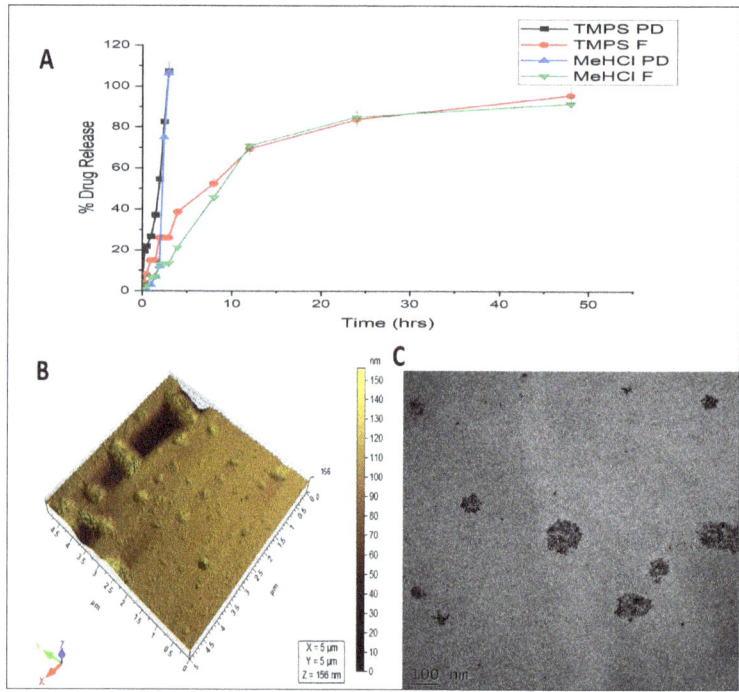

Figure 8. (**A**) Drug release profile of MeHCl & TMPS in pure form and SLNs where the data is represented in mean ± SD (n = 3) (**B**) AFM image of M + T SLN (**C**) TEM micrographs of M + T loaded SLNs.

3.5.4. In-Vitro Cumulative % Drug Release Study

As shown in Figure 8A, the In-vitro % drug release study was performed with pure drug mixture solutions and M + T SLNs formulation. The pure drug released 100 ± 6% of MeHCl and 100 ± 7% of TMPS within 3 h, but the M + T SLNs released 91.73 ± 1.5% of MeHCl and 95.90 ± 1.51% of TMPS. About 80% of MeHCl and TMPS were released from SLNs slowly up to 48 h.

3.5.5. AFM

AFM topography image (Figure 8B) further confirmed the particle size of SLNs in the range of 156nm. The morphology of the SLNs as per the AFM topography was irregularly spherical with a smooth surface. The different shapes of the nanoparticles may be attributed to the mechanism of formation of the nanoparticles.

3.5.6. Stability Studies

The effect of different storage conditions on the particle size and PDI of MeHCl + TMPS SLNs. MeHCl + TMPS SLNs stored at 4 ± 2 °C showed a slight increase in particle from 159.9 ± 0.0 nm to 162.35 ± 0.0707 nm, whereas the PDI also increased slightly from 0.154 ± 0.0 to 0.182 ± 0.0007 from day 1 to day 90, respectively.

Similarly, the storage condition of 25 ± 2 °C showed a slight but lesser increase in particle size when compared to 4 ± 2 °C. The particle size was 159.9 ± 0.0 nm on day 1 which increased gradually to 160.45 ± 0.070 nm on day 90. Furthermore, the PDI increased from 0.154 ± 0.0 to 0.161 ± 0.0007 on day 1 and day 90, respectively. The stability data revealed no significant changes in particle size and PDI in both 4 ± 2 °C and 25 ± 2 °C, which shows that the formulation is stable at both storage conditions (Figure 9).

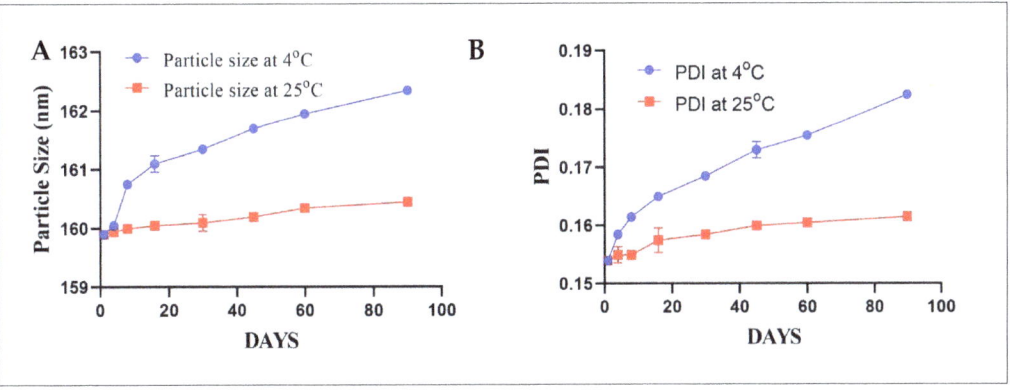

Figure 9. Effect of storage condition on particle size and PDI of M + T SLNs (**A**) Particle Size (**B**) PDI. The data is presented in mean ± SD (*n* = 3).

3.6. Pharmacokinetics

The results of the pharmacokinetic parameters with an i.p. injection of M + T PD and M + T SLNs are represented in Table 3 and Figure 10. While the M + T PD solution demonstrated a quick initial clearance rate from the blood within 1 h of administration, M + T SLNs still showed delayed blood clearance rates even after 4 h of administration. In comparison to M + T SLNs, the significant pharmacokinetics characteristics of M + T PD showed a shorter mean residence time (MRT). The peak plasma concentration (C_{max}) was found to be 144.601 ± 0.354 & 57.018 ± 0.2029 for M + T PD and 204.79 ± 0.042 and 65.618 ± 0.292 for M + T SLNs. The increase in the $AUC_{0-\infty}$ in M + T SLNs might be due to the avoidance of first-pass metabolism by lymphatic transport. Additionally, M + T SLNs had considerably lower plasma clearance than M + T PD (Table 3). Figure 10 shows the Pharmacokinetic graph of M + T PD & M + T SLNs administered intraperitoneally at 30 mg/kg body weight (1:3 molar ratio). These results suggest that M + T SLNs have improved pharmacokinetic profiles when compared to the pure drug.

3.7. Bio Distribution

The highest concentration was found in the brain after dosing with M + T SLNs i.e., 177.9598 ± 18.366291 & 30.29417 ± 2.012082 µg/mL of MeHCl & TMPS, respectively, which (Figure 11) might be because of the faster and better absorption by the brain. The concentration of both drugs was very minimal in the liver (62.35548836 ± 13.335808 & 13.79340481 ± 3.012082 µg/mL), spleen (36.345 ± 9.169307 & 3.621701 ± 1.912082 µg/mL) and kidneys (18.96022784 ± 12.036123 & 2.26547381 ± 1.012082) of MeHCl & TMPS respectively in comparison to that of the pure drugs.

Table 3. Pharmacokinetic parameters of MeHCl + TMPS PD & MeHCl + TMPS SLN were administered intraperitoneally at 30 mg/kg (1:3 molar ratio).

Parameters	M + T PD		M + T SLN	
	MeHCl PD *	TMPS PD *	MeHCl SLN *	TMPS SLN *
C_{max}	144.601 ± 0.354	57.018 ± 0.2029	204.79 ± 0.042	65.618 ± 0.292
T_{max}	1 ± 0	1 ± 0	4 ± 0	4 ± 0
Cl	7.509 ± 0.099	20.239 ± 0.1166	4.465 ± 0.134	12.05 ± 0.113
MRT	16.634 ± 0.475	10.437 ± 0.236	18.31 ± 0.241	15.22 ± 0.229
$AUC_{0-\infty}$	2635.268 ± 0.118	491.537 ± 0.731	4573.705 ± 0.12	835.45 ± 0.478
AUC_{0-48}	1854.468 ± 0.103	412.285 ± 0.502	3401.657 ± 0.289	614.376 ± 0.288
V_z	325.604 ± 0.113	798.56 ± 0.602	136.938 ± 0.101	538.887 ± 0.229

* Mean ± SD (n = 3).

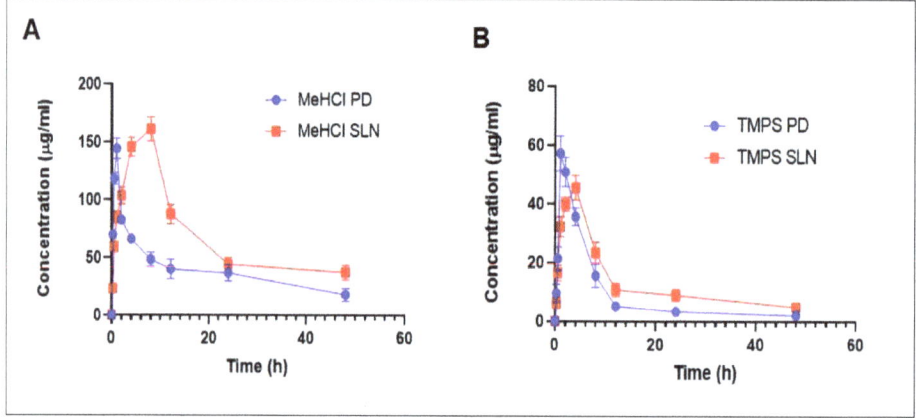

Figure 10. Plasma concentration-time profile of MeHCl + TMPS PD and MeHCl + TMPS SLNs administered intraperitoneally at 30 mg/kg (1:3 molar ratio) (**A**) Plasma concentration-time profile of MeHCl PD & MeHCl SLN (**B**) Plasma concentration-time profile of TMPS PD & TMPS SLN. The data is represented in mean ± SD (n = 3).

M + T PD, when delivered intraperitoneally, demonstrated considerably lower brain concentrations (48.07 ± 3.050 & 5.015 ± 7.031 µg/mL) than the drug-loaded SLNs. The pure drug concentration was very high in the liver (174.929 ± 3.505 & 31.650 ± 7.012 µg/mL) followed by other organs such as the spleen (61.239 ± 6.067 & 3.621 ± 2.012 µg/mL) and kidneys (50.467 ± 7.828 & 2.717 ± 2.012 µg/mL).

3.8. Pharmacodynamics

3.8.1. Morris Water Maze (MWM)

The impact of $AlCl_3$-induced AD in rats on hippocampal-dependent spatial memory was assessed by the MWM test. As shown in Figure 12E, $AlCl_3$-treated rats showed increased latency time to find the hidden platform ($p < 0.01$) when compared with normal rats. $AlCl_3$-treated rats spent significantly less time ($p < 0.05$), lesser number of entries ($p < 0.01$) and covered less distance ($p < 0.01$) in the target quadrant compared when compared with normal rats. This indicates that $AlCl_3$ successfully induces AD in rats. M + T SLNs (10 + 5 mg/kg) treated rats showed reduced latency time to find the hidden platform, increased number of entries in the target quadrant, spend more time, and covered more distance in the target quadrant (Figure 12A–E). These data indicate that M + T SLNs restores spatial memory.

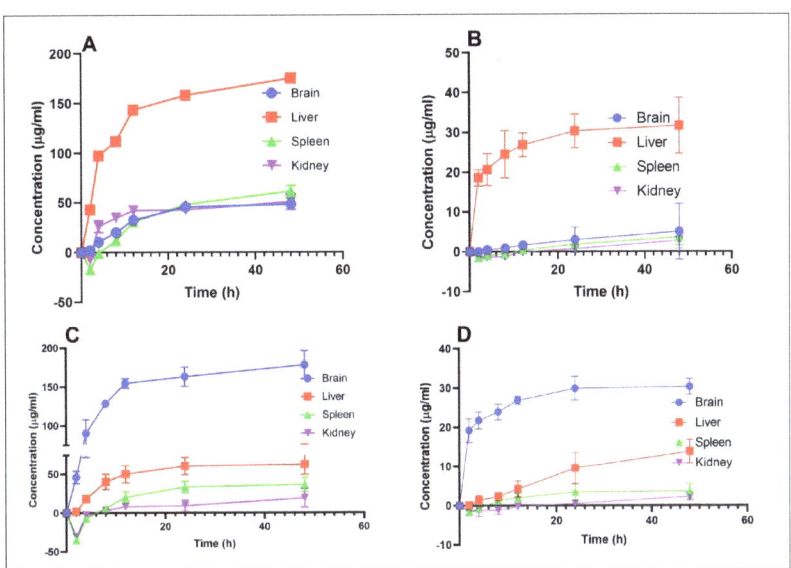

Figure 11. MeHCl and TMPS Concentration in major organs after intraperitoneal administration at 30 mg/kg body weight (1:3 molar ratio) (**A**) MeHCl PD (**B**) TMPS PD (**C**) MeHCl SLN (**D**) TMPS SLN. Data are represented in mean ± SD (n = 3).

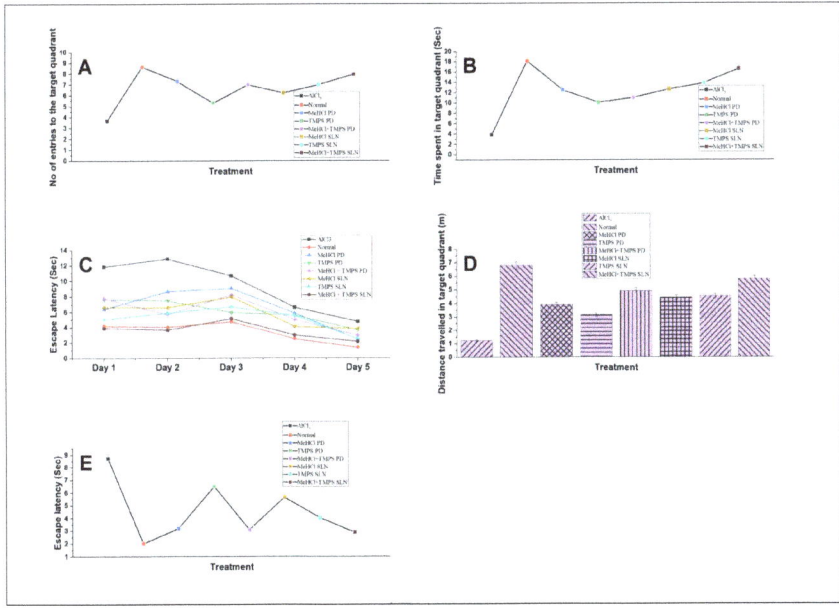

Figure 12. Daily administration of MeHCl & TMPS improved spatial memory in rats which was demonstrated by the (**A**) No. of entries in the target quadrant (**B**) Time spent in the target quadrant (**C**) Learning pattern in the training phase (**D**) Distance travelled in the target quadrant (**E**) Escape latency where all the results showed that $AlCl_3$ induced AD and M + T SLNs showed the best results in comparison with other treatment groups. All the data is represented in mean ± SD (n = 3) with $p < 0.01$.

3.8.2. ELISA

We performed an ELISA assay to determine the impact of AlCl$_3$, MeHCl & TMPS pure drug and M + T PD, MeHCl & TMPS SLNs, and M + T SLNs on the levels of Aβ in the hippocampal region of rat brain. Normal Rat hippocampus showed the lowest concentration of Aβ whereas the AlCl$_3$ treated with the highest concentration of Aβ. There was a significant decrease in the levels of Aβ ($p < 0.01$) in M + T SLNs when compared to that of M + T PD upon simultaneous induction of AD using AlCl$_3$ and treatment with the drugs (Figure 13).

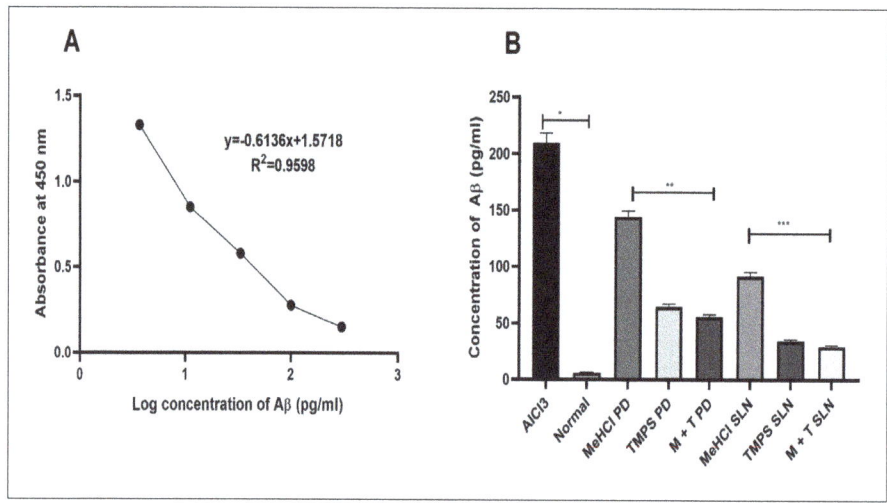

Figure 13. Determination of Aβ concentration in AlCl$_3$ induced AD in Rat brain (**A**) Aβ standard curve (**B**) Reduced Aβ concentration in MeHCl + TMPS treated rat brain with data represented as mean ± SD (n = 3). * indicates $p < 0.01$, ** indicates $p < 0.05$ and *** indicates $p < 0.001$.

3.8.3. Histopathology

Microscopic examination of CA1, CA2, and DG region of the hippocampus using congo red stain was carried out to examine the deposition of Aβ in various treatment groups. AlCl$_3$-induced AD showed marked deposition of Aβ in CA1, CA2, and DG regions of rat hippocampus, whereas the control group showed normal hippocampal neurons with no deposition of Aβ. Among the treatment groups, the SLN-treated groups showed the deposition of very few foci of Aβ in various regions of the hippocampus when compared to that of the pure drug groups which showed deposition of multiple foci of Aβ (Figure 14).

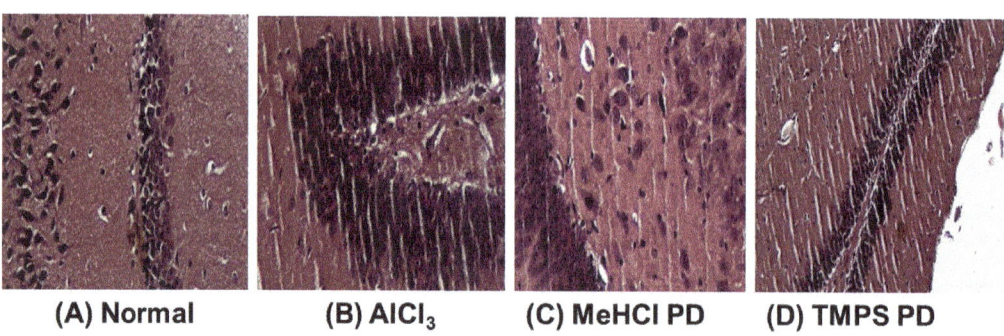

Figure 14. *Cont.*

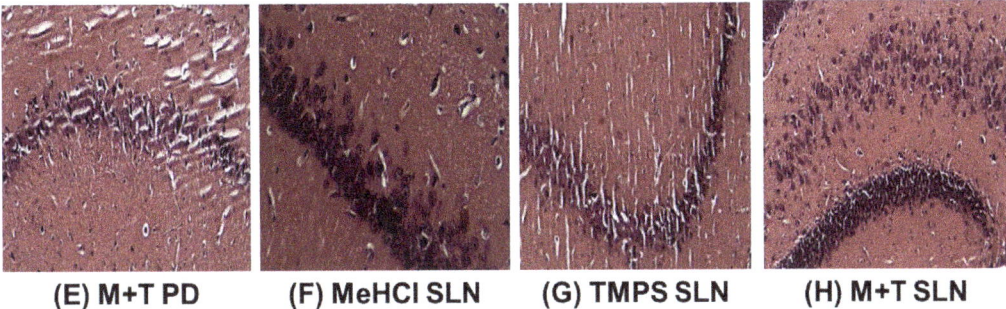

Figure 14. Histopathology of Hippocampal region of rat brain stained with congo red dye (**A**) Control group shows hippocampal neurons appeared normal without any deposition of Aβ (**B**) AlCl$_3$ represents the deposition of foci of Aβ in the CA1, CA2, DG region of hippocampus also adjacent ventricle is filled with Aβ (**C**) MeHCl PD shows birefringence deposition of multiple foci of Aβ in CA2 region of the hippocampus (**D**) TMPS PD shows deposition of few foci of Aβ in CA1 region of the hippocampus (**E**) M + T PD shows deposition of few foci of Aβ in CA1 region of the hippocampus (**F**) MeHCl SLN showed deposition of few foci of Aβ in hippocampus neurons of CA1 region (**G**) TMPS SLN showed very few depositions of Aβ in CA1 region of the hippocampus (**H**) M + T SLN showed deposition of very few foci of Aβ deposition in various regions of the hippocampus.

4. Discussion

The current study's objective was to develop and characterize solid lipid nanoparticles for the elimination of Aβ in Alzheimer's disease using the homogenization-ultrasonication technique. The use of SLNs can increase bioavailability without the use of high doses by passing physiological barriers, guiding the active compound towards the target site with a significant reduction in toxicity for the surrounding tissues, and protecting drugs from chemical and enzymatic degradation [34]. Memantine Hydrochloride (MeHCl) and tramiprosate (TMPS) were the drugs chosen to be administered in combination as both of them have shown potential in inhibiting Aβ aggregation. Previous research suggests that Memantine hydrochloride an NMDA antagonist has Aβ disaggregation activity [35] but showed no interaction with Aβ (2BEG) in molecular docking studies, however, in contrast, it showed 3.22% inhibition of aggregation in thioflavin-T-based in vitro assay. Tramiprosate showed good interaction with various amino acid residues of the Aβ protein [36] and inhibited 16.56% of Aβ aggregation thus proving its potential in Aβ sheet disaggregation.

The in vitro % cell viability studies of SHSY5Y cells in the treatment of Aβ, MeHCl PD, and SLNs, and TMPS PD and SLNs were evaluated by MTT assay. It was seen that as the concentration of Aβ increased the cell viability decreased. The IC$_{50}$ value for Aβ was 80.35μM ± 0.455 μM which was used for further cell viability studies. In the case of MeHCl PD and TMPS PD, as the concentration increased the cell viability decreased which may be attributed to the toxicity of the pure drug. In presence of Aβ, the cell viability increased as the concentration increased which suggests that the treatment is reducing the Aβ concentration with an IC$_{50}$ of 30.28 ± 4.196 for MeHCl PD + Aβ & 9.89 ± 1.56 for TMPS PD + Aβ. The drugs, when formulated into SLNs, showed an increase in cell viability with an increase in concentration up to 88% for MeHCl SLN + Aβ and 97% for TMPS SLN + Aβ. It can also be seen that the IC$_{50}$ of MeHCl SLN + Aβ was 10.67 ± 4.268 and TMPS SLN + Aβ was 9.535 ± 1.651 which was the lowest IC$_{50}$ when compared to that of the pure drug. Taking into consideration the obtained results, we conducted a simultaneous combination assay at a 3:1 molar ratio, which resulted in enhanced neuroprotection when compared to that of individual pure drug and SLNs, and also resulted in a much lower IC$_{50}$; 5.235 ± 0.41 for M + T PD and 3.627 ± 0.56 for M + T SLN. Hence, we considered the 3:1 molar ratio for further studies.

The M + T SLNs were prepared using the homogenization-ultrasonication method using Labrasol as liquid lipid and gelucire 43/04 (2:1) as solid lipid which was chosen based on the drug solubility in the respective lipids. The surfactants used were tween 80 and co-surfactant labrafil (3:1) was used which was selected by constructing ternary phase diagrams. The Box-behnken design was used to optimize M + T SLNs where homogenization time, homogenization speed, and smix ratio were independent variables and Particle size and PDI were dependent variables. The predicted response values for PS and PDI were 193.94nm and 0.146 respectively which is well in agreement with the experimental values having PS of 159.9 ± 0.081 and PDI of 0.154 ± 0.0036.

The particle size of less than 200nm will effectively cross the blood brain barrier [37] and lower the polydispersity index more uniform the particle distribution. A negative zeta potential of -6.4mV shows that the particles are neutral [38]. The % of entrapment efficiency ensures that the chosen lipids efficiently entrap the drugs. The spherical morphology was confirmed by both TEM and AFM. The in vitro drug release studies showed that the pure drugs released completely within 3hrs whereas the M + T SLNs showed a sustained release up to 48hrs which followed the Higuchi model for drug release. The improved formulation's excellent stability suggests that it can preserve integrity even when it is diluted in the body. The in-vitro characterization study was similar to earlier studies.

The in vivo pharmacokinetics and bio-distribution study in rats following a single i.p. dose was investigated using the HPLC technique. The maximum plasma concentration (C_{max}) and the time required to reach it (T_{max}) were directly calculated from the Plasma concentration-time profile. The non-compartmental model's calculation of the additional crucial pharmacokinetic parameters was carried out utilizing Phoenix winnonlin software. The M + T SLNs showed improved pharmacokinetic parameters when compared to the pure drug (Table 3), thus proving the efficiency of the formulation. Closely, there was a 4-fold increase in the concentration of SLNs in the brain compared with pure drug-treated brains in rats. The biodistribution pattern strongly suggests that MeHCl + TMPS is present in the lipid carrier in intact form, allowing the medication to pass the blood-brain barrier.

The pharmacodynamics study was carried out on $AlCl_3$-induced AD in rats. The effect of $AlCl_3$ on spatial memory was assessed using Morris water maze studies which showed that the M + T SLNs enhanced spatial memory. This was proven by the increased number of entries to the target quadrant, increased time spent, distance travelled, and decreased escape latency in M + T SLN treated group when compared with the control group. ELISA assay was used to quantify the Aβ protein in rat hippocampus in various treatment groups. Reduced concentration of Aβ in the M + T SLN treated group shows that the treatment is effective in reducing the Aβ concentration in rat hippocampus. The histopathological studies using congo red dye also confirmed the presence of Aβ plaques in the $AlCl_3$-induced group which decreased significantly in the M + T SLN-treated group.

All the in vitro and in vivo data confirmed that the M + T SLNs was superior when compared to that of pure drugs. This study also proved that the combinational therapy achieved the desired reduction of Aβ protein burden when compared to the individual pure drug and formulation. The currently available treatments do not focus on the pathological hallmarks of AD or reduce the protein burden in the brain [39]. The BBB would be one more major drawback in treating neuronal disorders which can be overcome by the use of lipid-based NPs [40,41]. The results of bio-distribution suggest that the M + T SLNs are capable of crossing the BBB. Based on the positive outcomes of the various in vitro characterizations of SLNs, we draw the conclusion that M + T SLNs can serve as an effective drug delivery system to cross BBB and manage AD. Treatments mainly targeting the patient's pathological hallmark burden would help in better management of the disease [42].

5. Summary and Conclusions

In the current investigation, homogenization-ultrasonication was used to prepare solid lipid nanoparticles (SLNs), which were then optimized utilizing the box-Behnken design approach in JMP pro software. The effect of the independent factors on the PS and PDI of M + T SLNs was effectively examined. The TEM and AFM results showed the SLNs being roughly spherical and having maximum entrapment efficiency which was stable over 60 days. Both medications were released steadily from SLNs, according to in vitro drug release experiments. Furthermore, the increased safety and effectiveness of M + T SLNs have been verified by in vitro cell-based assays. Based on the constructive results obtained from the various in vitro characterizations of SLNs we conclude that the M + T SLNs can be a useful carrier to deliver drugs across BBB.

Author Contributions: Conceptualization: M.G.S., S.P. and D.V.G. Methodology: M.G.S., S.P., U.H. and M.R. Software: M.G.S., Y.A. and A.S. Validation: M.G.S. and M.R. Formal Analysis: M.G.S., S.P., M.G., Y.A. and A.S. Investigation: M.G.S., U.H., M.R., M.G., Y.A., A.H.A. and R.A.M.O. Resources: D.V.G. and R.A.M.O. Data Curation: M.G.S., M.G., Y.A., S.P. and A.S. Writing—Original Draft Preparation: M.G.S., R.A.M.O., A.S. and M.R. Writing—Review & Editing: U.H., S.P., R.A.M.O., D.V.G., A.H.A. and A.S. Visualization: M.G. and Y.A. Supervision: D.V.G. and R.A.M.O. Project Administration: D.V.G. Funding Acquisition: M.G.S. and U.H. All authors have read and agreed to the published version of the manuscript.

Funding: The authors extend their appreciation to the Deanship of Scientific Research at King Khalid University, Saudi Arabia, for funding this work through the small Program (grant number RGP.1/30/43).

Institutional Review Board Statement: The study was conducted according to the guidelines of the Declaration of Helsinki and approved by the Institutional ethical committee of JSS Academy of Higher Education and Research (central animal facility) was approved on 12 February 2022 and the project proposal number is JSSAHER/CPT/IAEC/101/2022.

Informed Consent Statement: Not applicable.

Data Availability Statement: Data will be made available on request to the corresponding author.

Acknowledgments: The authors extend their appreciation to the Deanship of Scientific Research at King Khalid University, Saudi Arabia, for funding this work through the small Program (grant number RGP.1/30/43). Authors express a deep sense of gratitude towards the management and leadership of JSS College of Pharmacy, JSS Academy of Higher Education and Research (JSS AHER), Mysuru, Karnataka, India, for providing all the necessary facilities to carry out the research. M.G.S. would like to thank the Karnataka Science and Technology Promotion Society (KSTePS) for providing a Ph.D. fellowship. We would like to acknowledge Saravanababu Chidambaram, Centre for Experimental Pharmacology and Toxicology, Central Animal Facility, JSS Academy of Higher Education and Research, Mysuru 570015, India for providing guidance on animal study.

Conflicts of Interest: The authors declare no conflict of interest.

References

1. Sadigh-Eteghad, S.; Sabermarouf, B.; Majdi, A.; Talebi, M.; Farhoudi, M.; Mahmoudi, J. Amyloid-Beta: A Crucial Factor in Alzheimer's Disease. *Med. Princ. Pract.* **2015**, *24*, 1–10. [CrossRef]
2. Dementia. Available online: https://www.who.int/news-room/fact-sheets/detail/dementia (accessed on 17 July 2020).
3. Morley, J.E.; Farr, S.A.; Nguyen, A.D.; Xu, F. What Is the Physiological Function of Amyloid-Beta Protein? *J. Nutr. Health Aging* **2019**, *23*, 225–226. [CrossRef]
4. O'Brien, R.J.; Wong, P.C. Amyloid Precursor Protein Processing and Alzheimer's Disease. *Annu. Rev. Neurosci.* **2011**, *34*, 185–204. [CrossRef]
5. Scarpini, E.; Schelterns, P.; Feldman, H. Treatment of Alzheimer's Disease; Current Status and New Perspectives. *Lancet Neurol.* **2003**, *2*, 539–547. [CrossRef]
6. Nisticò, R.; Borg, J.J. Aducanumab for Alzheimer's Disease: A Regulatory Perspective. *Pharmacol. Res.* **2021**, *171*, 105754. [CrossRef]
7. Zenaro, E.; Piacentino, G.; Constantin, G. The Blood-Brain Barrier in Alzheimer's Disease. *Neurobiol. Dis.* **2017**, *107*, 41–56. [CrossRef]
8. Leszek, J.; Md Ashraf, G.; Tse, W.H.; Zhang, J.; Gasiorowski, K.; Fidel Avila-Rodriguez, M.; Tarasov, V.V.; Barreto, E.G.; Klochkov, G.S.; Bachurin, O.S.; et al. Nanotechnology for Alzheimer Disease. *Curr. Alzheimer Res.* **2017**, *14*, 1182–1189. [CrossRef]
9. Dara, T.; Vatanara, A.; Sharifzadeh, M.; Khani, S.; Vakilinezhad, M.A.; Vakhshiteh, F.; Nabi Meybodi, M.; Sadegh Malvajerd, S.; Hassani, S.; Mosaddegh, M.H. Improvement of Memory Deficits in the Rat Model of Alzheimer's Disease by Erythropoietin-Loaded Solid Lipid Nanoparticles. *Neurobiol. Learn. Mem.* **2019**, *166*, 107082. [CrossRef]

10. Vakilinezhad, M.A.; Amini, A.; Akbari Javar, H.; Baha'addini Beigi Zarandi, B.F.; Montaseri, H.; Dinarvand, R. Nicotinamide Loaded Functionalized Solid Lipid Nanoparticles Improves Cognition in Alzheimer's Disease Animal Model by Reducing Tau Hyperphosphorylation. *DARU J. Pharm. Sci.* **2018**, *26*, 165–177. [CrossRef]
11. Loureiro, J.A.; Andrade, S.; Duarte, A.; Neves, A.R.; Queiroz, J.F.; Nunes, C.; Sevin, E.; Fenart, L.; Gosselet, F.; Coelho, M.A.N.; et al. Resveratrol and Grape Extract-Loaded Solid Lipid Nanoparticles for the Treatment of Alzheimer's Disease. *Molecules* **2017**, *22*, 277. [CrossRef]
12. Campos, J.R.; Severino, P.; Santini, A.; Silva, A.M.; Shegokar, R.; Souto, S.B.; Souto, E.B. Chapter 1—Solid Lipid Nanoparticles (SLN): Prediction of Toxicity, Metabolism, Fate and Physicochemical Properties. In *Nanopharmaceuticals*; Shegokar, R., Ed.; Elsevier: Amsterdam, The Netherlands, 2020; pp. 1–15, ISBN 978-0-12-817778-5.
13. Scioli Montoto, S.; Muraca, G.; Ruiz, M.E. Solid Lipid Nanoparticles for Drug Delivery: Pharmacological and Biopharmaceutical Aspects. *Front. Mol. Biosci.* **2020**, *7*, 587997. [CrossRef] [PubMed]
14. Satapathy, M.K.; Yen, T.-L.; Jan, J.-S.; Tang, R.-D.; Wang, J.-Y.; Taliyan, R.; Yang, C.-H. Solid Lipid Nanoparticles (SLNs): An Advanced Drug Delivery System Targeting Brain through BBB. *Pharmaceutics* **2021**, *13*, 1183. [CrossRef]
15. Pizzol, C.D.; Filippin-Monteiro, F.B.; Restrepo, J.A.S.; Pittella, F.; Silva, A.H.; Alves de Souza, P.; Machado de Campos, A.; Creczynski-Pasa, T.B. Influence of Surfactant and Lipid Type on the Physicochemical Properties and Biocompatibility of Solid Lipid Nanoparticles. *Int. J. Environ. Res. Public. Health* **2014**, *11*, 8581–8596. [CrossRef]
16. Karn-orachai, K.; Smith, S.M.; Saesoo, S.; Treethong, A.; Puttipipatkhachorn, S.; Pratontep, S.; Ruktanonchai, U.R. Surfactant Effect on the Physicochemical Characteristics of γ-Oryanol-Containing Solid Lipid Nanoparticles. *Colloids Surf. Physicochem. Eng. Asp.* **2016**, *488*, 118–128. [CrossRef]
17. Sonkusare, S.K.; Kaul, C.L.; Ramarao, P. Dementia of Alzheimer's Disease and Other Neurodegenerative Disorders—Memantine, a New Hope. *Pharmacol. Res.* **2005**, *51*, 1–17. [CrossRef] [PubMed]
18. Kocis, P.; Tolar, M.; Yu, J.; Sinko, W.; Ray, S.; Blennow, K.; Fillit, H.; Hey, J.A. Elucidating the Aβ42 Anti-Aggregation Mechanism of Action of Tramiprosate in Alzheimer's Disease: Integrating Molecular Analytical Methods, Pharmacokinetic and Clinical Data. *CNS Drugs* **2017**, *31*, 495–509. [CrossRef]
19. Sathya, S.; Shanmuganathan, B.; Saranya, S.; Vaidevi, S.; Ruckmani, K.; Pandima Devi, K. Phytol-Loaded PLGA Nanoparticle as a Modulator of Alzheimer's Toxic Aβ Peptide Aggregation and Fibrillation Associated with Impaired Neuronal Cell Function. *Artif. Cells Nanomed. Biotechnol.* **2017**, *46*, 1719–1730. [CrossRef]
20. Gobbi, M.; Re, F.; Canovi, M.; Beeg, M.; Gregori, M.; Sesana, S.; Sonnino, S.; Brogioli, D.; Musicanti, C.; Gasco, P.; et al. Lipid-Based Nanoparticles with High Binding Affinity for Amyloid-Beta1-42 Peptide. *Biomaterials* **2010**, *31*, 6519–6529. [CrossRef]
21. Akel, H.; Ismail, R.; Csóka, I. Progress and Perspectives of Brain-Targeting Lipid-Based Nanosystems via the Nasal Route in Alzheimer's Disease. *Eur. J. Pharm. Biopharm.* **2020**, *148*, 38–53. [CrossRef]
22. Greenberg, S.M.; Rosand, J.; Schneider, A.T.; Creed Pettigrew, L.; Gandy, S.E.; Rovner, B.; Fitzsimmons, B.-F.; Smith, E.E.; Edip Gurol, M.; Schwab, K.; et al. A Phase 2 Study of Tramiprosate for Cerebral Amyloid Angiopathy. *Alzheimer Dis. Assoc. Disord.* **2006**, *20*, 269–274. [CrossRef]
23. Jokar, S.; Erfani, M.; Bavi, O.; Khazaei, S.; Sharifzadeh, M.; Hajiramezanali, M.; Beiki, D.; Shamloo, A. Design of Peptide-Based Inhibitor Agent against Amyloid-β Aggregation: Molecular Docking, Synthesis and in Vitro Evaluation. *Bioorg. Chem.* **2020**, *102*, 104050. [CrossRef] [PubMed]
24. Giannousi, K.; Geromichalos, G.; Kakolyri, D.; Mourdikoudis, S.; Dendrinou-Samara, C. Interaction of ZnO Nanostructures with Proteins: In Vitro Fibrillation/Antifibrillation Studies and in Silico Molecular Docking Simulations. *ACS Chem. Neurosci.* **2020**, *11*, 436–444. [CrossRef] [PubMed]
25. Tarozzi, A.; Merlicco, A.; Morroni, F.; Franco, F.; Cantelli-Forti, G.; Teti, G.; Falconi, M.; Hrelia, P. Cyanidin 3-O-Glucopyranoside Protects and Rescues SH-SY5Y Cells against Amyloid-Beta Peptide-Induced Toxicity. *NeuroReport* **2008**, *19*, 1483–1486. [CrossRef] [PubMed]
26. Xiao, Z.; Huang, C.; Wu, J.; Sun, L.; Hao, W.; Leung, L.K.; Huang, J. The Neuroprotective Effects of Ipriflavone against H2O2 and Amyloid Beta Induced Toxicity in Human Neuroblastoma SH-SY5Y Cells. *Eur. J. Pharmacol.* **2013**, *721*, 286–293. [CrossRef] [PubMed]
27. Abdul Manap, A.S.; Wei Tan, A.C.; Leong, W.H.; Yin Chia, A.Y.; Vijayabalan, S.; Arya, A.; Wong, E.H.; Rizwan, F.; Bindal, U.; Koshy, S.; et al. Synergistic Effects of Curcumin and Piperine as Potent Acetylcholine and Amyloidogenic Inhibitors With Significant Neuroprotective Activity in SH-SY5Y Cells via Computational Molecular Modeling and in Vitro Assay. *Front. Aging Neurosci.* **2019**, *11*, 206. [CrossRef]
28. Aljaeid, B.M.; Hosny, K.M. Miconazole-Loaded Solid Lipid Nanoparticles: Formulation and Evaluation of a Novel Formula with High Bioavailability and Antifungal Activity. *Int. J. Nanomed.* **2016**, *11*, 441–447. [CrossRef]
29. Taylor, E.N.; Kummer, K.M.; Dyondi, D.; Webster, T.J.; Banerjee, R. Multi-Scale Strategy to Eradicate Pseudomonas Aeruginosa on Surfaces Using Solid Lipid Nanoparticles Loaded with Free Fatty Acids. *Nanoscale* **2013**, *6*, 825–832. [CrossRef]
30. Rao, R.N.; Maurya, P.K.; Shinde, D.D.; Khalid, S. Precolumn Derivatization Followed by Liquid Chromatographic Separation and Determination of Tramiprosate in Rat Plasma by Fluorescence Detector: Application to Pharmacokinetics. *J. Pharm. Biomed. Anal.* **2011**, *55*, 282–287. [CrossRef]

31. Jalalizadeh, H.; Raei, M.; Tafti, R.F.; Farsam, H.; Kebriaeezadeh, A.; Souri, E. A Stability-Indicating HPLC Method for the Determination of Memantine Hydrochloride in Dosage Forms through Derivatization with 1-Fluoro-2,4-Dinitrobenzene. *Sci. Pharm.* **2014**, *82*, 265–279. [CrossRef]
32. Chen, X.; Zhang, M.; Ahmed, M.; Surapaneni, K.M.; Veeraraghavan, V.P.; Arulselvan, P. Neuroprotective Effects of Ononin against the Aluminium Chloride-Induced Alzheimer's Disease in Rats. *Saudi J. Biol. Sci.* **2021**, *28*, 4232–4239. [CrossRef]
33. Scearce-Levie, K. Monitoring Spatial Learning and Memory in Alzheimer's Disease Mouse Models Using the Morris Water Maze. *Methods Mol. Biol. Clifton NJ* **2011**, *670*, 191–205. [CrossRef]
34. Yakupova, E.I.; Bobyleva, L.G.; Vikhlyantsev, I.M.; Bobylev, A.G. Congo Red and Amyloids: History and Relationship. *Biosci. Rep.* **2019**, *39*, BSR20181415. [CrossRef] [PubMed]
35. Cacciatore, I.; Ciulla, M.; Fornasari, E.; Marinelli, L.; Di Stefano, A. Solid Lipid Nanoparticles as a Drug Delivery System for the Treatment of Neurodegenerative Diseases. *Expert Opin. Drug Deliv.* **2016**, *13*, 1121–1131. [CrossRef] [PubMed]
36. Alley, G.M.; Bailey, J.A.; Chen, D.; Ray, B.; Puli, L.K.; Tanila, H.; Banerjee, P.K.; Lahiri, D.K. Memantine Lowers Amyloid-Beta Peptide Levels in Neuronal Cultures and in APP/PS1 Transgenic Mice. *J. Neurosci. Res.* **2010**, *88*, 143–154. [CrossRef] [PubMed]
37. Gervais, F.; Paquette, J.; Morissette, C.; Krzywkowski, P.; Yu, M.; Azzi, M.; Lacombe, D.; Kong, X.; Aman, A.; Laurin, J.; et al. Targeting Soluble Aβ Peptide with Tramiprosate for the Treatment of Brain Amyloidosis. *Neurobiol. Aging* **2007**, *28*, 537–547. [CrossRef]
38. Neves, A.R.; Queiroz, J.F.; Weksler, B.; Romero, I.A.; Couraud, P.-O.; Reis, S. Solid Lipid Nanoparticles as a Vehicle for Brain-Targeted Drug Delivery: Two New Strategies of Functionalization with Apolipoprotein E. *Nanotechnology* **2015**, *26*, 495103. [CrossRef]
39. Clogston, J.D.; Patri, A.K. Zeta Potential Measurement. *Methods Mol. Biol. Clifton NJ* **2011**, *697*, 63–70. [CrossRef]
40. Se Thoe, E.; Fauzi, A.; Tang, Y.Q.; Chamyuang, S.; Chia, A.Y.Y. A Review on Advances of Treatment Modalities for Alzheimer's Disease. *Life Sci.* **2021**, *276*, 119129. [CrossRef]
41. Han, L.; Jiang, C. Evolution of Blood–Brain Barrier in Brain Diseases and Related Systemic Nanoscale Brain-Targeting Drug Delivery Strategies. *Acta Pharm. Sin. B* **2021**, *11*, 2306–2325. [CrossRef]
42. Ju, Y.; Tam, K.Y. Pathological Mechanisms and Therapeutic Strategies for Alzheimer's Disease. *Neural Regen. Res.* **2021**, *17*, 543–549. [CrossRef]

Disclaimer/Publisher's Note: The statements, opinions and data contained in all publications are solely those of the individual author(s) and contributor(s) and not of MDPI and/or the editor(s). MDPI and/or the editor(s) disclaim responsibility for any injury to people or property resulting from any ideas, methods, instructions or products referred to in the content.